Applications of Liquid Chromatography in Analysis of Pharmaceuticals and Natural Products

Applications of Liquid Chromatography in Analysis of Pharmaceuticals and Natural Products

Editors

Jan Oszmianski
Sabina Lachowicz-Wiśniewska

MDPI • Basel • Beijing • Wuhan • Barcelona • Belgrade • Manchester • Tokyo • Cluj • Tianjin

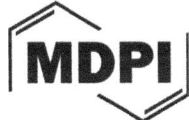

Editors

Jan Oszmianski
Departament of Fruit,
Vegetable and Plant
Nutraceutical Technology
Wroclaw University of
Environmental and
Life Sciences
Wrocław
Poland

Sabina
Lachowicz-Wiśniewska
Department of Health
Sciences
Calisia University
Kalisz
Poland

Editorial Office
MDPI
St. Alban-Anlage 66
4052 Basel, Switzerland

This is a reprint of articles from the Special Issue published online in the open access journal *Pharmaceuticals* (ISSN 1424-8247) (available at: www.mdpi.com/journal/pharmaceuticals/special_issues/Liquid_Chromatography_Natural_Products).

For citation purposes, cite each article independently as indicated on the article page online and as indicated below:

LastName, A.A.; LastName, B.B.; LastName, C.C. Article Title. *Journal Name* **Year**, *Volume Number*, Page Range.

ISBN 978-3-0365-4468-7 (Hbk)
ISBN 978-3-0365-4467-0 (PDF)

Contents

About the Editors

Jan Oszmianski

Jan Oszmiański, Professor Dr., Retired Professor, completed his Ph.D. degree at Agricultural Academy August Cieszkowski in Poznań in the area of enzymatic transformations of phenolic compounds in model systems and fruit extracts and subsequently carried out postdoctoral research at the Wroclaw University of Environmental and Life Sciences in the area of polyphenolic compounds and functional food. His main research interest is in the phenolic compounds, isolation and qualitative and quantitative determination of polyphenols and technique chromatography as UV-VIS, HPLC-MS-MS. He is a member of the committee of Food Sciences and Nutrition of the Polish Academy of Sciences.

Sabina Lachowicz-Wiśniewska

Sabina Lachowicz-Wiśniewska, Dr., Assistant Professor, completed her Ph.D. degree in Wrocław University of Environmental and Life Sciences under the direction of Professor Jan Oszmiański in the area of natural product technology and chemistry. Nowadays, she is carrying out postdoctoral research at the Calisia University in the Kalisz Microbiota Research Team under the direction of Professor Ireneusz Kapusta in the area of prebiotic functional food and bioavailability of their bioactive compounds in the prevention of oxidative stress and inflammation. Her research experience is in the general area of functional food, and pharmaceutical and medicinal plant chemistry, with over 74 peer-reviewed scientific papers covering research field such as (i) production of innovatiwe functional food with designed for health promotion properties; (ii) bioavailability and digestibility of bioactive compounds in the simulated digestive system by in vitro method; (iii) determination of the antioxidant, anti-diabetic, anti-obesity, and anti-inflammatory potential; and (iv) identification and assessment of health-promoting properties of bioactive compounds from plant materials based on chromatographic techniques. Research collaborations have been established within Dekaban Fundation with Prof. Anubhav Pratap Singh (Faculty of Land and Food Systems (LFS), University of British Columbia), Prof. Antonio J. Meléndez-Martínez in the Food Colour and Quality Laboratory, Universidad de Sevilla and also with many European research centres.

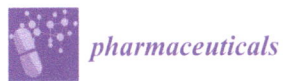

Article

Quantification of Degradation Products Formed during Heat Sterilization of Glucose Solutions by LC-MS/MS: Impact of Autoclaving Temperature and Duration on Degradation

Sarah Leitzen [1,2], Matthias Vogel [2], Michael Steffens [2], Thomas Zapf [2], Christa Elisabeth Müller [3] and Martin Brandl [1,*]

1   Department of Physics, Chemistry and Pharmacy, University of Southern Denmark, 5230 Odense, Denmark; sarah.leitzen@bfarm.de
2   Federal Institute for Drugs and Medical Devices, 53175 Bonn, Germany; matthias.vogel@bfarm.de (M.V.); michael.steffens@bfarm.de (M.S.); thomas.zapf@bfarm.de (T.Z.)
3   PharmaCenter Bonn, Pharmaceutical Institute, Pharmaceutical & Medicinal Chemistry, University of Bonn, 53121 Bonn, Germany; christa.mueller@uni-bonn.de
*   Correspondence: mmb@sdu.dk

Citation: Leitzen, S.; Vogel, M.; Steffens, M.; Zapf, T.; Müller, C.E.; Brandl, M. Quantification of Degradation Products Formed during Heat Sterilization of Glucose Solutions by LC-MS/MS: Impact of Autoclaving Temperature and Duration on Degradation. *Pharmaceuticals* **2021**, *14*, 1121. https://doi.org/10.3390/ph14111121

Academic Editors: Jan Oszmianski, Sabina Lachowicz and Daniela de Vita

Received: 22 September 2021
Accepted: 26 October 2021
Published: 1 November 2021

Publisher's Note: MDPI stays neutral with regard to jurisdictional claims in published maps and institutional affiliations.

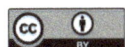

Abstract: Heat sterilization of glucose solutions can lead to the formation of various glucose degradation products (GDPs) due to oxidation, hydrolysis, and dehydration. GDPs can have toxic effects after parenteral administration due to their high reactivity. In this study, the application of the F0 concept to modify specific time/temperature models during heat sterilization and their influence on the formation of GDPs in parenteral glucose solutions was investigated using high-performance liquid chromatography-tandem mass spectrometry (LC-MS/MS). Glucose solutions (10%, w/v) were autoclaved at 111 °C, 116 °C, and 121 °C for different durations. The GDPs glyoxal, methylglyoxal, glucosone, 3-deoxyglucosone/3-deoxygalactosone, 3,4-dideoxyglucosone-3-ene, and 5-hydroxymethylfurfural were quantified after derivatization with o-phenylenediamine by an optimized LC-MS/MS method. For all GDPs, the limit of detection was <0.078 µg/mL, and the limit of quantification was <0.236 µg/mL. The autoclaving time of 121 °C and 15 min resulted in the lowest levels of 3-DG/3-DGal and 5-HMF, but in the highest levels of GO and 2-KDG. The proposed LC-MS/MS method is rapid and sensitive. So far, only 5-HMF concentrations are limited by the regulatory authorities. Our results suggest reconsidering the impurity limits of various GDPs, especially the more toxic ones such as GO and MGO, by the Pharmacopoeias.

Keywords: F0 concept; steam sterilization; sterilization safety; glucose degradation products; α-dicarbonyl compounds; derivatization; tandem mass spectrometry; *Geobacillus stearothermophilus*

1. Introduction

Sterile glucose infusion solutions for parenteral administration are commonly used as reconstitution solvents or diluents for injectable drugs and for peritoneal dialysis [1]. The sterility of the parenteral glucose solutions is a crucial prerequisite for their safety. Sterility can be achieved via several methods and conditions. Whenever possible, a process is chosen in which the product is sterilized in its final container (final sterilization). In order to guarantee the sterility of steam-sterilized glucose solutions, the European Pharmacopoeia stipulates that the products to be steam-sterilized must be heated to at least 121 °C for 15 min (reference sterilization procedure). Other combinations of time and temperature may be used if they achieve a sterility assurance level (SAL) of 10^{-6} or less. This process is to be controlled with the guide germ *Geobacillus stearothermophilus* [2]. The F0 concept is considered to be an equivalent sterilization process; this refers to processes that achieve a comparably lethal effect with different temperature and time combinations as the reference sterilization process described in the European Pharmacopoeia. Sterilization procedures carried out according to the F0 concept have the advantage that sterilization temperatures below 121 °C may be more suitable for temperature-sensitive products and containers offering comparable effects when combined with extended sterilization times [3]. However, reducing the temperature results in a longer autoclaving time. F0 indicates the specified time in minutes to which the solution to be autoclaved is exposed in its final container [4]. During the heat sterilization process of glucose solutions, glucose degradation products (GDPs) can be formed [5–7]. So far, some monocarbonyl as well as dicarbonyl degradation products have been identified [8–10]. Most GDPs are formed by oxidative and dehydrative processes (Figure 1).

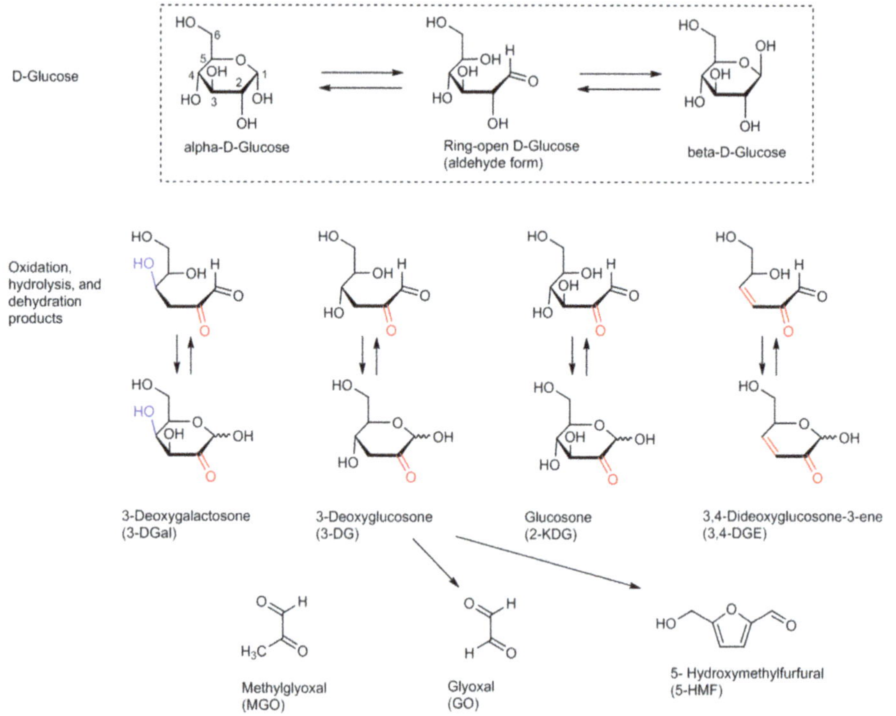

Figure 1. Reaction products of D-glucose due to oxidation, hydrolysis, and dehydration reactions observed during autoclaving of aqueous glucose solutions.

Figure 1 shows the potential GDPs of D-glucose that can be formed by oxidation, hydrolysis, and dehydration.

These are promoted by the hydrolytic activity of the aqueous solvent and by heat. It has been shown that high levels of GDPs may result in the formation of Advanced Glycation End products (AGEs) that have an impact on cellular homeostasis and health in general [1]. Parenteral administration of glucose solutions is expected to lead to an accumulation of these AGEs on the walls of blood vessels [11].

To date, only a few studies have been published that have focused on reducing the formation of GDPs in heat sterilized glucose solutions for parenteral use by the application of appropriate sterilization procedures [12–14] and determining the quality and quantity of GDPs in these solutions [1,5,15–17].

Due to the frequent use of glucose infusion solutions in practice [1,5] and the discussed possible toxicity of some GDPs such as glyoxal (GO) [18] and methylglyoxal (MGO) [19], this work deals with a current and highly sensitive topic. It is particularly important to closely examine glucose solutions for parenteral administration [11] and to reduce the amount of GDPs generated during the heat sterilization process to a minimum using appropriate methods such as the F0 concept.

In order to investigate parameters that influence heat sterilized glucose solutions potentially leading to different concentrations of formed GDPs such as the α-dicarbonyl (α-DC) compounds GO, MGO, glucosone (2-KDG), 3-deoxyglucosone (3-DG), 3-deoxygalactosone (3-DGal), 3,4-dideoxyglucosone-3-ene (3,4-DGE), and the monocarbonylic compound 5-hydroxymethylfurfural (5-HMF), 10% (*w/v*) glucose solutions in water were prepared. These were heat sterilized using the F0 concept at adapted temperature/time ratios in final containers, and the GDP concentrations were subsequently quantified by LC-MS/MS. In addition, a validation of the method developed for the quantitative measurements was carried out. The success of the autoclaving process was controlled in terms of the inactivation of the bacterial spores of *Geobacillus stearothermophilus*, which is used as a typical key germ.

2. Results

Since the 10% (*w/v*) glucose solutions are of particular interest with regard to their use as carrier solutions for electrolytes and drugs, we wanted to examine these solutions in more detail [20]. The objective of this study was to show the influence of the heating time when the required autoclaving times (scheme A) are not exactly observed and the glucose solutions are heated for too long (scheme B) (Table 1).

Table 1. Autoclaving schemes A/B.

Temperature [°C]	Scheme A (Overkill Conditions) Autoclaving Time (F0) [min]	Scheme B Autoclaving Time (F0) [min]
111	180	233
116	57	85
121	18	30

The basis for calculating the sterilization cycles according to schemes A and B can be found in the methods Section 4.2.2.

It is of enormous importance to validate the autoclaving procedure well, especially when working with temperature-sensitive substances such as glucose. For this purpose, an LC-MS/MS method according to Mittelmaier et al. [8], but further modified and optimized, was used to identify and quantify major GDPs in form of α-DCs, in particular GO, MGO, 2-KDG, 3-DG, 3-DGal, 3,4-DGE, and 5-HMF from freshly autoclaved glucose solutions.

2.1. Autoclaving under Germicidal Control

This experiment demonstrated that all temperature/time combinations presented by means of the F0 concept in Table 1 were suitable in practice to kill the lead germ *Geobacillus stearothermophilus* used in steam sterilization in the prepared 10% (*w/v*) glucose solutions described in Section 4.2.1. If the autoclaving time or temperature had not been sufficient to kill the germ, the germ would have survived the sterilization and secreted acid metabolites in the culture medium after incubation, causing a color change from purple to yellow. This color change did not happen, which can be seen in Figure S1 in the Supplementary Materials. As a control, a non-autoclaved EZ-Test® was co-incubated at 60 °C for 24 h. The test was incubated in the nutrient medium. The "Test/Control" figure clearly shows the color change of the indicator bromocresol purple from purple, at a pH of 6.8 to yellow at more acidic pH values around 5.2 [21]. The results of the autoclaving procedure are additionally described in Table 2.

Table 2. Overview of the autoclaving results with regard to the germ *Geobacillus stearothermophilus*.

Temperature [°C]	F0 [min] (Scheme A)	*Geobacillus stearothermophilus* Killed (Scheme A/Scheme B)?
111	180	yes
116	57	yes
121	18	yes

2.2. Measuring of the pH Values of the Autoclaved and Non-Autoclaved Glucose Solutions

The solutions listed in Table 3 were all cooled down to room temperature after heat sterilization, which took place at 111 °C, 116 °C, and 121 °C, and then the pH of these solutions was determined at room temperature.

Table 3. Overview of the obtained pH-values ± SD (= standard deviation) in different temperatures/sterilization-times/vessels.

Temperature [°C]	10% Glucose Solution (n = 3 for Each Scheme A/B)		Control Values of Autoclaved Water without Glucose (n = 3 for Each Scheme A/B)	
	10% PP Bottle (Scheme A) pH ± SD	10% PP Bottle (Scheme B) pH ± SD	Water, PP Bottle (Scheme A) pH ± SD	Water, PP Bottle(Scheme B) pH ± SD
111	5.17 ± 0.0	4.08 ± 0.0	7.03 ± 0.0	6.80 ± 0.0
116	4.67 ± 0.0	4.12 ± 0.0	6.77 ± 0.0	6.53 ± 0.0
121	4.36 ± 0.0	4.15 ± 0.0	6.68 ± 0.0	6.11 ± 0.0
non-autoclaved (room temperature)	4.98 ± 0.0		6.81 ± 0.0	

In Table 3 it can clearly be seen that with increasing heat sterilization temperature from 111 °C to 121 °C, the pH value decreases. In the non-autoclaved glucose solution, the pH value is clearly higher than in the autoclaved one. This can be explained by the fact that the amount of acidic GDPs formed during heat sterilization increases with increasing exposure time and with increased uptake of CO_2 from the ambient air. The effect of the temperature increase during heat sterilization does not seem to contribute significantly to a reduction of the pH value. Compared to the 10% (w/v) glucose solution, the pH values of autoclaved water are higher, even those of the non-autoclaved solutions.

2.3. Content of GDPs in Autoclaved 10% (w/v) Glucose Solutions in PP Bottles

Next, we determined the GDP contents in 10% (w/v) glucose solutions in PP bottles that had been prepared and autoclaved within this study ($n = 27$ measurements each within scheme A/B; for each temperature, 3 bottles per autoclave run were autoclaved in 3 autoclave runs. Each of these 9 bottles was measured 3 times in total). The results are shown in Table 4.

Table 4. Concentrations of GDPs in 10% (w/v) glucose solution in PP bottles autoclaved according to scheme A ($n = 27$).

	Temp [°C]	GO [µg/mL] ± SD	MGO [µg/mL] ± SD	2-KDG [µg/mL] ± SD	3-DG/3-DGal [µg/mL] ± SD	3,4-DGE [µg/mL] ± SD	5-HMF [µg/mL] ± SD
Scheme A	111	4.4 ± 2.7	3.0 ± 0.3	5.9 ± 2.2	56.0 ± 10.2	59.6 ± 14.5	81.9 ± 29.5
	116	4.2 ± 0.7	2.5 ± 0.2	7.1 ± 0.6	55.0 ± 1.6	50.9 ± 1.7	31.6 ± 0.5
	121	5.6 ± 1.3	2.6 ± 0.2	7.5 ± 1.4	52.2 ± 4.0	55.5 ± 1.7	17.4 ± 3.9
Scheme B	111	18.0 ± 9.7	12.9 ± 3.2	5.2 ± 0.3	72.9 ± 10.5	66.2 ± 6.2	94.0 ± 4.0
	116	20.6 ± 1.7	11.8 ± 0.4	6.5 ± 0.8	65.2 ± 6.7	73.6 ± 2.8	56.3 ± 7.4
	121	23.2 ± 0.9	11.5 ± 0.8	6.9 ± 0.7	60.3 ± 6.8	59.5 ± 2.8	37.2 ± 0.8

The results of autoclaving the glucose solutions according to scheme A show that the concentrations of GDPs formed decrease with increasing temperature, except for GO and 2-KDG and 3,4-DGE. In comparison, the highest concentrations of GDPs formed are present for 3-DG/3-DGal, 3,4-DGE, and 5-HMF.

The 10% (*w/v*) glucose solutions autoclaved according to scheme B also show the same trend as described above: the concentrations of GO and 2-KDG increase with increasing temperature, whereas the concentrations of MGO, 3-DG/3-DGal, 3,4-DGE and especially 5-HMF decrease with increasing temperature. These results are shown in Figures 2 and 3.

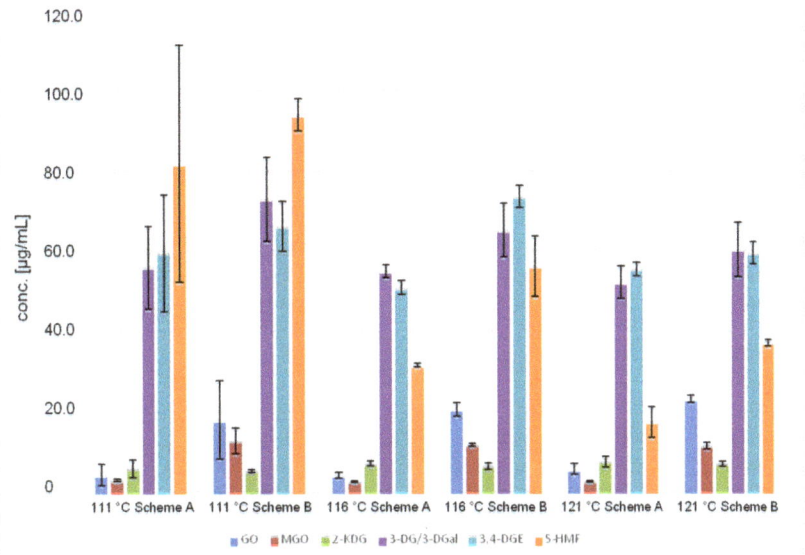

Figure 2. Comparison of the concentrations of GDPs according to the autoclaving scheme (**A/B**) and temperature (111 °C, 116 °C, 121 °C) (*n* = 27).

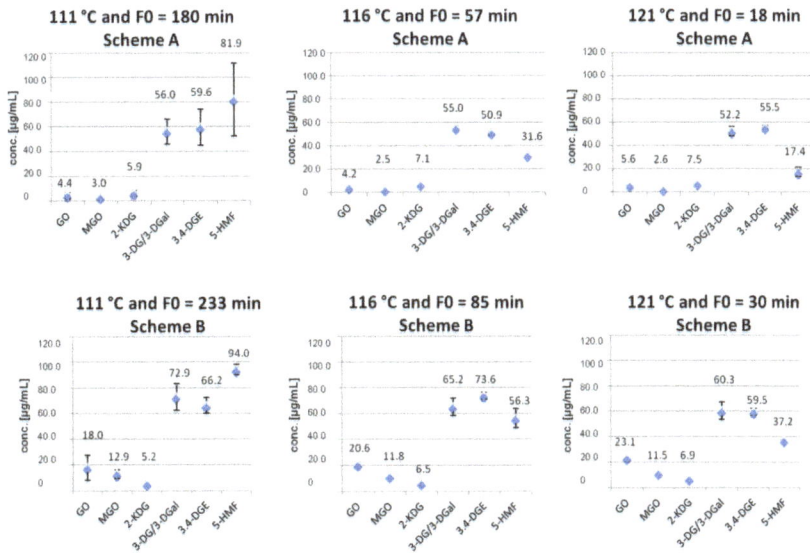

Figure 3. Comparison of the concentrations of GDPs formed at 111–116 °C autoclaved according to scheme A and according to scheme B (*n* = 27).

Figure 2 shows the different concentrations of GDPs formed at the respective temperatures according to scheme A versus scheme B. In comparison, it can be seen that higher concentrations of GDPs are formed in scheme B. The highest concentrations could be observed for the GDPs 3-DG/3-DGal and 5-HMF. The following Figure 3 shows an alternative representation.

Further figures showing the different concentrations of GDPs at the selected temperatures 111 °C, 116 °C, and 121 °C (schemes A and B) can be found in the Supplementary Materials (Figures S2–S13).

When the 10% (w/v) glucose solution is autoclaved at the standard autoclaving temperature of 121 °C for a much longer time (F0 = 202 min versus F0 = 18 min), thus exposing it to the high energy level for a much longer time, it can be observed that compared to scheme A, the concentrations of MGO, 2-KDG, 3-DG/3-DGal, and 3,4-DGE decrease by up to 85.3%, but the concentrations of GO and 5-HMF increase by up to 136.2% (Table 5).

Table 5. Concentrations of GDPs in 10% (w/v) glucose solutions in PP bottles heat sterilized at 121 °C for 350 min (F0 = 202 min). 3 batches with 3 bottles each were analyzed ($n = 9$).

Temp [°C]	GO [µg/mL] ± SD	MGO [µg/mL] ± SD	2-KDG [µg/mL] ± SD	3-DG/3-DGal [µg/mL] ± SD	3,4-DGE [µg/mL] ± SD	5-HMF [µg/mL] ± SD
121	8.3 ± 0.0	1.2 ± 0.1	1.1 ± 0.1	13.7 ± 0.1	12.5 ± 0.3	41.1 ± 0.1

In Table 5 it can be clearly seen that there are significantly lower concentrations of MGO, 2-KDG, 3-DG/3-DGal, and 3,4-DGE compared to the 10% glucose solution prepared at the standard autoclaving time (121 °C and F0 = 18 min). Table 5 is also shown in the Supplementary Materials (Figure S14).

The non-autoclaved 10% (w/v) glucose solution served as a reference value. Small amounts of GDPs (especially GO and MGO) were also observed (Table 6).

Table 6. Concentrations of GDPs in 10% (w/v) glucose solutions in PP bottles that were not heat sterilized (reference value). Three bottles were analyzed ($n = 3$).

Temp [°C]	GO [µg/mL] ± SD	MGO [µg/mL] ± SD	2-KDG [µg/mL] ± SD	3-DG/3-DGal [µg/mL] ± SD	3,4-DGE [µg/mL] ± SD	5-HMF [µg/mL] ± SD
121	1.0 ± 0.5	0.9 ± 0.1	0.1 ± 0.0	n.d.	n.d.	0.1 ± 0.0

n.d. = not detectable.

2.4. Content of GDPs in Commercially Available Aqueous Glucose Solutions (5–50%) in Different Types of Vessels from Three Different Manufacturers

In the following part of the experiment, different high concentrations of glucose solutions from three manufacturers A–C were investigated with regard to the occurrence and concentrations of GDPs. The glucose solutions had been autoclaved by the manufacturers A–C according to scheme A (F0 value of 18 min at 121 °C). Three measurements per batch were determined (Tables 7–9).

Table 7. Concentrations of GDPs. Manufacturer A ($n = 3$).

MAH/Conc	GO [µg/mL] ± SD	MGO [µg/mL] ± SD	2-KDG [µg/mL] ± SD	3-DG/3-DGal [µg/mL] ± SD	3,4-DGE [µg/mL] ± SD	5-HMF [µg/mL] ± SD
5% PP	35.9 ± 2.5	0.8 ± 0.3	0.5 ± 0.6	8.5 ± 0.7	1.2 ± 1.0	0.4 ± 0.6
10% PP	42.1 ± 8.5	0.8 ± 0.3	1.1 ± 0.9	11.3 ± 1.0	1.5 ± 1.3	0.7 ± 0.6
20% PP	39.2 ± 3.4	0.8 ± 0.2	18.9 ± 4.8	1.3 ± 0.1	0.1 ± 0.1	2.1 ± 0.2
40% PP	47.3 ± 2.6	0.9 ± 0.2	23.0 ± 0.3	0.4 ± 0.1	0.0 ± 0.0	4.6 ± 0.4
50% Glass	43.6 ± 3.9	0.9 ± 0.4	11.1 ± 1.0	31.4 ± 2.4	3.5 ± 0.3	5.6 ± 0.9

Table 8. Concentrations of GDPs. Manufacturer B (*n* = 3).

MAH/Conc	GO [µg/mL] ± SD	MGO [µg/mL] ± SD	2-KDG [µg/mL] ± SD	3-DG/3-DGal [µg/mL] ± SD	3,4-DGE [µg/mL] ± SD	5-HMF [µg/mL] ± SD
5% PP	0.6 ± 0.1	0.5 ± 0.1	1 ± 0.9	14.2 ± 3.4	3.4 ± 1.0	1.6 ± 0.3
10% PP	11.1 ± 0.5	0.6 ± 0.1	1.7 ± 0.1	18.4 ± 2.1	3.6 ± 0.4	2.6 ± 0.4
20% PP	13.7 ± 1.3	0.7 ± 0.3	5.1 ± 2.7	20.2 ± 0.4	3.3 ± 0.3	5.0 ± 0.3
40% PP	16.1 ± 3.6	0.8 ± 0.5	17.5 ± 8.8	20.4 ± 0.4	1.6 ± 0.0	9.5 ± 1.2
50% Glass	15.9 ± 0.9	0.9 ± 0.2	10.1 ± 2.6	34.6 ± 0.5	4.0 ± 0.3	7.9 ± 1.0

Table 9. Concentrations of GDPs. Manufacturer C (*n* = 3).

MAH/Conc	GO [µg/mL] ± SD	MGO [µg/mL] ± SD	2-KDG [µg/mL] ± SD	3-DG/3-DGal [µg/mL] ± SD	3,4-DGE [µg/mL] ± SD	5-HMF [µg/mL] ± SD
5% Glass	20.9 ± 5.1	0.7 ± 0.3	0.3 ± 0.6	12.3 ± 0.7	2.9 ± 0.2	1.2 ± 0.1
10% Glass	31.9 ± 3.2	0.7 ± 0.2	0.9 ± 0.9	13.3 ± 1.4	2.5 ± 0.2	2.9 ± 0.2
20% Glass	33.0 ± 0.8	0.7 ± 0.1	7.6 ± 4.2	14.2 ± 0.6	1.2 ± 0.2	14.1 ± 1.1
40% PP	32.4 ± 6.5	0.8 ± 0.4	15.3 ± 2.3	10.8 ± 1.1	0.8 ± 0.1	4.6 ± 0.1
50% Glass	40.5 ± 3.3	0.9 ± 0.3	6.7 ± 4.5	31.8 ± 3.0	2.9 ± 0.2	12.9 ± 0.5

Comparing manufacturers A and B, it is noticeable that manufacturer A contains more GO and manufacturer B contains more 5-HMF in all glucose solutions (5–50%). Manufacturer C also has a comparatively very high proportion of GO and 5-HMF in relation to the 50% solution compared with manufacturers A and B.

With reference to the characteristics of the vessels of the marketed glucose solutions, it can be observed that in glass containers there are lower concentrations of GO and 2-KDG compared to PP bottles (50% glass versus 40% PP), despite the higher concentration of the glucose solutions. In return, there is a significant increase in 3-DG/3-DGal in the 50% glucose solutions autoclaved in glass vessels.

2.5. Method Validation via LC-MS/MS

The optimized method was validated according to the ICH Q2(R1) guideline [22].

2.5.1. Selectivity

The LC-MS/MS method developed is selective for the GDPs investigated in this study. The glucose matrix did not affect the AUCs of the derivatized GDPs. Glucose was not derivatized at all and its presence did not affect the quantitative analysis of the GDPs. However, a limitation in terms of selectivity is that the method does not adequately separate 3-DG from 3-DGal.

2.5.2. Linearity

All analytes could be well analyzed and evaluated and showed linear regression.

The 5-HMF concentration-dependent curve exhibited good correlation with $R^2 = 0.993$. 3,4-DGE exhibited very good correlation with $R^2 = 0.998$. GO, MGO, 2-KDG and 3-DG/3-DGal had excellent correlation coefficients with $R^2 = 0.999$. 3,4-DGE and 3-DG/3-DGal and 5-HMF were weighted $\frac{1}{x}$. Other GDPs were not weighted.

2.5.3. Range

All GDP derivatives GO, MGO, 2-KDG, 3-DG/3-DGal, 3,4-DGE and 5-HMF provided adequate regression levels in the tested interval 0.5–100 µg/mL. The range was calculated as a compromise including all expected GDP concentrations.

2.5.4. LOD

All derivatized GDPs had a LOD between 0.004 µg/mL and 0.078 µg/mL:

$$LOD = 3.3 * standard\ deviation\ of\ the\ response/slope\ of\ the\ calibration\ curve. \quad (1)$$

2.5.5. LOQ

All derivatized GDPs had a LOQ between 0.012 µg/mL and 0.236 µg/mL:

$$LOQ = 10 * standard\ deviation\ of\ the\ response/slope\ of\ the\ calibration\ curve. \quad (2)$$

2.5.6. Accuracy

Accuracy was reported as % recovery and tested in order to exclude possible systematic errors. The mean recovery (in%) was performed at three concentrations with six replicates each for the concentration levels 0.5, 25, and 100 µg/mL after a 16 h derivatization period with 0.75 mg/mL OPD. It ranged from 89.8 to 109.0%.

2.5.7. Precision

The intraday precision was evaluated by analyzing three different concentrations with three replicates of each concentration. Intraday precision was calculated as RSD% for peak area. It ranged from 0.7 to 2.5% for GO, 0.7 to 1.4% for MGO, 0.5 to 2.9% for 2-KDG, 0.7 to 4.9% for 3-DG/3-DGal, 1.1 to 4.3% for 3,4-DGE and 1.0 to 3.4% for 5-HMF. All values of the RSD% are below 5%.

The validation results show that the method described here is a precise and reliable method for the quantification of GDPs in glucose solutions in the range indicated. All parameters of the method validation are presented in Tables 10 and 11.

Table 10. Method validation parameters.

Analyte	Regression	R^2	Weighting	Range [µg/mL]	LOD [µg/mL] ([1] calc.)	LOQ [µg/mL] ([1] calc.)
GO	$y = 1.01040x + 4.55224e^{-4}$	0.999	none	0.5–100	0.078	0.236
MGO	$y = 3.30991x + 0.00154$	0.999	none	0.5–100	0.023	0.070
2-KDG	$y = 1.98896x - 2.01261e^{-5}$	0.999	none	0.5–100	0.053	0.161
3-DG/3-DGal	$y = 13.02104x + 0.00448$	0.999	$\frac{1}{x}$	0.5–100	0.004	0.012
3,4-DGE	$y = 5.15815x + 5.56583e^{-4}$	0.998	$\frac{1}{x}$	0.5–100	0.015	0.046
5-HMF	$y = 11.23859x + 0.01012$	0.993	$\frac{1}{x}$	0.5–100	0.010	0.031

[1] calc. = calculated according to ICH Q2(R1) guideline [22].

Table 11. Precision in terms of % relative standard deviation (RSD) for replicate measurements ($n = 3$) at three different levels, and accuracy reported as percent recovery for three concentrations/six replicates each of the total analytical procedure.

GDP	GDP conc. [µg/mL]	Precision (as% RSD) Mean [µg/mL] ± SD	RSD%	Accuracy (% Recovery) Mean [µg/mL] ± SD	% Recovery
GO	0.5	0.5 ± 0.0	2.5	0.5 ± 0.0	98.8
	25	23.0 ± 0.3	1.2	24.6 ± 0.7	98.3
	100	98.5 ± 0.7	0.7	98.2 ± 3.0	98.2
MGO	0.5	0.7 ± 0.0	0.8	0.5 ± 0.0	109.0
	25	24.0 ± 0.3	1.4	25.5 ± 0.7	102.1
	100	98.5 ± 0.7	0.7	99.5 ± 2.4	99.5

Table 11. *Cont.*

GDP	GDP conc. [µg/mL]	Precision (as% RSD)		Accuracy (% Recovery)	
		Mean [µg/mL] ± SD	RSD%	Mean [µg/mL] ± SD	% Recovery
2-KDG	0.5	0.6 ± 0.0	2.9	0.5 ± 0.0	103.7
	25	24.7 ± 0.6	2.4	26.0 ± 0.9	103.9
	100	101.5 ± 0.5	0.5	103.6 ± 3.7	103.6
3-DG/ 3-DGal	0.5	0.4 ± 0.0	4.9	0.4 ± 0.0	89.8
	25	26.4 ± 0.2	0.7	25.1 ± 1.8	100.2
	100	99.3 ± 2.0	2.0	100.5 ± 3.1	100.5
3,4-DGE	0.5	0.5 ± 0.0	4.3	0.5 ± 0.0	106.9
	25	25.9 ± 0.5	2.0	26.0 ± 2.0	104.2
	100	92.3 ± 1.1	1.1	96.1 ± 4.0	96.1
5-HMF	0.5	0.5 ± 0.0	3.1	0.5 ± 0.0	94.8
	25	26.9 ± 0.3	1.4	27.0 ± 0.7	107.9
	100	103.4 ± 3.6	0.5	102.5 ± 4.5	102.5

2.6. Statistical Analysis

Finally, a statistical analysis of the differences in concentrations of the individual GDPs autoclaved according to schemes A and B was carried out to evaluate the significance of the measured values (Table 12). The concentrations of the GDPs were compared per temperature and per GDP after they had been autoclaved either via scheme A or via scheme B.

Table 12. Comparison of the two autoclaving schemes A and B with regard to the influence of temperature on the resulting GDP concentrations.

GDP Temp [°C]			F0 Scheme A vs. F0 Scheme B		
			p-Value	Significance Level	Degrees of Freedom
GO	111 °C		0.008012	*	
	116 °C		1.512×10^{-12}	*/**	
	121 °C		1.516×10^{-13}	*/**	
MGO	111 °C		0.3065	not significant	
	116 °C		6.058×10^{-14}	*/**	
	121 °C		2.938×10^{-13}	*/**	
2-KDG	111 °C		0.5692	not significant	
	116 °C		0.1991	not significant	
	121 °C		0.4838	not significant	16
3-DG/ 3-DGal	111 °C		0.05203	not significant	
	116 °C		0.003162	*	
	121 °C		0.01666	*	
3,4-DGE	111 °C		0.4311	not significant	
	116 °C		6.311×10^{-8}	*/**	
	121 °C		0.02456	*	
5-HMF	111 °C		0.3691	not significant	
	116 °C		1.03×10^{-6}	*/**	
	121 °C		4.946×10^{-9}	*/**	

* $p \leq 0.05$: significant on nominal significance level ** $p \leq 0.003$ (0.05/18): significant after Bonferroni correction for multiple testing.

A two sample *t*-tests was used to investigate if there was a significant difference between the two selected autoclaving schemes A and B (Table 1). Here, the content of each GDP per temperature of scheme A was compared with the content of each GDP within scheme B.

Subsequently, a two-sample t-test was performed based on the standard temperature of 121 °C, which was compared against the two alternative temperatures 111 °C and 116 °C with respect to the concentrations that occurred according to autoclaving scheme A (Table 13).

Table 13. Comparison of GDP concentrations at 121 °C versus the two alternative autoclaving temperatures 116 °C and 121 °C in autoclaving scheme A.

GDP	121 °C versus 111 °C and 116 °C				
	Standard Autoclaving Temperature	Alternative Autoclaving Temperature	*p*-Value	Significance Level	Degrees of Freedom
GO	121 °C	111 °C	0.3051	not significant	
	121 °C	116 °C	0.05448	not significant	
MGO	121 °C	111 °C	0.1987	not significant	
	121 °C	116 °C	0.6584	not significant	
2-KDG	121 °C	111 °C	0.2506	not significant	
	121 °C	116 °C	0.6102	not significant	
3-DG/ 3-DGal	121 °C	111 °C	0.6078	not significant	16
	121 °C	116 °C	0.1801	not significant	
3,4-DGE	121 °C	111 °C	0.6067	not significant	
	121 °C	116 °C	0.01357	*	
5-HMF	121 °C	111 °C	1.256×10^{-4}	*/**	
	121 °C	116 °C	5.134×10^{-7}	*/**	

* $p \leq 0.05$: significant on nominal significance level ** $p \leq 0.004$ (0.05/12): significant after Bonferroni correction for multiple testing.

The two-sample t-test was performed in order to investigate if there is a significant difference between the standard autoclaving temperature 121 °C and the two alternative autoclaving temperatures, 111 °C and 116 °C, within scheme A. A clear significance can be seen for the GDPs 3,4-DGE (121 °C versus 116 °C) and 5-HMF (121 °C versus 111 °C and 121 °C versus 116 °C). At 121 °C, significantly lower concentrations of these GDPs are formed. This is in line with the graphical representation from Figures 2 and 3.

3. Discussion

Known factors that can influence the content of GDPs are glucose concentration [7,17], pH [7], the chosen container [1,23,24], storage conditions [7], temperature [7], and heating time [12–14]. The last two influencing factors were examined in detail in this paper as they seem to be important components. A number of studies have already been carried out on different degradation products that have occurred in marketed medicinal products as well as in self-autoclaved glucose solutions after heat sterilization [12–14].

The objective of this work was to investigate the effect of different temperatures and autoclaving times on 10% (*w/v*) glucose solutions with regard to the formation of the six α-dicarbonyls GO, MGO, 2-KDG, 3-DG/3-DGal and 3,4-DGE as well as the aldehyde 5-HMF that occur after heat sterilization. In addition, suitable conditions to produce the lowest possible GDP concentrations were analyzed.

Due to possibly different activation energies and degradation kinetics of the various degradation reactions, the type and amount of GDPs obtained differ. The F0 value is derived on the basis of a first-order reaction and offers the possibility of comparing different heat treatment processes with one another or setting limit values for them [25–27]. The sterilization value is often used to optimize heat treatment processes, since most heat-related chemical degradation or formation reactions and predominantly also the killing of microorganisms can be described with the first-order reaction [25–27]. The killing of microorganisms takes place during heating phase, holding time, and cooling phase. The holding time is the variable part of heat sterilization. By autoclaving at higher temperatures, the required F0 value is achieved with a shorter total time. The holding time of the sterilization process can thus be shortened.

In Table 1, the calculated autoclaving times of the autoclaving schemes A and B were presented. The duration of the autoclaving procedure according to autoclaving scheme A was calculated according to the described formulae from the European Pharmacopoeia [4]. The equation used with its respective parameters is described in Section 4.2.2. In autoclaving scheme B, the calculated F0 time of scheme A was set as the holding time in the autoclave. Since the heating and cooling phases were added to the holding time, the autoclaving times for scheme B were significantly longer than for scheme A. Scheme B was used to investigate whether exceeding the recommended autoclaving time has a significant influence on the concentration of the resulting degradation products. The bioindicator *Geobacillus stearothermophilus* was used to check the effectiveness of killing all spores during the autoclaving process [28]. The successful killing of the germ during the autoclaving process was shown in Figure S1 (Supplementary Materials). Subsequently, the GDP concentrations obtained from the 10% glucose solutions autoclaved according to scheme A were compared with those obtained from scheme B for the temperatures 111 °C, 116 °C, and 121 °C. In addition, marketed 10% glucose solutions from different manufacturers A–C were analyzed and a validation of the LC–MS/MS method was carried out.

The glucose solutions exposed to scheme A with the shorter autoclaving times show lower concentration of GDPs (except for 2-KDG) than the glucose solutions autoclaved according to scheme B (longer autoclaving times). 2-KDG is apparently formed more preferentially at higher temperatures than at lower temperatures. However, in comparison from the longer to the shorter autoclaving time, it is more likely to be degraded with longer heat sterilization than with shorter autoclaving time. This was to be expected, as glucose degrades by oxidation, hydrolysis and dehydration, as shown in Figure 1. The longer moist heat is applied to glucose, the greater the proportion of GDPs formed. Comparing the concentrations of the GDPs at increasing temperatures within scheme A and scheme B, respectively, it is noticeable that the concentrations of GO and 2-KDG increase slightly with increasing temperature, whereas the concentrations of MGO, 3-DG/3-DGal, 3,4-DGE (exception 116 °C) and 5-HMF decrease.

Haybrard et al. describe glucose being degraded to 3-DG (and presumably also to its diastereomer 3-DGal) by enolization and dehydration [1]. From this, in turn, the α-DC MGO can be formed by breaking of bond (cleavage). Cyclisation of 3-DG (and 3-DGal) also produces 3,4-DGE. 3,4-DGE dehydrates further to 5-HMF. GO is an intermediate reactant, which is formed directly from glucose. This reaction sequence suggests that at higher temperatures and shorter autoclaving times, as shown in scheme A, slightly more intermediate reactants such as GO are formed from glucose, but all degradation products that depend on the intermediate 3-DG/3-DGal decrease. This means that enolization and dehydration of glucose decrease with increasing temperature and shorter autoclaving time.

In general, the concentrations of the GDPs 3-DG/3-DGal, 3,4-DGE, and 5-HMF (scheme A: 17.4–81.9 µg/mL; scheme B: 37.2–94.0 µg/mL) are many times higher than those of GO, MGO and 2-KDG (scheme A: 2.5–7.5 µg/mL; scheme B: 5.2–23.1 µg/mL), which is in line with the description of Haybrard et al. [1]. This means that the enolization and dehydration of glucose to 3-DG/3-DGal, its subsequent cyclization to 3,4-DGE and the subsequent dehydration to 5-HMF take place preferentially because they are energetically favored compared to the formation of GO, MGO and 2-KDG.

The standard autoclaving time of 121 °C and F0 = 18 min appears to produce the lowest levels of 3-DG/3-DGal and 5-HMF, but the highest levels of GO and 2-KDG.

Almost all GDPs (except 2-KDG) show lower concentrations in scheme A (=shorter autoclaving time). While GO, MGO, and 3,4-DGE show the significantly lowest concentrations in scheme A at 116 °C, the concentrations of 3-DG/3-DGal as well as of 5-HMF are lowest at 121 °C in scheme A. 2-KDG achieved the lowest values in scheme B at 111 °C (Table 4). Furthermore, the concentration of 5-HMF decreases with increasing temperature. Tao et al. assumed that this is due to the hydrolytic degradation of 5-HMF to levulinic acid and formic acid [29]. Mannermaa et al. observed that the same applies to Ringer solutions: the use of the shortest sterilization cycle leads to the lowest 5-HMF concentrations in Ringer glucose solutions. Additional studies by Mannermaa et al. showed that at the same F0 value, the concentration of 5-HMF decreases the most at the highest temperatures [12–14]. Sturgeon et al. analyzed the breakdown of 10% dextrose solutions under simulated sterilization conditions. They investigated the autoclaved solutions at 102–132 °C and found that at all temperatures of heating, the formation rates of 5-HMF gradually increased with heating time [30]. We can confirm this finding with our results. Comparing the concentrations for 5-HMF within the schemes A and B, respectively, we found that less 5-HMF was formed at higher temperatures where heating was shorter compared to colder autoclaving temperatures where autoclaving was longer (e.g., 121 °C versus 111 °C).

When comparing the self-autoclaved glucose solutions according to scheme A (121 °C, F0 = 18 min) with the industrially produced counterpart of manufacturers A, B, and C, it is noticeable that generally for manufacturers A–C the values for GO are clearly higher than our determined values. For MGO, 2-KDG, 3-DG/3-DGal, 3,4-DGE, and 5-HMF, the 10% (w/v) glucose solutions of manufacturers A–C showed significantly lower contents, regardless of the nature of the vessels. Looking at the 5–50% (w/v) glucose solutions from manufacturers A–C, we see that all manufacturers have the highest GDP values for GO and 3-DG/3-DGal (Tables 7–9). MGO has the lowest concentrations in all solutions. Compared to our autoclaved solutions corresponding to scheme A, it is noticeable that we obtain much lower values of GO in the 10% (w/v) glucose solution, but slightly higher values for MGO, 2-KDG, and significantly higher values for 3-DG/3-DGal, 3,4-DGE, and 5-HMF. This may be due to the different autoclaving devices or possibly also additives that the manufacturers used to adjust the pH of their glucose solutions. In accordance with the national monograph, we did not use such additives here. The rate-determining step in the formation of GDPs is not solely dependent on the respective glucose concentration and this process is not based on a linear reaction mechanism. This can be seen from the fact that, for example, the 20% glucose solutions from manufacturers A–C do not have twice the content of GDPs compared to the 10% glucose solution.

The examination of the glucose solutions autoclaved at the standard temperature of 121 °C for 350 min (F0 = 202 min) with a significantly longer heat exposure, showed an increase in the concentrations of GO and 5-HMF and a decrease in the concentrations of MGO, 2-KDG, 3-DG/3-DGal, and 3,4-DGE (Table 5). This means that the formation of GO and 5-HMF is favored with long heat exposure, while the other degradation products decompose.

Regarding the pH values, it can be concluded that the non-autoclaved 10% (w/v) glucose solution measured at room temperature with pH = 4.976 has a significantly more acidic pH value than double distilled water (pH = 6.812). A clear trend was seen that with increasing temperature and also with increasing autoclaving time, the pH becomes more acidic. Since GDPs have an acidic pH [31,32], it is reasonable to assume that many acidic GDPs are produced due to the influence of temperature and autoclaving time. The comparison of autoclaved double-distilled water also showed this trend, which is due to the fact that CO_2 from the air is absorbed and bound by the double-distilled water and carbonic acid is formed. Mannermaa et al. found, that the pH of the solutions decreases during sterilization, with the exception of F0 values at 5–15 min [12]. With 20% glucose solutions, stored at room temperature for 30 days, the pH value decreases by approx. 0.20 units [12]. This is also the same in our study. A possible explanation might be that more GDPs are formed, which are acidic by their nature. This phenomenon is also observed with longer storage times [1]. Haybrard et al. have conducted an analysis of covariance (ANCOVA). They showed that there is a significant influence of storage time and oxygen permeability on the formation rates of 5-HMF in sterile glucose solutions for infusion [1]. This is in line with observations from Kjellstrand et al. who have reported that the most important factor determining the rate of GDP production during storage was temperature [7]. The GDPs created by heat sterilization promoted further degradation. They stated, that at a storage temperature of 20 °C and a pH of 3.2, degradation was almost negligible. They found that after 2 years at 40 °C, the concentrations of GDPs produced during storage were of the same magnitude as those caused by heat sterilization.

The validation of the method presented in this work confirms that the investigated parameters were all within the required ranges of the ICH guideline. Compared with the work of Mittelmaier et al. [8], it can be stated that in the present study somewhat higher values for LOD and LOQ were determined for the GDPs GO, MGO, 2-KDG (LOD: 0.30–1.34 µM, LOQ: 0.90–4.07 µM). When investigating marketed single- and double-chamber peritoneal dialysis (PD) fluids, Mittelmaier et al. [8] achieved values for LOD from 0.13 to 0.19 µM and for LOQ from 0.40 to 0.57 µM. However, more sensitive detection and quantification values were obtained for 3-DG/3-DGal as well as for 3,4-DGE and 5-HMF (LOD: 0.02–0.10 µM and LOQ 0.07–0.32 µM).

A useful factor to add to the assessment of the ideal autoclave condition is the fact of toxicity. There are many divergent studies on 5-HMF, which examined the possible genotoxic or carcinogenic potential of 5-HMF [33]. Janzowski et al. found that 5-HMF induced moderate cytotoxicity. DNA damage was not measurable. 5-HMF was weakly mutagenic at concentrations between 80 and 140 mM [34]. This corresponds to a concentration of 10.1–17.7 mg/mL. Ulbricht et al. found that very high levels of 5-HMF exceeding 75 mg/kg body weight may lead to acute toxicity [35].

According to the German national monograph of glucose solutions for parenteral use, however, the limits for 5-HMF are significantly lower, with a maximum of 44 µg/mL. Thus, the possible toxicity level is not reached by far. Although the toxic potential of 5-HMF has been much discussed in the past, it has been classified as not harmful to health according to the safety data sheet and by the German Federal Institute for Risk Assessment (BfR) [36].

After classification of the seven investigated degradation products according to EU Chemicals Regulation (EC) No 1272/2008 [37] it can be stated that especially GO and MGO were classified as potentially germ cell mutagenic (category 2, H341) and that sensitization by skin contact (category 1, H317) is possible [18,19]. In addition, for 3,4-DGE there is a risk of skin corrosion/irritation (category 2) as well as for serious eye damage/eye irritation (category 2) [38]. For 5-HMF there is a potential irritant effect on the skin (category 2), H315 as well as for eye irritation (category 2), H319 [39]. 2-KDG, 3DG, and 3-DGal are not evaluated as hazardous substances or mixtures according to Directive (EC) No 1272/2008 [40–42]. Since a health risk may arise in particular from the GDPs GO and MGO [18,19], it would be useful to set limits here for the presence of these GDPs in glucose infusion solutions.

However, we already found approximately 1 µg/mL for GO and MGO in the non-autoclaved 10% glucose solution that served as reference solution. The fact that a small amount of glucose is enolized and dehydrated even without heat sterilization (Table 6) should be further observed due to the different information on toxicity.

Disadvantages for the human health status result mainly from the further reaction of GDPs in the human body, as it is known that GDPs are highly reactive molecules that bind to serum proteins and lead to the formation of advanced glycation end products (AGEs) [1,6,43]. AGEs increase the oxidative stress of cells [44,45] and accumulate in vessels [11]. They affect the cardiovascular system [44,46–48] and are associated with an increase in cardiovascular morbidity [49] and strokes [50]. They also play a causative role in vascular complications of diabetes mellitus [51], Alzheimer's disease [52], and deterioration of kidney function [5,10,53].

4. Materials and Methods

4.1. Reagents and Chemicals

For all experiments, freshly prepared ultrapure water was taken from Sartorius arium®
pro UV water treatment system (Sartorius AG, Göttingen, Germany). All chemicals were
of analytical grade, unless noted otherwise. Acetonitrile, OPD, 2,3-dimethylquinoxaline,
MGO, GO, 2-KDG, 3-DG, 5-HMF, D-(+)-glucose monohydrate, methanol and ammonium
acetate were purchased from Sigma (Sigma-Aldrich Chemie GmbH, Steinheim, Germany).
3-DGal was obtained from Cayman (Cayman Chemical Company, Ann Arbor, MI, USA).
3,4-DGE was purchased from Carbosynth (Carbosynth Ltd., Compton, Berkshire, UK).

The aqueous phase during LC-MS/MS measurement was a 5 mM ammonium acetate
buffer solution adjusted to pH = 3.5 using 0.1% (v/v) acetic acid. It was freshly prepared in
accordance to Thomas et al. [54]. The EZ-Test® [55] Biological Indicator from MesaLabs
was used in order to test sterility.

4.2. Experimental Overview

In order to investigate the effects of heat and exposure time on heat sterilized glucose
solutions, which can lead to different concentrations of GDPs formed, 10% (w/v) glucose
solutions were prepared and heat sterilized according to the F0 concept, which describes the
sum of all lethal effects acting on a population of the key germ *Geobacillus stearothermophilus*
in the course of heating. Furthermore, the identity and amount of these GDPs were
analyzed using a slightly modified LC-MS/MS method described by Mittelmaier [8].
The autoclaving process was performed in polypropylene (PP) bottles that were heat
resistant up to 121 °C. The amounts of GDPs formed in the different temperature/time
constellations were determined and compared, as were the pH values of the autoclaved and
non-autoclaved solutions. In addition, 10% (w/v) aqueous glucose solutions in PP bottles
from a finished drug manufacturer were tested for the presence of GDPs and compared to
the extent of GDPs formed from the self-autoclaved glucose solutions at 121 °C.

4.2.1. Preparation of Glucose Solutions

A total of 11 L of a 10% (w/v) glucose solution were prepared according to the German
standard approval monograph [20]. Double distilled water and glucose monohydrate
were used for this purpose. The solution was then sterile filtered through pre-sterilized
Stericup and Steritop® Vaccuum Driven Disposable Filtration System with 0.22 μm filter
membranes (Merck Milipore Express PLUS). Filtration was performed directly into the
final containers, which were sterilized by autoclaving. The final containers to be sterilized
were 225 mL PP bottles (Kautex™), each filled with 200 mL glucose solution.

4.2.2. Calculation of the Required Steam Sterilization Time

The reference cycle for steam sterilization is 15 min at 121 °C in saturated steam, with
the temperature measured at the coldest point of the chamber [2]. The calculation of the
sterilization efficiency with the F0 concept was performed by the following equation

$$F0 = (\log N0 - \log Nt) * \left(D2 * 10^{\frac{(T2-T1)}{z}} \right), \tag{3}$$

which is described in the general text of the European Pharmacopoeia [4].

N0 is the assumed initial germ load of 10^6. Nt is the target final germ load after the
autoclaving process 10^{-6}. The D2 value of the reference germ *Bacillus stearothermophilus*
at 121 °C is 1.5. The D-value (or decimal reduction value) is the value of a sterilization
parameter (duration or absorbed dose) required to reduce the number of reproducible units
to 10 percent of the initial value. T2 is the standard temperature of 121 °C. T1 is the selected
temperature (111 °C; 116 °C) and z is the temperature change necessary to change the D
value by a factor of 10. The value 10 was assumed for z.

The F0 value thus obtained is now the new autoclaving time at the selected temperature and for the corresponding germ (= overkill condition). F0 can be described most simply

as the equivalent time required in minutes at 121 °C to produce the same microbiological killing effect as the process used [56].

The calculated F0 values for the overkill procedure according to scheme A were shown in Table 1. The total F0 value of a process (unit: minutes) takes into account the heating and cooling phases of the cycle. The 10% (w/v) glucose solutions calculated and autoclaved in accordance with the F0 concept (scheme A) were also to be compared with solutions that were specifically autoclaved for too long (scheme B), in order to investigate not only the influence of the temperature but also that of the exposure time.

For the calculations of the F0 times of scheme B, the F0 times for heating up and cooling down the glucose solutions were added to the F0 times from A. This is also shown in Table 1. Three batches per selected temperature from schemes A and B were autoclaved, each batch consisting of three bottles, which were processed after cooling. In addition, three batches with three bottles ($n = 9$) of 10% (w/v) glucose solution were heat sterilized at 121 °C for 350 min (F0 = 202 min). The purpose of this experiment was to investigate an extreme situation in terms of autoclaving time with respect to the concentrations of GDPs occurring at the standard temperature of 121°C. Three bottles of a non-autoclaved 10% (w/v) glucose solution were also analyzed (reference value).

4.2.3. Autoclaving under Germicidal Control

The Varioklav EC from Thermo Scientific was used for heat sterilization. The 10% (w/v) glucose solutions in PP bottles were autoclaved at 111 °C, 116 °C, and 121 °C in their final container. To each autoclave run, an ampoule of EZ-Test® from Mesa Labs containing the heat sterilization lead germ *Geobacillus stearothermophilus*, culture 7953, at a concentration of approximately 1×10^5 to 1×10^6 was added to check for successful bacterial kill. In addition to the germ *Geobacillus stearothermophilus*, the ampoule EZ-Test® contains a nutrient solution based on soybean casein digest, as well as the violet pH indicator bromocresol purple. The ampoule was placed in another container filled with water, which was analogous to the final container to be autoclaved (e.g., when autoclaving the PP bottles, the EZ-Test® was placed in another PP bottle filled with water to mimic the conditions in the final container to be sterilized).

After the autoclaved EZ-Test® ampoules had cooled in the fume hood for 10 min, the culture medium and the indicator were activated. For this, the ampoules were placed in an upright position and gently squeezed to break the glass ampoules by hand. The growth media was allowed to come in contact with the spores of *Geobacillus stearothermophilus*.

These ampoules were then placed in an incubator rack in a GFL 3032 incubator and incubated together with an unsterilized ampoule, which was also crushed. The ampoules were incubated at 60 °C for 24 h and afterwards observed for color change.

4.2.4. Measuring of the pH Values

To evaluate the influence of the pH value on the formation of GDPs formed by heat sterilization, the pH value was determined in all autoclaved and non-autoclaved glucose solutions as well as in the control samples.

4.2.5. Preparation of Calibration Solutions

A stock solution containing GO, MGO, 2-KDG, 3-DG, 3-DGal, 3,4-DGE, and 5-HMF, each with a concentration of 100 µg/mL per GDP, was prepared in bi-distilled water in amber vials. This stock solution was diluted with bi-distilled water to obtain a concentration of 2 µg/mL. From this solution, a dilution series was prepared ranging from 0.005 to 0.85 µg/mL. All solutions of the calibration series also contained 0.1 mg/mL glucose, as well as 0.75 mg/mL OPD and 5 µg/mL of the internal standard 2,3-dimethylquinoxaline.

4.2.6. Derivatization of Autoclaved Glucose Solutions

The heat sterilized glucose solutions described in Section 4.2.1. and those from the manufacturers A–C were diluted with water in a ratio of 1:1000. The diluted solutions also contained 0.75 mg/mL OPD and 5 μg/mL of the internal standard (2,3-dimethylquinoxaline).

All solutions were left in the dark for 16 h and were subsequently analyzed via LC-MS/MS. The suitability of the chosen derivatization procedure in terms of OPD concentration and derivatization time has been shown elsewhere [57].

4.2.7. LC-MS/MS Analysis

The development of an LC-MS/MS method was based on the process reported by Mittelmaier et al. [8], which we optimized. Qualitative analysis and structure elucidation was performed by LC-MS/MS. The respective LC-MS/MS parameters and ion transitions are shown in Table 14.

Table 14. Parameters of the LC-MS/MS analysis.

ID	Q1 [m/z]	Q3 [m/z]	Dwell Time [msec]	CE [eV]	DP [eV]	R_t [min]
GO	131.1	76.7	50	40	100	6.95
MGO	145.1	77	50	40	100	7.80
2-KDG	251.1	173.2	50	20	100	3.51
3-DG/3-DGal	235.1	199.1	50	25	100	4.79
3.4-DGE	217.1	169.1	50	20	100	6.37
5-HMF	215.1	197.1	50	25	100	6.46
IS	159.1	118.1	50	40	100	8.48

ID = Identity of analyte, Q1 = Quadrupole 1, Q3 = Quadrupole 3, CE = Collision energy, DP = Declustering Potential, R_t = Retention time.

Liquid chromatography was performed on a Shimadzu Nexera ultra-fast liquid chromatograph (UFLC) equipped with an analytical C18 column (Nucleoshell RP 18, 100 mm × 3 mm, 2.7 μm particle size, Macherey-Nagel, Dueren, Germany). The UHPLC system (degasser, binary pump, autosampler, column oven) was coupled to a SCIEX QTrap6500 triple quadrupole mass spectrometer (Sciex, Darmstadt, Hessen, Germany) and operated under positive electrospray ionization (ESI) conditions with a needle voltage of 5500 V at 450 °C and nitrogen as drying gas.

The collision energies were 40 eV for the internal standard (2,3-Dimethylquinoxaline), MGO- and GO- and 20 eV for 2-KDG- and 3,4-DGE- and 25 eV for 3-DG-, 3-DGal- and 5-HMF-derivatives, respectively. Mobile phase A consisted of a 5 mM ammonium acetate buffer solution adjusted to pH 3.5 using 0.1% (v/v) acetic acid, and mobile phase B consisted of acetonitrile. The total flow rate was 0.35 mL/min. The gradient started at 5% solvent B, remained isocratic for 0.2 min, and increased to 50% B within 10 min. From 10.00 to 10.01 it increased to 100% B, remaining there for 1 min. The column was re-equilibrated from 11.01 min to 14.00 min at 5% B. The overall run time was 14 min. The injection volume was 5 μL. System control, data acquisition, and processing were performed by Analyst 1.6.2 software.

4.2.8. Method Validation

To validate the method, all parameters listed in the ICH Q2 (R1) guideline [22] were considered: Accuracy (reported as percent recovery), precision, linearity, range, limit of detection (LOD), and limit of quantitation (LOQ) were determined.

In order to calculate the accuracy (reported as% recovery), an unheated 10% (w/v) glucose solution fluid was spiked with 0.5, 25, and 100 μg/mL of each GDP, 5 μg/mL internal standard (2,3-dimethylquinoxaline) and 0.75 mg/mL OPD (i.e., three concentrations/six replicates). These samples and an unspiked fluid were analyzed via LC-MS/MS as described in Section 4.2.7. after 16 h of derivatization. The mean recovery of three experiments for each concentration level was determined and expressed as: (GDP concentration-GDP concentration of the unspiked sample)/added GDP concentration×100% (Table 11). Precision was expressed as standard deviation and coefficients of variation (% RSD). Nine determinations covering the specified range for the procedure (three concentrations/three replicates each) were made. The mean value, the standard deviation, and the precision were calculated (Table 11). The LOD was expressed as (3.3 × standard deviation of the response)/slope of calibration curve and LOQ was expressed as (10 × standard deviation of the response)/slope of calibration curve [22]. LOD and LOQ are shown in Table 10. An eight-point-calibration curve in order to determine linearity was prepared in three replicates (0.5–100 µg/mL each GDP in water as well as 10% glucose, 5 µg/mL 2,3-dimethylquinoxaline and 0.75 mg/mL OPD). The calibration curve was obtained by plotting the quotient of the peak areas of the derivatized GDPs and the internal standard (ordinate) against the concentration of the derivatized GDPs (abscissa). Calibration lines are shown in Table 10. Linear regression analysis was used to assess the linearity of the calibration curve. Regression parameters were computed using Excel (Microsoft Office Professional Plus 2016).

4.2.9. Statistical Analysis

The GDP concentrations that occurred at the three temperatures 111 °C, 116 °C, and 121 °C in scheme A should be compared with the analogously measured GDP concentrations of scheme B in order to test for differences in the mean GDP concentration.

In addition, the standard temperature of 121 °C was to be tested against the two temperatures 111 °C and 116 °C with respect to the differences in the measured GDP concentration within scheme A. For this purpose, we used the classical t-test analysis.

The degree of freedom for each of the two-sample tests was 16, since each group consisted of exactly 9 samples. To account for multiple testing, we calculated Bonferroni-corrected *p*-values in addition to the nominal values for each test. All tests were performed by the use of the statistic software environment R-4.0.2.

5. Conclusions

A previously described LC-MS/MS method for quantitative analysis of GDPs typically formed during heat sterilization of glucose solutions was slightly modified and validated according to the ICH Q2(R1) guideline [22]. The modified method was demonstrated to be precise, sensitive, and reproducible and thus suited to screen and simultaneously quantify the content of all 7 GDPs.

After analyzing marketed 10% glucose solutions from manufacturers A–C, as well as 10% glucose solutions prepared and autoclaved according to autoclaving schemes A/B, and taking into account factors such as toxicity, it may be appropriate to change the standard conditions from 121 °C and 15 min to 116 °C and F0 = 57 min. The main reason for this recommendation is that the lowest concentrations of the toxic GDPs GO and MGO occurred when the autoclaving temperature and duration were changed to 116 °C and F0 = 57 min. In this autoclaving scheme, the concentration of 5-HMF was 31.6 µg/mL, still well below the limit of 44 µg/mL required by the national monograph.

Another advantage for industry in the large-scale production of glucose solutions could also be that the proposed new autoclaving temperature of 116 °C is 5 °C below the temperature of the reference process, thus possibly saving energy costs. However, the autoclaving time would also be longer compared to 121 °C and 15 min. The actual energy costs would have to be determined in further trials.

Supplementary Materials: The following are available online at https://www.mdpi.com/article/10.3390/ph14111121/s1, Figure S1: EZ-Test® for the control of germ killing of the lead germ Geobacillus stearothermophilus after heat sterilization, Figure S2: Concentrations of GO after heat sterilization of 10% glucose solutions at 111 °C, 116°C, and 121 °C autoclaved according to scheme A (*n* = 27), Figure S3: Concentrations of MGO after heat sterilization of 10% glucose solutions at 111 °C, 116 °C, and 121 °C autoclaved according to scheme A (*n* = 27), Figure S4: Concentrations of 2-KDG after heat sterilization of 10% glucose solutions at 111 °C, 116 °C, and 121 °C autoclaved according to scheme A (*n* = 27), Figure S5: Concentrations of 3-DG/3-DGal after heat sterilization of 10% glucose solutions at 111 °C, 116 °C, and 121 °C autoclaved according to scheme A (n = 27), Figure S6: Concentrations of 3,4-DGE after heat sterilization of 10% glucose solutions at 111 °C, 116 °C, and 121 °C autoclaved according to scheme A (n = 27), Figure S7: Concentrations of 5-HMF after heat sterilization of 10% glucose solutions at 111 °C, 116 °C, and 121 °C autoclaved according to scheme A (n = 27), Figure S8: Concentrations of GO after heat sterilization of 10% glucose solutions at 111 °C, 116 °C, and 121 °C autoclaved according to scheme B (n = 27), Figure S9: Concentrations of MGO after heat sterilization of 10% glucose solutions at 111 °C, 116 °C and 121 °C autoclaved according to scheme B (n = 27), Figure S10: Concentrations of 2-KDG after heat sterilization of 10% glucose solutions at 111 °C, 116 °C, and 121 °C autoclaved according to scheme B (n = 27), Figure S11: Concentrations of 3-DG/3-DGal after heat sterilization of 10% glucose solutions at 111 °C, 116 °C, and 121 °C autoclaved according to scheme B (n = 27), Figure S12: Concentrations of 3,4-DGE after heat sterilization of 10% glucose solutions at 111 °C, 116 °C, and 121 °C autoclaved according to scheme B (n = 27), Figure S13: Concentrations of 5-HMF after heat sterilization of 10% glucose solutions at 111 °C, 116 °C, and 121 °C autoclaved according to scheme B (n = 27), Figure S14: Concentrations of GDPs in 10% (w/v) glucose solutions in PP bottles heat sterilized at 121 °C for 350 min (F0 = 202 min) (n = 9).

Author Contributions: Conceptualization, S.L., T.Z. and M.B.; data curation, M.V. and M.S.; formal analysis, S.L., M.V. and M.S.; investigation, S.L.; methodology, S.L., M.V., T.Z. and M.B.; project administration, S.L., M.V., T.Z. and M.B.; software, S.L. and M.V.; supervision, M.V., T.Z., C.E.M. and M.B.; validation, S.L. and T.Z.; visualization, S.L. and C.E.M.; writing—original draft, S.L.; writing—review and editing, C.E.M. and M.B. All authors have read and agreed to the published version of the manuscript.

Funding: This research did not receive any dedicated grant from funding agencies in the public, commercial, or not-for-profit sectors.

Institutional Review Board Statement: Not applicable.

Informed Consent Statement: Not applicable.

Data Availability Statement: All data are contained within the article.

Acknowledgments: The authors would like to thank Serag-Wiessner for providing glucose solutions of various batches as well as giving us insight into their autoclaving protocols. Furthermore, we thank BfArM's Pharmacopoeia Unit for their advice in carrying out qualitative and quantitative analysis and the entire BfArM for financial support and the supply of chemicals and equipment.

Conflicts of Interest: The authors have no conflict of interest to declare.

References

1. Haybrard, J.; Simon, N.; Danel, C.; Pinçon, C.; Barthélémy, C.; Tessier, F.J.; Décaudin, B.; Boulanger, E.; Odou, P. Factors Generating Glucose Degradation Products in Sterile Glucose Solutions for Infusion: Statistical Relevance Determination of Their Impacts. *Sci. Rep.* **2017**, *7*, 11932. [CrossRef] [PubMed]
2. Council of Europe. 5.1.1 Methods of Preparation of Sterile Products. In *European Pharmacopoeia 10.0*; EDQM: Strasbourg, France, 2020; pp. 995–1000.
3. Boehringer Ingelheim Pharma KG F0-Concept in Steam Sterilization and the Connected Sterilization Safety. Available online: https://ecv.de/suse_item.php?suseId=Z%7Cpi%7C1762&susePattern (accessed on 19 October 2021).
4. Council of Europe. 5.1.5. Application of the F0 concept to Steam Sterilization of Aqueous Preparations. In *European Pharmacopoeia 10.0*; EDQM: Strasbourg, France, 2020; p. 1009.
5. Bryland, A.; Broman, M.; Erixon, M.; Klarin, B.; Linden, T.; Friberg, H.; Wieslander, A.; Kjellstrand, P.; Ronco, C.; Carlsson, O.; et al. Infusion fluids contain harmful glucose degradation products. *Intensive Care Med.* **2010**, *36*, 1213–1220. [CrossRef] [PubMed]
6. Linden, T.; Forsbäck, G.; Deppisch, R.; Henle, T.; Wieslander, A. 3-Deoxyglucosone, a promoter of advanced glycation end products in fluids for peritoneal dialysis. *Perit. Dial. Int.* **1998**, *18*, 290–293.
7. Kjellstrand, P.; Erixon, M.; Wieslander, A.; Lindén, T.; Martinson, E. Temperature: The Single Most Important Factor for Degradation of Glucose Fluids during Storage. *Perit. Dial. Int.* **2004**, *24*, 385–391. [CrossRef] [PubMed]
8. Mittelmaier, S.; Fünfrocken, M.; Fenn, D.; Berlich, R.; Pischetsrieder, M. Quantification of the six major α-dicarbonyl contaminants in peritoneal dialysis fluids by UHPLC/DAD/MSMS. *Anal. Bioanal. Chem.* **2011**, *401*, 1183–1193. [CrossRef]
9. Ledebo, I.; Wieslander, A.; Kjellstrand, P. Can we prevent the degradation of glucose in peritoneal dialysis solutions? *Perit. Dial. Int.* **2000**, *20*, 48–51. [CrossRef]
10. Frischmann, M.; Spitzer, J.; Fünfrocken, M.; Mittelmaier, S.; Deckert, M.; Fichert, T.; Pischetsrieder, M. Development and validation of an HPLC method to quantify 3,4-dideoxyglucosone-3-ene in peritoneal dialysis fluids. *Biomed. Chromatogr.* **2009**, *23*, 843–851. [CrossRef]

11. Nakayama, M.; Kawaguchi, Y.; Yamada, K.; Hasegawa, T.; Takazoe, K.; Katoh, N.; Hayakawa, H.; Osaka, N.; Yamamoto, H.; Ogawa, A.; et al. Immunohistochemical detection of advanced glycosylation end-products in the peritoneum and its possible pathophysiological role in CAPD. *Kidney Int.* **1997**, *51*, 182–186. [CrossRef]
12. Mannermaaa, J.P.; Yliruusic, J.; Kanerva, U. Optimization of Moist Heat Sterilization of Glucose Infusions—The effect of different Fo-values on the pH and 5-hydroxymethyl 2-furaldehyde content of the solutions. *Pharm. Ind.* **1992**, *54*, 729–732.
13. Mannermaaa, J.P.; Yliruusic, J.; Muttonen, E. Optimization of Moist Heat Sterilization of Glucose Infusions—The effect of sterilization parameters on the number of particles released from different rubber stoppers. *Pharm. Ind.* **1992**, *54*, 639–642.
14. Mannermaa, J.P.; Muttonen, E.; Yliruusi, J.; Määttänen, L. The use of different time/temperature combinations in the optimization of sterilization of Ringers/glucose infusion solution. *J. Pharm. Sci. Technol.* **1992**, *46*, 184–191.
15. Hung, C.T.; Selkirk, A.B.; Taylor, R.B. A chromatographic quality control procedure based on HPLC for 5-hydroxymethylfurfural in autoclaved D-glucose infusion fluids. *J. Clin. Pharm. Ther.* **1982**, *7*, 17–23. [CrossRef] [PubMed]
16. Cook, A.P.; Macleod, T.M.; Appleton, J.D.; Fell, A.F. Reversed-phase high-performance liquid chromatographic method for the quantification of 5-hydroxymethylfurfural as the major degradation product of glucose in infusion fluids. *J. Chromatogr. A* **1989**, *467*, 395–401. [CrossRef]
17. Postaire, E.; Pradier, F.; Postaire, M.; Pradeau, D.; Matchoutsky, L.; Prognon, P.; Hamon, M. Various techniques for the routine evaluation of the degradation of glucose in parenteral solutions—A critical study. *J. Pharm. Biomed. Anal.* **1987**, *5*, 309–318. [CrossRef]
18. Sigma-Aldrich. Taufkirchen (Germany), Safety Data Sheet. Glyoxal Solution. Product Number 128465. 2020. Available online: https://www.sigmaaldrich.com/DE/de/sds/sial/128465 (accessed on 27 October 2021).
19. Sigma-Aldrich. Taufkirchen (Germany), Safety Data Sheet. Methylglyoxal Solution. Product Number M0252. 2019. Available online: https://www.sigmaaldrich.com/DE/de/sds/sigma/m0252 (accessed on 27 October 2021).
20. Braun, R. Glucose-Lösungen 5 bis 50%. In *Standardzulassungen für Fertigarzneimittel*; Deutscher Apotheker Verlag: Eschborn, Germany, 2010; Volume 16.
21. National Library of Medicine. Compund Summary. Bromocresol Purple. PubChem CID 8273. Available online: https://pubchem.ncbi.nlm.nih.gov/compound/Bromocresol-purple (accessed on 27 October 2021).
22. European Medicines Agency ICH Topic Q 2 (R1) Validation of Analytical Procedures: Text and Methodology. Available online: https://www.ema.europa.eu/en/documents/scientific-guideline/ich-q-2-r1-validation-analytical-procedures-text-methodology-step-5_en.pdf (accessed on 19 October 2021).
23. Pohloudek-Fabini, R.; Martin, E. The effect of the gas permeability of plastics on the stability of thiomersal. Part 49: Contributions to problems concerning the use of plastic receptacles for liquid pharmaceuticals (author's transl). *Pharmazie* **1981**, *36*, 683–685.
24. Allwood, M.C.; Kearney, M.C. Compatibility and stability of additives in parenteral nutrition admixtures. *Nutrition* **1998**, *14*, 697–706. [CrossRef]
25. Ball, C.O. Thermal process time for canned food. *Bull. Natl. Res. Counc.* **1923**, *7*, 1–76.
26. Reuter, H. Bewertung der thermischen Wirksamtkeit von UHT-Anlagen, Teil I: Reaktionskinetische Grundlagen. *Dtsch. Molk.-Ztg.* **1980**, *101*, 362–370.
27. Burton, H. *Ultra-High-Temperature Processing of Milk and Milk Products*; Elsevier Applied Science: London, UK, 1988.
28. Miorini, T. Grundlagen der Sterilisation. Available online: https://wfhss.com/wp-content/uploads/wfhss-training-2-03_de.pdf (accessed on 19 October 2021).
29. Tao, F.-R.; Zhuang, C.; Cui, Y.-Z.; Xu, J. Dehydration of glucose into 5-hydroxymethylfurfural in SO3H-functionalized ionic liquids. *Chin. Chem. Lett.* **2014**, *25*, 757–761. [CrossRef]
30. Sturgeon, R.J.; Athanikar, N.K.; Harbison, H.A.; Henry, R.S.; Jurgens, R.W.; Welco, A.D. Degradation of Dextrose during Heating under Simulated Sterilization. *PDA J. Pharm. Sci. Technol.* **1980**, *34*, 175–182.
31. Qian, X.; Nimlos, M.R.; Johnson, D.K.; Himmel, M.E. Acidic sugar degradation pathways. *Appl. Biochem. Biotechnol.* **2005**, *124*, 989–997. [CrossRef]
32. Kjellstrand, P.; Martinson, E.; Wieslander, A.; Kjellstrand, K.; Jeppsson, E.; Svensson, E.; Järkelid, L.; Linden, T.; Olsson, L.F. Degradation in peritoneal dialysis fluids may be avoided by using low pH and high glucose concentration. *Perit. Dial. Int.* **2001**, *21*, 338–344. [CrossRef]
33. Capuano, E.; Fogliano, V. Acrylamide and 5-hydroxymethylfurfural (HMF): A review on metabolism, toxicity, occurrence in food and mitigation strategies. *LWT Food Sci. Technol.* **2011**, *44*, 793–810. [CrossRef]
34. Janzowski, C.; Glaab, V.; Samimi, E.; Schlatter, J.; Eisenbrand, G. 5-Hydroxymethylfurfural: Assessment of mutagenicity, DNA-damaging potential and reactivity towards cellular glutathione. *Food Chem. Toxicol.* **2000**, *38*, 801–809. [CrossRef]
35. Ulbricht, R.J.; Northup, S.J.; Thomas, J.A. A review of 5-hydroxymethylfurfural (HMF) in parenteral solutions. *Fundam. Appl. Toxicol.* **1984**, *4*, 843–853. [CrossRef]
36. Bundesinstitut für Risikobewertung 5-HMF-Gehalte in Lebensmitteln Sind Nach Derzeitigem Wissenschaftlichen Kenntnisstand Gesundheitlich Unproblematisch. Available online: https://www.bfr.bund.de/cm/343/5_hmf_gehalte_in_lebensmitteln_sind_nach_derzeitigem_wissenschaftlichen_kenntnisstand_gesundheitlich_unproblematisch.pdf (accessed on 19 October 2021).

37. European Parliament and of the Council Regulation (EC) No 1272/2008 of the European Parliament and of the Council of 16 December 2008 on Classification, Labelling and Packaging of Substances and Mixtures, Amending and Repealing Directives 67/548/EEC and 1999/45/EC, and Amending Regulation (EC) No 1907/2006 (Text with EEA Relevance). Available online: https://eur-lex.europa.eu/eli/reg/2008/1272/oj (accessed on 19 October 2021).
38. Carbosynth Ltd. Compton (UK), Safety Data Sheet. 3,4-Dideoxyglucosone-3-ene. Product Number MD44643. 2021. Available online: https://www.carbosynth.com/80257AD2003D1CDB/0/64654136FF2B356548257F64000E36D2/$file/MSDS_MD44643_5000_EN.pdf (accessed on 27 October 2021).
39. Sigma-Aldrich. Taufkirchen (Germany), Safety Data Sheet. 5-(Hydroxymethyl)-furfural. Product Number 53407. 2019. Available online: https://www.sigmaaldrich.com/DE/de/sds/sial/53407 (accessed on 27 October 2021).
40. Sigma-Aldrich. Taufkirchen (Germany), Safety Data Sheet. 2-Keto-D-glucose. Product Number 61793. 2019. Available online: https://www.sigmaaldrich.com/DE/de/sds/sigma/61793 (accessed on 27 October 2021).
41. Cayman Chemical. Ann Arbor. Michigan (US), Safety Data Sheet. 3-deoxy Galactosone. Product Number 16801. 2020. Available online: https://www.caymanchem.com/msdss/16801m.pdf (accessed on 27 October 2021).
42. Sigma-Aldrich. Taufkirchen (Germany), Safety Data Sheet. 3-Deoxyglucosone. Product Number 75762. 2019. Available online: https://www.sigmaaldrich.com/DE/de/sds/sigma/75762 (accessed on 27 October 2021).
43. Zeier, M.; Schwenger, V.; Deppisch, R.; Haug, U.; Weigel, K.; Bahner, U.; Wanner, C.; Schneider, H.; Henle, T.; Ritz, E. Glucose degradation products in PD fluids: Do they disappear from the peritoneal cavity and enter the systemic circulation? *Kidney Int.* **2003**, *63*, 298–305. [CrossRef]
44. García–López, E.; Carrero, J.J.; Suliman, M.E.; Lindholm, B.; Stenvinkel, P. Risk Factors for Cardiovascular Disease in Patients Undergoing Peritoneal Dialysis. *Perit. Dial. Int.* **2007**, *27*, 205–209. [CrossRef]
45. Kandarakis, S.A.; Piperi, C.; Topouzis, F.; Papavassiliou, A.G. Emerging role of advanced glycation-end products (AGEs) in the pathobiology of eye diseases. *Prog. Retin. Eye Res.* **2014**, *42*, 85–102. [CrossRef] [PubMed]
46. Himmele, R.; Sawin, D.-A.; Diaz-Buxo, J.A. GDPs and AGEs: Impact on cardiovascular toxicity in dialysis patients. *Adv. Perit. Dial.* **2011**, *27*, 22–26.
47. Müller-Krebs, S.; Kihm, L.; Zeier, B.; Gross, M.; Wieslander, A.; Haug, U.; Zeier, M.; Schwenger, V. Glucose degradation products result in cardiovascular toxicity in a rat model of renal failure. *Perit. Dial. Int.* **2010**, *30*, 35–40. [CrossRef] [PubMed]
48. Simm, A.; Wagner, J.; Gursinsky, T.; Nass, N.; Friedrich, I.; Schinzel, R.; Czeslik, E.; Silber, R.E.; Scheubel, R.J. Advanced glycation endproducts: A biomarker for age as an outcome predictor after cardiac surgery? *Exp. Gerontol.* **2007**, *42*, 668–675. [CrossRef]
49. Cho, Y.; Johnson, D.W.; Vesey, D.A.; Hawley, C.M.; Pascoe, E.M.; Clarke, M.; Topley, N. Baseline serum interleukin-6 predicts cardiovascular events in incident peritoneal dialysis patients. *Perit. Dial. Int.* **2015**, *35*, 35–42. [CrossRef]
50. Zimmerman, G.A.; Meistrell, M.; Bloom, O.; Cockroft, K.M.; Bianchi, M.; Risucci, D.; Broome, J.; Farmer, P.; Cerami, A.; Vlassara, H. Neurotoxicity of advanced glycation endproducts during focal stroke and neuroprotective effects of aminoguanidine. *Proc. Natl. Acad. Sci. USA* **1995**, *92*, 3744–3748. [CrossRef]
51. Chawla, D.; Bansal, S.; Banerjee, B.; Madhu, S.; Kalra, O.P.; Tripathi, A. Role of advanced glycation end product (AGE)-induced receptor (RAGE) expression in diabetic vascular complications. *Microvasc. Res.* **2014**, *95*, 1–6. [CrossRef]
52. Srikanth, V.; Maczurek, A.; Phan, T.; Steele, M.; Westcott, B.; Juskiw, D.; Münch, G. Advanced glycation endproducts and their receptor RAGE in Alzheimer's disease. *Neurobiol. Aging* **2011**, *32*, 763–777. [CrossRef] [PubMed]
53. Sarafidis, P.A.; Whaley-Connell, A.; Sowers, J.R.; Bakris, G.L. Cardiometabolic syndrome and chronic kidney disease: What is the link? *J. CardioMetab. Syndr.* **2006**, *1*, 58–65. [CrossRef] [PubMed]
54. Thomas, A.; Vogel, M.; Piper, T.; Krug, O.; Beuck, S.; Schänzer, W.; Thevis, M. Quantification of AICAR-ribotide concentrations in red blood cells by means of LC-MSMS. *Anal. Bioanal. Chem.* **2013**, *405*, 9703–9709. [CrossRef]
55. MesaLabs EZ-Test® Steam. Geobacillus Stearothermophilus. Technical Report. Available online: https://biologicalindicators.mesalabs.com/wp-content/uploads/sites/31/2013/11/EZTest-Steam-TIR-003.pdf (accessed on 19 October 2021).
56. Cook, A.P.; MacLeod, T.M.; Appleton, J.D.; Fell, A.F. HPLC studies on the degradation profiles of glucose 5% solutions subjected to heat sterilization in a microprocessor-controlled autoclave. *J. Clin. Pharm. Ther.* **1989**, *14*, 189–195. [CrossRef]
57. Leitzen, S.; Vogel, M.; Engels, A.; Zapf, T.; Brandl, M. Identification and quantification of glucose degradation products in heat-sterilized glucose solutions for parenteral use by thinlayer chromatography. *PLoS ONE* **2021**, *16*, e0253811. [CrossRef] [PubMed]

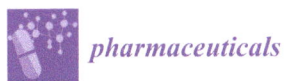

Article

Application of High-Performance Liquid Chromatography for Simultaneous Determination of Tenofovir and Creatinine in Human Urine and Plasma Samples

Patrycja Olejarz, Grażyna Chwatko, Paweł Kubalczyk, Krystian Purgat, Rafał Głowacki and Kamila Borowczyk *

Department of Environmental Chemistry, Faculty of Chemistry, University of Lodz, 163 Pomorska Str., 90-236 Łódź, Poland; patrycja.olejarz@o2.pl (P.O.); grazyna.chwatko@chemia.uni.lodz.pl (G.C.); pawel.kubalczyk@chemia.uni.lodz.pl (P.K.); krystianpurgat@gmail.com (K.P.); rafal.glowacki@chemia.uni.lodz.pl (R.G.)
* Correspondence: kamila.borowczyk@chemia.uni.lodz.pl; Tel.: +48-4263-558-44

Received: 30 September 2020; Accepted: 4 November 2020; Published: 5 November 2020

Abstract: Tenofovir disoproxil fumarate is widely used in the therapy of human immunodeficiency virus and hepatitis B virus; however, a high concentration of the prodrug effects kidney function damage. To control the effectiveness of kidney functions in treated patients, the level of creatinine in the body must be controlled. This work describes a simple, fast, and "plastic-waste" reducing method for the simultaneous determination of tenofovir and creatinine in human urine and plasma. In both assays, only 50 µL of body fluid was required. The tests were carried out by reversed phase high-performance liquid chromatography with UV detection. In urine samples, the limits of detection for tenofovir and creatinine were 4 µg mL^{-1} and 0.03 µmol mL^{-1}, respectively. In plasma samples, the limits of detection were 0.15 µg mL^{-1} for tenofovir and 0.0003 µmol mL^{-1} for creatinine. The method was applied for the determination of tenofovir and creatinine in human urine and plasma samples. The biggest advantage of the elaborated method is the possibility to determine tenofovir and creatinine in one analytical run in both urine and plasma sample collected from HIV and HBV patients. The possibility to reduce the level of laboratory waste in a sample preparation protocol is in the mainstream of a new trend of analytical chemistry which is based on green chemistry.

Keywords: tenofovir; creatinine; HPLC-UV; hepatitis B virus; human immunodeficiency virus

1. Introduction

The report presented by the Joint United Nations Program on HIV/AIDS (UNAIDS) in 2018 shows that 36.9 million people globally are living with human immunodeficiency virus (HIV) [1]. The World Health Organization (WHO) found that, worldwide, 257.0 million persons were living infected with hepatitis B virus (HBV) in 2016, and 1.3 million deaths were caused by the virus in 2015 alone. Both viruses are major public health problems that require an urgent response [2].

HBV infection is caused by the virus belonging to the hepadnavirus family, one of the smallest viruses known to infect humans. The enveloped DNA virus infects liver cells, causing hepatocellular necrosis and inflammation [2,3]. HIV infects immune system cells and is able to destroy or impair their functions [1].

To stop the worldwide transmission of HBV and HIV, the WHO recommends the use of antiretroviral (ARV) treatment for infected people and the application of ARV drugs to prevent the mother-to-child transmission of HIV [2–5]. Currently, to treat patients with chronic hepatitis B

(CHB), HBV or HIV, or people living with HBV-HIV coinfection, seven antiviral agents have been recommended. One of those is tenofovir disoproxil fumarate, which is an orally available bioactive prodrug of tenofovir (TFV) [6]. TFV is a nucleotide analog of reverse transcriptase, which is very effective in therapy against retroviruses and hepadnaviruses [7]. It was approved by the US Food and Drug Administration for the treatment of infections: HIV in 2001 and CHB in 2008. Currently, TFV is recommended as one of the first drugs in monotherapy of CHB [8]. Statistical data presented by the WHO have shown a crucial delay in the progression of cirrhosis, reduction in the incidence of CHB and improvement of long-term survival in people living with HBV treated with TFV [3]. Generally, TFV is well tolerated. However, some evidence of a decrease in bone mineral density, changes in kidney functions and in the rate of tubular dysfunction after treatment with TFV has been reported [9,10]. TFV treatment has been confirmed to be associated with a higher risk of nephrotoxicity in clinical cohorts [11,12]. Several studies have shown a raised prevalence of proximal renal tubular dysfunction in TFV-treated patients, attributed to increased intracellular TFV concentrations and direct mitochondrial toxicity in the proximal tubule cells [13,14].

The first case of nephrotoxicity induced by TFV in a patient with HIV was reported in 2002 [15]. Since that time, severe or symptomatic nephrotoxicity has also been reported in CHB patients treated with TFV [16–20]. That was proven that even short-term therapy with this drug results in severe renal dysfunction [20]. Due to the nephrotoxicity of TFV, every initiation of the drug treatment must be preceded by renal function control. Additionally, more frequent monitoring of TFV level and kidney functions in TFV-treated patients at higher risk of renal dysfunction is recommended by the WHO [3].

The guideline on TFV monitoring in HBV patients published by the European Liver Research Association recommends an estimation of glomerular filtration rate (eGFR) before starting the TFV therapy. The eGFR control is based on comparison of levels of creatinine (Crn) in plasma and urine. Monitoring of eGFR in all patients treated with TFV every 1–3 months during the first year of treatment and then every 3–6 months is recommended by the WHO [3,21].

The renal clearance of Crn is one of the most used and commonly accepted tests of renal function [22]. Since TFV is mainly excreted by tubular secretion and it is active on the tubular cells, its urinary concentration could be a useful marker of TFV-associated tubular toxicity and a reasonable candidate for clinical use [21]. Additional tests for Crn concentration in urine and plasma are helpful to control the bodily absorption, distribution, metabolism and TFV excretion.

Since HIV and HBV infections are possible through blood samples, the use of urine in place of plasma for body TFV monitoring seems to be safer, more significant and deeply required [2,3,22]. Utilization of urine samples significantly reduces the risk of random infections associated with the transport, storage or disposal of infected samples compared to plasma. Moreover, for studying the effect of antiviral therapy on kidney functions, it is necessary to determine the Crn content in urine.

The lack of information about analytical protocols dedicated for simultaneous quantitation of TFV and Crn indicates the need to develop an essential assay for the measurement of side-effects/interactions and optimization of treatment protocols of HIV and HBV/CHB patients. In this paper, we present a new analytical tool based on reversed-phase high-performance liquid chromatography (RP-HPLC) with UV detection for the direct and simultaneous determination of Crn and TFV in urine samples collected from CHB patient treated with TFV and plasma samples spiked with this drug.

2. Results

2.1. Chromatpgraphy

RP-HPLC is one of the most common analytical techniques dedicated to biological sample analysis. The choice of chromatographic conditions directly affects the quality of analyte separation. The amounts of organic and inorganic solvents in a mobile phase are crucial from the chromatographic, economic and environmental points of view. To reduce the amount of toxic waste in this analysis, we decided to use low-concentration phosphate buffer (PB) and a small amount of acetonitrile (MeCN).

The mobile-phase pH can be a powerful tool to control retention and selectivity. Hence, we studied concentrations of PB in the range from 0.01 to 0.05 mol L^{-1} and its pH in the range from 7.0 to 7.6 (Figure 1). The results were obtained using a urine sample spiked with Crn and TFV. The analysis was performed at 25 °C with a mobile phase flow rate equal to 1 mL min^{-1}.

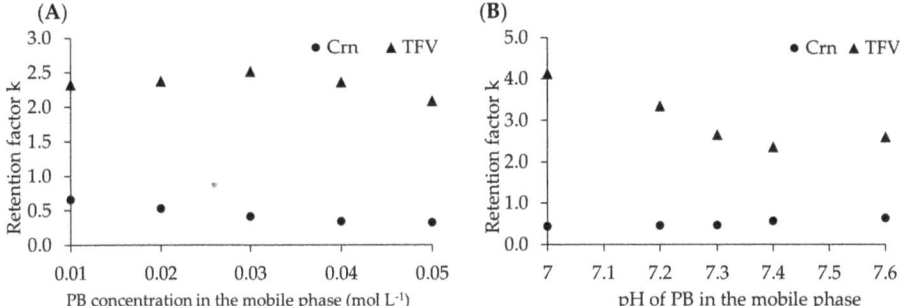

Figure 1. The influence of phosphate buffer (PB) concentration (**A**) and pH (**B**) in the mobile phase on the retention factors of creatinine (Crn) and tenofovir (TFV). Chromatographic conditions in Section 4.5.

In the case of chromatographic methods based on UV detection, utilization of the most proper wavelengths is crucial for detection of the analyte and the method sensitivity. For this reason, we considered application of two different wavelengths. Detection was carried out by using 234 nm from 0 to 3 min for Crn monitoring and 260 nm from 3 to 8 min for TFV detection. Representative chromatograms of urine and plasma samples have been presented on Figure 2.

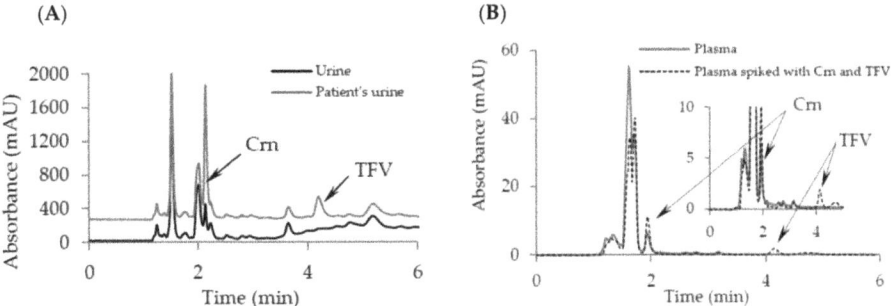

Figure 2. Representative chromatograms of: (**A**) urine, patient's urine and patient's urine spiked with TFV; (**B**) plasma and plasma spiked with Crn and TFV. Chromatographic conditions in Section 4.5.

2.2. Method Validation

2.2.1. Method Calibration

For method calibration, 50 μL of urine samples were placed in glass vials and spiked with 10 μL of growing amounts of working standard solution containing the analytes at seven levels of concentration. The calibration ranges were 10.0–300.0 μg mL^{-1} urine and 0.1–30 μmol mL^{-1} urine for TFV and Crn, respectively. Plasma samples (50 μL) were spiked with the increasing amounts of working solutions of TFV and Crn to provide the final concentration of TFV from 0.5 to 5 μg mL^{-1} plasma and for Crn from 0.001 to 0.04 μmol mL^{-1} plasma. Then, the samples were processed according to the procedures described in Section 4.4. The calibration solutions were prepared in triplicate. The calibration curves were obtained by plotting the peak areas against the analyte concentrations. Regression equations and correlation coefficients have been presented in Table 1.

Table 1. Calibration data.

Analyte (n = 3)	Linear Ranges	Regression Equation	R^2	RSD (%)		Recovery (%)	
				Min	Max	Min	Max
TFV (μg mL^{-1} urine)	10.0–300.0	$y = 2.02x + 0.47$	0.999	1.1	6.1	96.0	108.0
TFV (μg mL^{-1} plasma)	0.5–5.0	$y = 4.12x - 0.06$	0.999	2.1	8.4	99.0	100.3
Crn (μmol mL^{-1} urine)	0.1–30.0	$y = 415.88x + 514.96$	1.000	0.4	3.1	99.3	111.1
Crn (μmol mL^{-1} plasma)	0.001–0.04	$y = 1086.71x + 24.19$	0.999	0.3	4.9	93.6	107.4

2.2.2. LOD and LOQ

The limit of detection (LOD) and limit of quantification (LOQ) were defined as the concentrations with a signal-to-noise (S/N) ratio of 3 and 10, respectively [23]. Peaks of the analytes were identified by comparison of spectrum and retention time with parameters obtained for authentic standards. In the method dedicated to urine, LODs were 4 μg mL^{-1} and 0.03 μmol mL^{-1}, while LOQs were 8 μg mL^{-1} and 0.1 μmol mL^{-1} for TFV and Crn, respectively. In the method dedicated to the determination of TFV and Crn in plasma, LODs and LOQs were 0.15 and 0.2 μg mL^{-1} for TFV and 0.0003 and 0.001 μmol mL^{-1} for Crn, respectively.

2.2.3. Precision and Accuracy

Precision and accuracy were calculated using the results of the analysis of urine and plasma samples spiked with known amounts of these analytes, analyzed in triplicate. The procedure followed the guidelines for biological sample analysis [23,24]. Precision was expressed in terms of relative standard deviation (RSD), whereas accuracy was considered as the percentage of analyte recovery calculated by expressing the mean measured amount as a percentage of the added amount. The estimated validation parameters for analytes were satisfying. The detailed data are presented in Table 2.

Table 2. Accuracy and precision.

Analyte	Concentrations	Precision (%)		Accuracy (%)	
		Intra-Day	Inter-Day	Intra-Day	Inter-Day
TFV (μg mL^{-1} urine)	10	2.3	5.8	95.9	105.7
	40	4.1	8.1	97.5	113.4
	300	1.9	4.3	100.3	96.1
TFV (μg mL^{-1} plasma)	0.5	4.7	5.6	91.1	93.8
	2	4.1	3.6	91.5	93.5
	5	3.7	4.5	93.3	97.2
Crn (μmol mL^{-1} urine)	0.1	4.2	6.8	111.4	120.1
	2.5	1.7	5.4	100.6	104.4
	30	3.7	6.1	99.3	108.9
Crn (μmol mL^{-1} plasma)	0.001	1.9	4.0	91.3	102.8
	0.01	0.6	5.1	100.9	99.6
	0.04	0.5	1.4	100.7	99.3

2.3. Stability Study

To confirm the usefulness of the elaborated method, the analyte stability studies were also performed. Urine and plasma samples were spiked with known amounts of analytes and prepared according to protocols described in Section 4.4. Samples were kept at 4 °C—the temperature used during sample storing—and at 37 °C—the temperature close to the human body temperature. Samples were analyzed in 30 min intervals over 3 h for plasma and 4 h for urine. Urine and plasma samples dedicated for stability studies were prepared in triplicate. The obtained data are presented in Figure 3.

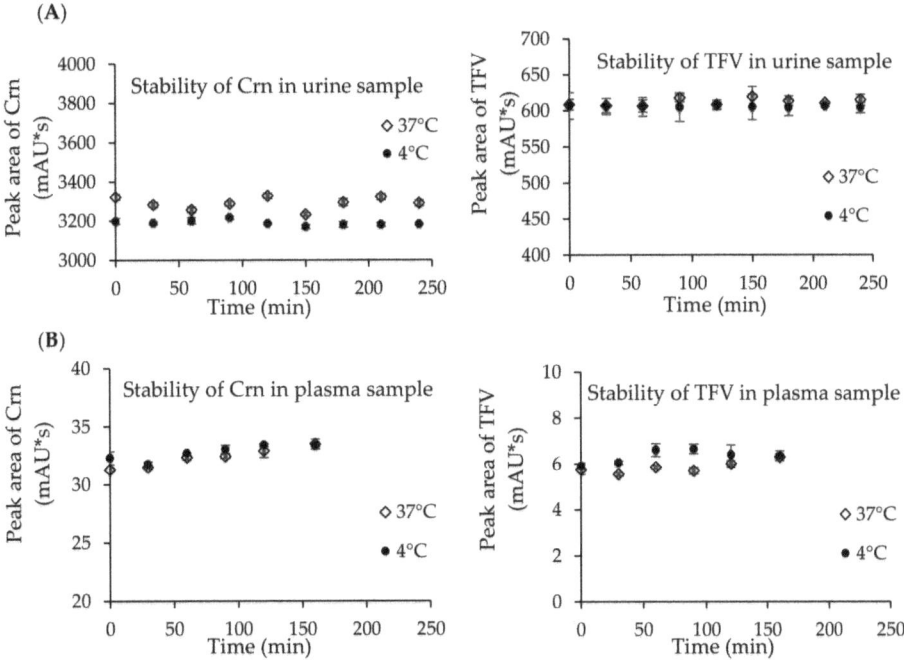

Figure 3. Stability of Crn and TFV in urine (**A**) and plasma (**B**) samples kept at 4 °C and 37 °C; $n = 3$ for each time point.

2.4. Urinary Excretion of TFV

The method was applied to control the urinary excretion of TFV in one CHB patient treated with TFV in form of Viread 123 mg film-coated tablets. Urine samples were collected after one, two, four, six and eight hours after taking the pharmaceutical dose, prepared in triplicate and analyzed. The concentration of TFV in each sample was simultaneously normalized to Crn. The obtained results are presented in Figure 4.

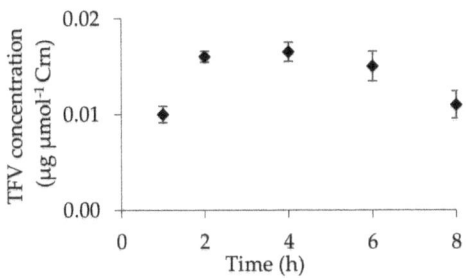

Figure 4. Urinary excretion of TFV after drug intake in dose 123 mg. TFV concentration normalized against Crn; $n = 3$ for each time point.

2.5. Carry-Over Assay

To confirm the possibility of the application of reusable/washed HPLC glass vials, the carry-over assay was performed. Carry-over was assessed by injecting two blank proxy matrix placed in glass vials used previously for storage the high concentrated solutions of standards (300 μg mL^{-1} for TFV and 30 μmol mL^{-1} for Crn). No peaks at the retention times of the analytes were found. Since Crn is an endogenous compound present in human urine, in this experiment we used a proxy matrix as the blank samples.

3. Discussion

Due to high individual variability of pharmacokinetic in different patients treated with the same dose of TFV monitoring of TFV level in HIV and HBV patient's body fluids is recommended by the WHO [3,25]. The dissimilarity is related to the quality and speed of metabolism and interactions between drugs. TFV concentration in plasma affects its action in the human body. Too low a level of the drug may lead to immunization of the virus, while too high concentration significantly increases its renal toxicity [9,10]. Monitoring of TFV in HIV patients is required in controlling the therapeutic dose and in relation to the control of normal renal functions [26,27]. In patients with impaired renal function, it is necessary to adjust the dose of the drug, due to its potential toxicity. The control is performed by Crn clearance study [28,29].

Testing of TFV level in human peripheral blood might be painful for patients and carries the risk of additional HIV/HBV infections. Methods created for TFV determination in non-infected matrices, such as urine [28,30] or hair [31,32], do not provide the possibility for simultaneous monitoring concentration of Crn. Previously published reports mainly described methods for the determination of TFV in plasma [25,26,29,33–40], which determines a higher risk of infection. These assays were based on a solid phase extraction [35,41–43] or derivatization [37].

Additional steps in analytical protocols usually increase the number of used tubes, tips, polypropylene vials or columns for solid phase extraction. We proposed the preparation of urine samples directly in HPLC glass vials. To confirm if this can produce a carry-over effect, we performed an additional test. Using the same glass vial for the analysis of standard solutions and next for proxy matrix analysis, we did not observe peaks at the retention times of the analytes in the blank samples. Additionally, precision and accuracy presented in Table 2 show the low possibility of a carry-over effect for the method. We confirmed that even at the highest concentration, there were no adsorption issues related to glass and it was possible to evaluate the LOQ level. This indicates that the goals of the reduction in plastic waste and the possibility to reuse the glass vials have been obtained. In the literature, only two methods are known to be useful for the determination of TFV in urine samples [28,30]; however, none of these allow for the determining of Crn. For decreasing the hazardous properties of the matrix collected from HIV or HBV/CHB patients, analysis of urine samples is more desirable. The acquisition and preparation of urine are safer and do not pose a threat of HIV infection.

Previously described assays dedicated for TFV determination are based on RP-HPLC, usually coupled with mass spectrometry [25,29,32,37,39,40]. Methods requiring commonly available detectors such as spectrophotometric [35,36] or spectrofluorimetric [33,34] detectors are used rarely.

To obtain the most acceptable results of chromatographic separation, various analytical columns, including Aeris WIDEPORE XB-C18 (150 × 4.6 mm, 5 μm), Poroshell (75 × 4.6 mm, 2.7 μm), Kinetex HILIC (100 × 4.6 mm, 2.6 μm) and Zorbax SB C-18 (150 × 4.6 mm, 5 μm) were tested. The choice was based on information that Aeris WIDEPORE column enables the analysis of plasma samples without previous deproteinization [44]. HILIC is one of the most commonly applied methods to solve retention problems of highly polar analytes [45]. Due to the high polarity of the tested compounds, we evaluated the use of a HILIC column. A typical mobile phase for HILIC chromatography includes water-miscible polar organic solvents such as MeCN with a small amount of water [45]. Alcohols can also be adopted, although a higher concentration is needed to achieve the same degree of retention of the analyte relative to an aprotic solvent–water combination [46]. HILIC separations are performed either in isocratic mode with a high percentage of organic solvent or with gradients starting with a high percentage of organic solvent and ending with a high proportion of aqueous solvent [47]. To obtain the best resolution of the analytes for each column, several mobile phase variations were investigated, and initially the effect of organic modifiers such as methanol and MeCN was evaluated. Our aim was to obtain sharp peaks within an acceptable analysis time and to minimize the amount of organic modifier in the mobile phase. The best separation with the symmetrical peak shapes was performed using the Zorbax SB C-18 (150 × 4.6 mm, 5 μm) column. To provide optimal separation between eluted compounds, MeCN was selected as an organic modifier and the gradient mode of separation was performed.

To the best of our knowledge, the HPLC-UV method described herein is the first that makes it possible to determine both Crn and TFV in urine or plasma samples in one analytical run. The total time for urine sample preparation and analysis is less than 10 min, and is shorter than in previous assays [25,30,35,36]. The proposed assay provides quick determination of TFV and simultaneous normalization against Crn concentration. This significantly shortens the entire time of the analytical procedure. The proposed analytical conditions allow good separation of analytes from the matrix components. For Crn, the retention time was 2.3 min, and for TFV, it was 4.5 min. Detection was carried out by using two different wavelengths in one analytical run. The gradient of wavelengths improved specificity and sensitivity of the method.

The proposed analytical procedure has been fully validated. The process was based on recommendations of the EMA Guideline on Bioanalytical Method Validation (2015) [23] and the FDA Guidance for Industry Bioanalytical Method Validation (2018) [24]. The obtained data meet the validation requirements (Tables 1 and 2). To confirm the precision and accuracy of the elaborated assay, we have compared parameters of the new assay to methods published before, using data indicated for urine and plasma samples (Tables 3 and 4). As shown in Tables 3 and 4, the obtained validation data are satisfying. The presented method requires only 50 μL of the sample, while in the previously published methods, much higher volumes of urine or plasma (Tables 3 and 4) were demanded [30,35,36,38].

Table 3. Comparison of validation parameters methods for determination of TFV in urine sample.

Parameters	LC-DAD * [30]	LC-MS * [28]	Proposed Method
Sample volume (mL)	0.5	1.0	0.05
Linear range (μg mL^{-1})	1–100	-	10–300
R^2	0.999	0.999	0.999
LOD (μg mL^{-1})	0.14	0.19	4.0
LOQ (μg mL^{-1})	0.42	0.39	8.0
Intra-day (RSD%)	0.54	6.69	2.8
Inter-day (RSD%)	0.89	9.38	6.1

* The method cannot be applied for the determination of creatinine in urine samples.

Table 4. Comparison of validation parameters methods for determination of TFV in plasma sample.

Parameters	LC-DAD * [35]	LC-UV * [36]	Proposed Method
Sample volume (mL)	0.1	1.00	0.05
Linear range (μg mL^{-1})	0.02–10.0	0.01–4.0	0.5–5
R^2	0.999	-	0.999
LOD (μg mL^{-1})	0.02	0.003	0.15
LOQ (μg mL^{-1})	0.06	0.01	0.5
Intra-day (RSD%)	3.8	5.9	3.7
Inter-day (RSD%)	4.6	8.6	5.6

* The method cannot be applied for the determination of creatinine in plasma samples.

The sensitivity of our assay is lower when compared to previously elaborated methods (Tables 3 and 4); however, we must remember that Crn as a breakdown product of creatine phosphate from muscle and protein metabolism is a typical metabolite present in the human body [21,22]. TFV is a drug administered to HIV and HBV patients. In patients treated with this drug, both compounds are present in quite high concentrations [21,22]. As it was indicated in a previously published method dedicated to the determination of TFV in urine samples, the concentration of the drug was in the range from 0.453 to 43.576 μg mL^{-1} [28]. These data show that our method would be useful for the analysis of those samples and confirm that higher sensitivity would be more required in the case of trace analytes. For this reason, we decided to pay more attention to making it possible to determine both TFV and Crn in one analytical run. That can help us to observe the negative influence of the drug on kidney functions.

For the stability studies, urine and plasma samples were prepared according to the protocols described in Section 4.4. The experiments have proven that TFV and Crn are stable over 180 min in plasma and 240 min in urine at 4 and 37 °C without a noticeable change in the concentration in both cases (Figure 3). RSD for Crn in plasma samples store at 40 and 37 °C was 2.0% and 2.6%, and for TFV, it was 4.7% and 4.5%, respectively. In the case of urine samples kept at 4 and 37 °C, RSD for Crn was 0.4% and 1.0%, and for TFV it was 0.2% and 0.4%, respectively.

The newly elaborated analytical method was used to analyze urine samples collected from CHB patient treated with 123 mg drug dose. The study was mainly focused on the verification of TFV pharmacokinetic. The obtained results clearly indicate that the largest amount of TFV was excreted within 2 to 4 h after taking the drug, and gradually decreased to the eighth hour (Figure 4). Eight hours after the drug was administered, the amount of TFV became constant. It must be highlighted that having a limited number of patients, we cannot provide statistical data to discuss and clearly show a good trend of urinary TFV excretion. However, the validation data clearly indicate that the elaborated method would be useful to carry out this kind of study.

4. Materials and Methods

4.1. Chemicals

TFV and Crn standards were received from Sigma Aldrich Company (St. Louis, MO, USA). HPLC gradient grade MeCN, sodium hydrogen phosphate heptahydrate, sodium dihydrogen phosphate dihydrate and sodium hydroxide were from J.T. Baker (Deventer, The Netherlands). Perchloric acid was from Merck (Darmstadt, Germany). Deionized water was produced in our laboratory.

4.2. Instrumentation

The analyses were performed on 1220 Infinity LC system from Agilent equipped with a binary pump integrated with a two-channel degasser, autosampler, column oven and diode array detector. The samples were injected using the autosampler. Chromatographic separation was achieved on the Zorbax SB C-18 (150 × 4.6 mm, 5 μm) column from Agilent Technologies (Waldbronn, Germany). For instrument control, data acquisition and analysis, OpenLAB software was applied. Water was purified using Milli-QRG system (Millipore, Vienna, Austria). For pH measurement, an HI 221 (Hanna Instruments, Woonsocket, RI, USA) pH meter was used. Precipitated proteins were removed from the sample using Hettich Mikro 200R (Hettich Zentrifugen, Tuttlingen, Germany) centrifuge.

4.3. Stock Solutions

Stock solution of 0.3 mg mL^{-1} TFV was prepared in 0.1 mol L^{-1} NaOH [35] and kept at 4 °C for several days without significant changes in the analyte content. A stock solution of Crn 30 μmol mL^{-1} was prepared in deionized water and kept at 4 °C for several days as well. The working solutions were prepared by dilution with deionized water as needed.

4.4. Biological Matrices

The urine samples were collected both from healthy people and from CHB patients treated with TFV in the form of Viread 123 mg film-coated tablets. Optimization of analytical conditions were performed on plasma and urine samples collected from healthy volunteers. All samples were stored at −80 °C.

Written informed consent forms were obtained from all volunteers and this study was approved by the Bioethics Committee of the University of Lodz (12/KBBN-UL/I/2015).

4.4.1. Urine Sample Preparation

To reduce the amount of laboratory waste, such as polypropylene tubes or tips, urine samples were prepared directly in reusable HPLC glass vials. For the determination of TFV and Crn to 50 µL of urine, 450 µL of 0.015 mol L^{-1} (pH 7.4) PB was added. Ten microliters of the final analytical solution was injected into the chromatographic column.

4.4.2. Plasma Sample Preparation

The samples were prepared in polypropylene tubes. Fifty microliters of plasma was diluted with 380 µL of 0.015 mol L^{-1} (pH 7.4) PB and spiked with 10 µL of increasing concentrations of TFV. To precipitate plasma proteins, 50 µL of 3 mol L^{-1} perchloric acid was added into the tube. Next, an appropriate amount of deionized water was added to obtain the final volume of 500 µL. The precipitated proteins were removed by centrifugation (15,000× *g*, 10 min, 10 °C). Ten microliters of the supernatant was injected into the chromatographic column.

4.5. HPLC Conditions for the Determination of TFV and Crn

4.5.1. Urine Analysis

For chromatographic separation of TFV and Crn in urine, a reversed-phase Zorbax SB C-18 (150 × 4.6mm, 5 µm) column was applied. The analytes were eluted by a mobile phase containing 0.015 mol L^{-1} PB, pH 7.4 and MeCN using gradient as follows: 0–6 min 2–4% MeCN, 6–7 min 4–2% MeCN, 7–8 min 2% MeCN. The flow rate of the mobile phase was 1 mL min^{-1}. For the detection of TFV and Crn, two different wavelengths were used—260 and 234 nm, respectively. The total time of the chromatographic analysis was 8 min. For the column reconditioning, 2 min post time was required. The analysis was performed at 25 °C.

4.5.2. Plasma Analysis

The chromatographic separation of TFV and Crn in plasma was obtained in 6 min. The analytes were eluted using isocratic elution with the mobile phase containing 98% of 0.015 mol L^{-1} PB pH 7.4 and 2% MeCN. The flow rate of the mobile phase was 1 mL min^{-1}. Similarly to urine analysis, for the detection of TFV and Crn, we used the following wavelength gradient: 0.0–2.5 min 234 nm for Crn and 2.5–6.0 min 260 nm for TFV. The column temperature was 25 °C. Identification of TFV and Crn peaks was based on the comparison of spectrum and retention time of signals with corresponding set of data obtained for authentic compounds.

5. Conclusions

For monitoring an adverse reaction of TFV, new analytical tools based on simultaneous separation and quantitation of TFV and Crn in urine and plasma samples have been developed. These assays allow a direct study of correlation between TFV concentration in plasma and urine and an indirect study on the influence of TFV therapy on kidney damage. The assays were fully validated and successfully applied to test urine samples donated by CHB patients treated with TFV administrated as Viread 123 mg.

The most important reason for the application of our assay in laboratories is the possibility to determine TFV and Crn in one analytical run in both urine and plasma samples. The other advantages of the assay, such as (i) the possibility for normalization of the drug concentration against Crn, (ii) a small plasma or urine volume required for analysis, (iii) the total time of the assay for urine analysis less than 10 min, (iv) a reduced amount of laboratory waste, such as tubes/tips/polypropylene vials, and (v) reduction in the amount of toxic organic solvents in the mobile phase, are the added values of the method. The elaborated procedures can be applied for the analysis of samples collected from HIV and HBV/CHB patients and are in the mainstream of new trend of analytical chemistry which is based on green chemistry.

Author Contributions: Conceptualization, P.O., K.B.; methodology, P.O., G.C., K.B.; validation, formal analysis, data curation, P.O.; writing—original draft preparation, P.O., K.B.; writing—review and editing, P.O., K.B., G.C., P.K.; visualization, P.K. and K.P.; supervision, G.C. and R.G. All authors have read and agreed to the published version of the manuscript.

Funding: This work was supported in part by grants from University of Lodz.

Acknowledgments: Special thanks for the CHB patient for participating in the study.

Conflicts of Interest: The authors declare no conflict of interest.

References

1. *Joint United Nations Programme on HIV/AIDS*; UNAIDS: Geneva, Switzerland, 2018; Available online: https://www.unaids.org/sites/default/files/media_asset/unaids-data-2018_en.pdf (accessed on 8 July 2020).
2. World Health Organization. *Global Hepatitis Report*; WHO: Geneva, Switzerland, 2017. Available online: https://apps.who.int/iris/bitstream/handle/10665/255016/9789241565455-eng.pdf;jsessionid=8A50620A8C4FF608C64807B9DC760DB6?sequence=1 (accessed on 8 July 2020).
3. World Health Organization. *Guidelines for the Prevention, Care and Treatment of Persons with Chronic Hepatitis B Infection*; WHO: Geneva, Switzerland, 2015; ISBN 978-92-4-154905-9. Available online: https://www.who.int/hiv/pub/hepatitis/hepatitis-b-guidelines/en/ (accessed on 18 September 2020).
4. World Health Organization. *Scaling up Antiretroviral Therapy in Resource, Guidelines for a Public Health Approach*; WHO: Geneva, Switzerland, 2002; ISBN 92-4-154570-4. Available online: https://www.who.int/hiv/pub/guidelines/pub18/en/ (accessed on 20 September 2020).
5. World Health Organization. *Guideline on when to Start Antiretroviral Therapy and on Pre-Exposure Prophylaxis for HIV*; WHO: Geneva, Switzerland, 2015; ISBN 978-92-4-150956-5. Available online: https://www.who.int/hiv/pub/guidelines/earlyrelease-arv/en/ (accessed on 9 September 2020).
6. Gallant, J.E.; Deresinski, S. Tenofovir disoproxil fumarate. *Clin. Infect. Dis.* **2003**, *37*, 944–950. [CrossRef]
7. Kearney, B.P.; Flaherty, J.F.; Shah, J. Tenofovir disoproxil fumarate: Clinical pharmacology and pharmacokinetics. *Clin. Pharmacokinet.* **2004**, *43*, 595–612. [CrossRef]
8. Yuen, M.F.; Lai, C.L. Treatment of chronic hepatitis B: Evolution over two decades. *J. Gastroenterol. Hepatol.* **2011**, *26*, 138–143. [CrossRef] [PubMed]
9. Woodward, C.L.; Hall, A.M.; Williams, L.G.; Madge, S.; Copas, A.; Nair, D.; Edwards, S.G.; Johnson, M.A.; Connolly, J.O. Tenofovir-associated renal and bone toxicity. *HIV Med.* **2009**, *10*, 482–487. [CrossRef] [PubMed]
10. Casado, J.L.; Del Rey, J.M.; Bañón, S.; Santiuste, C.; Rodriguez, M.; Moreno, A.; Perez-Elías, M.J.; Liaño, F.; Moreno, S. Changes in kidney function and in the rate of tubular dysfunction after tenofovir withdrawal or continuation in HIV-infected patients. *JAIDS* **2016**, *72*, 416–422. [CrossRef] [PubMed]
11. Scherzer, R.; Estrella, M.; Li, Y.; Deeks, S.G.; Grunfeld, C.; Shlipak, M.G. Association of tenofovir exposure with kidney disease risk in HIV infection. *AIDS* **2012**, *26*, 867–875. [CrossRef] [PubMed]
12. Ryom, L.; Mocroft, A.; Kirk, O.; Worm, S.W.; Kamara, D.A.; Reiss, P.; Ross, M.; Fux, C.A.; Morlat, P.; Moranne, O.; et al. Association Between Antiretroviral Exposure and Renal Impairment Among HIV-Positive Persons With Normal Baseline Renal Function: The D:A:D Study. *J. Infect. Dis.* **2013**, *207*, 1359–1369. [CrossRef] [PubMed]
13. Labarga, P.; Barreiro, P.; Martin-Carbonero, L.; Rodriguez-Novoa, S.; Solera, C.; Medrano, J.; Rivas, P.; Albalater, M.; Blanco, F.; Moren, V. Kidney tubular abnormalities in the absence of impaired glomerular function in HIV patients treated with tenofovir. *AIDS* **2009**, *23*, 689–696. [CrossRef] [PubMed]

14. Dauchy, F.A.; Lawson-Ayayi, S.; De La Faille, R.; Bonnet, F.; Rigothier, C.; Mehsen, N.; Miremont-Salam, G.; Cazanave, C.; Greib, C.; Dabis, F.; et al. Increased risk of abnormal proximal renal tubular function with HIV infection and antiretroviral therapy. *Kidney Int.* **2011**, *80*, 302–309. [CrossRef]

15. Verhelst, D.; Monge, M.; Meynard, J.L.; Fouqueray, B.; Mougenot, B.; Girard, P.M. Fanconi syndrome and renal failure induced by tenofovir: A first case report. *Am. J. Kidney Dis.* **2002**, *40*, 1331–1333. [CrossRef]

16. Hall, A.M.; Hendry, B.M.; Nitsch, D.; Connolly, J.O. Tenofovir-associated kidney toxicity in HIV-infected patients: A review of the evidence. *Am. J. Kidney Dis.* **2011**, *57*, 773–780. [CrossRef]

17. Fontana, R.J. Side effects of long-term oral antiviral therapy for hepatitis B. *Hepatology* **2009**, *49*, 185–195. [CrossRef] [PubMed]

18. Gracey, D.M.; Snelling, P.; McKenzie, P.; Strasser, S.I. Tenofovir-associated Fanconi syndrome in patients with chronic hepatitis B monoinfection. *Antivir. Ther.* **2013**, *18*, 945–948. [CrossRef] [PubMed]

19. Viganò, M.; Brocchieri, A.; Spinetti, A.; Zaltron, S.; Mangia, G.; Facchetti, F.; Fugazza, A.; Castelli, F.; Colombo, M.; Lampertico, P. Tenofovir-induced Fanconi syndrome in chronic hepatitis B monoinfected patients that reverted after tenofovir withdrawal. *J. Clin. Virol.* **2014**, *61*, 600–603. [CrossRef] [PubMed]

20. Cho, H.; Cho, Y.; Cho, E.J.; Lee, J.H.; Yu, S.J.; Oh, K.H.; Lee, K.; Mustika, S.; Yoon, J.H.; Kim, Y.J. Tenofovir-associated nephrotoxicity in patients with chronic hepatitis B: Two cases. *Clin. Mol. Hepatol.* **2016**, *22*, 286–291. [CrossRef] [PubMed]

21. European Association For The Study Of The Liver EASL clinical practice guidelines: Management of chronic hepatitis B virus infection. *J. Hepatol.* **2012**, *57*, 167–185. [CrossRef]

22. Perrone, R.D.; Madias, N.E.; Levey, A.S. Serum creatinine as an index of renal function: New insights into old concepts. *Clin. Chem.* **1992**, *38*, 1933–1953. [CrossRef]

23. European Medicines Agency. Committee for Medicinal Products for Human Use, Guideline on Bioanalytical Method Validation. Available online: https://www.ema.europa.eu (accessed on 1 June 2020).

24. FDA Guidance for Industry Bioanalytical Method Validation. Available online: https://www.fda.gov (accessed on 19 June 2020).

25. Djerada, Z.; Feliu, C.; Tournois, C.; Vautier, D.; Binet, L.; Robinet, A.; Marty, H.; Gozalo, C.; Lamiable, D.; Millart, H. Validation of a fast method for quantitative analysis of elvitegravir, raltegravir, maraviroc, etravirine, tenofovir, boceprevir and 10 other antiretroviral agents in human plasma samples with a new UPLC-MS/MS technology. *J. Pharmaceut. Biomed.* **2013**, *86*, 100–111. [CrossRef] [PubMed]

26. Delahunty, T.; Bushman, L.; Fletcher, C.V. Sensitive assay for determining plasma tenofovir concentrations by LC/MS/MS. *J. Chromatogr. B* **2006**, *830*, 6–12. [CrossRef]

27. Jansen, R.S.; Rosing, H.; Kromdijk, W.; Heine, R.T.; Schellens, J.H.M.; Beijnen, J.H. Simultaneous quantification of emtricitabine and tenofovir nucleotides in peripheral blood mononuclear cells using weak anion-exchange liquid chromatography coupled with tandem mass spectroscopy. *J. Chromatogr. B* **2010**, *878*, 621–627. [CrossRef]

28. Simiele, M.; Carcieri, C.; De Nicolò, A.; Ariaudo, A.; Sciandra, M.; Calcagno, A.; Bonora, S.; Perri, G.D.; D'Avolio, A. A LC-MS method to quantify tenofovir urinary concentrations in treated patients. *J. Pharmaceut. Biomed.* **2015**, *114*, 8–11. [CrossRef]

29. De Nicolò, A.; Simiele, M.; Pensi, D.; Boglione, L.; Allegra, S.; Perri, G.D.; D'Avolio, A. UPLC-MS/MS method for the simultaneous quantification of anti-HBV nucleos(t)ides analogs: Entecavir, lamivudine, telbivudine and tenofovir in plasma of HBV infected patients. *J. Pharmaceut. Biomed.* **2015**, *114*, 127–132. [CrossRef]

30. Gumustas, M.; Caglayan, M.G.; Onur, F.; Ozkan, S.A. Simultaneous determination and validation of emtricitabine, rilpivirine and tenofovir from biological samples using LC and CE methods. *Biomed. Chromatogr.* **2018**, *32*, e4158. [CrossRef]

31. Shah, S.A.B.; Mullin, R.; Jones, G.; Shah, I.; Baker, J.; Petroczi, A.; Naughton, D.P. Simultaneous analysis of antiretroviral drugs abacavir and tenofovir in human hair by liquid chromatography-tandem mass spectrometry. *J. Pharmaceut. Biomed.* **2013**, *74*, 308–313. [CrossRef]

32. Wu, Y.; Yang, J.; Duan, C.; Chu, L.; Chen, S.; Qiao, S.; Li, X.; Deng, H. Simultaneous determination of antiretroviral drugs in human hair with liquid chromatography-electrospray ionization-tandem mass spectrometry. *J. Chromatogr. B* **2018**, *1083*, 209–221. [CrossRef] [PubMed]

33. Jullien, V.; Tréluyer, J.M.; Pons, G.; Rey, E. Determination of tenofovir in human plasma by high-performance liquid chromatography with spectrofluorimetric detection. *J. Chromatogr. B* **2003**, *785*, 377–381. [CrossRef]

34. Sparidans, R.W.; Crommentruyn, K.M.L.; Schellens, J.H.M.; Beijnen, J.H. Liquid chromatographic assay for the antiviral nucleotide analogue tenofovir in plasma using derivatization with chloroacetaldehyde. *J. Chromatogr. B* **2003**, *791*, 227–233. [CrossRef]

35. Rezk, N.L.; Crutchley, R.D.; Kashuba, A.D.M. Simultaneous quantification of emtricitabine and tenofovir in human plasma using high-performance liquid chromatography after solid phase extraction. *J. Chromatogr. B* **2005**, *822*, 201–208. [CrossRef]

36. El Barkil, M.; Gagnieu, M.C.; Guitton, J. Relevance of a combined UV and single mass spectrometry detection for the determination of tenofovir in human plasma by HPLC in therapeutic drug monitoring. *J. Chromatogr. B* **2007**, *854*, 192–197. [CrossRef]

37. Podany, A.T.; Sheldon, C.; Grafelman, D.; Ohnmacht, C.M. Assay development for determination of tenofovir in human plasma by solid phase analytical derivatization and LC–MS/MS. *Bioanalysis* **2015**, *7*, 3085–3095. [CrossRef]

38. Yamada, E.; Takagi, R.; Sudo, K.; Kato, S. Determination of abacavir, tenofovir, darunavir, and raltegravir in human plasma and saliva using liquid chromatography coupled with tandem mass spectrometry. *J. Pharmaceut. Biomed.* **2015**, *114*, 390–397. [CrossRef]

39. Ocque, A.J.; Hagler, C.E.; Morse, G.D.; Letendre, S.L.; Ma, Q. Development and validation of an LC–MS/MS assay for tenofovir and tenofovir alafenamide in human plasma and cerebrospinal fluid. *J. Pharm. Biomed. Anal.* **2018**, *156*, 163–169. [CrossRef]

40. Wiriyakosol, N.; Puangpetch, A.; Manosuthi, W.; Tomongkon, S.; Sukasem, C.; Pinthong, D. A LC/MS/MS method for determination of tenofovir in human plasma and its application to toxicity monitoring. *J Chromatogr. B* **2018**, *1085*, 89–95. [CrossRef]

41. Nóvoa, R.; Labarga, S.; D'Avolio, P.; Barreiro, A.; Albalate, P.; Vispo, M.; Solera, E.; Siccardi, C.; Bonora, M.; Di Perri, S.; et al. Impairment in kidney tubular function in patients receiving tenofovir is associated with higher tenofovir plasma concentrations. *AIDS* **2010**, *24*, 1064–1066. [CrossRef]

42. Calcagno, A.; De Requena, G.; Simiele, M.; Avolio, A.D.; Nielson, M.; Tettoni, M.; Salassa, B.; Bramato, G. Tenofovir plasma concentration according to companion drugs: A cross-sectional study of HIV-positive patients with normal renal function. *Antimicrob. Agents Chemother.* **2013**, *57*, 1840–1843. [CrossRef]

43. Phipps, K. *LC-MS/MS Method for the Determination of Tenofovir from Plasma*; Application Note No. 20687; Thermo Scientific: Waltham, MA, USA, 2013.

44. Borowczyk, K.; Wyszczelska-Rokiel, M.; Kubalczyk, P.; Głowacki, R. Simultaneous determination of albumin and low-molecular-massthiols in plasma by HPLC with UV detection. *J. Chromatogr. B* **2015**, *981–982*, 57–64. [CrossRef]

45. Alpert, A.J. Hydrophilic-interaction chromatography for the separation of peptides, nucleic acids and other polar compounds. *J. Chromatogr. A* **1990**, *499*, 177–196. [CrossRef]

46. Hemström, P.; Irgum, K. Hydrophilic interaction chromatography. *J. Sep. Sci.* **2006**, *29*, 1784–1821. [CrossRef]

47. Buszewski, B.; Noga, S. Hydrophilic interaction liquid chromatography (HILIC)—A powerful separation technique. *Anal. Bioanal. Chem.* **2012**, *402*, 231–247. [CrossRef]

Publisher's Note: MDPI stays neutral with regard to jurisdictional claims in published maps and institutional affiliations.

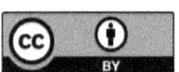

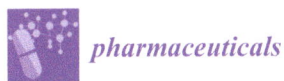 *pharmaceuticals*

Article

Profile and Content of Phenolic Compounds in Leaves, Flowers, Roots, and Stalks of *Sanguisorba officinalis* L. Determined with the LC-DAD-ESI-QTOF-MS/MS Analysis and Their In Vitro Antioxidant, Antidiabetic, Antiproliferative Potency

Sabina Lachowicz [1,*] , **Jan Oszmiański** [2] , **Andrzej Rapak** [3] **and Ireneusz Ochmian** [4]

1   Department of Fermentation and Cereals Technology, Wrocław University of Environmental and Life Science, 51-630 Wrocław, Poland

2   Department of Fruit, Vegetables and Nutraceutical Technology, Wrocław University of Environmental and Life Science, 51-630 Wrocław, Poland; jan.oszmianski@upwr.edu.pl

3   Laboratory of Tumor Molecular Immunobiology, Ludwik Hirszfeld Institute of Immunology and Experimental Therapy, Polish Academy of Sciences, 53-114 Wrocław, Poland; andrzej.rapak@hirszfeld.pl

4   Department of Horticulture, West Pomeranian University of Technology in Szczecin, 71-434 Szczecin, Poland; ireneusz.ochmian@zut.edu.pl

*   Correspondence: Sabina.lachowicz@upwr.edu.pl

Received: 8 July 2020; Accepted: 3 August 2020; Published: 12 August 2020

Abstract: The aim of this study was to accurately determine the profile of polyphenols using the highly sensitive LC-DAD-ESI-QTOF-MS/MS technique and to determine in vitro antioxidant activity, the ability of inhibition of α-amylase, α-glucoamylase, and pancreatic lipase activity, and antiproliferative activity in leaves, flowers, roots, and stalks of medical plant *Sanguisorba officinalis* L. The results of the analysis of the morphological parts indicated the presence of 130 polyphenols, including 62 that were detected in *S. officinalis* L. for the first time. The prevailing group was tannins, with contents ranging from 66.4% of total polyphenols in the flowers to 43.3% in the stalks. The highest content of polyphenols was identified in the flowers and reached 14,444.97 mg/100 g d.b., while the lowest was noted in the stalks and reached 4606.33 mg/100 g d.b. In turn, the highest values of the antiradical and reducing capacities were determined in the leaves and reached 6.63 and 0.30 mmol TE/g d.b, respectively. In turn, a high ability to inhibit activities of α-amylase and α-glucoamylase was noted in the flowers, while a high ability to inhibit the activity of pancreatic lipase was demonstrated in the leaves of *S. officinalis* L. In addition, the leaves and the flowers showed the most effective antiproliferative properties in pancreatic ductal adenocarcinoma, colorectal adenocarcinoma, bladder cancer, and T-cell leukemia cells, whereas the weakest activity was noted in the stalks. Thus, the best dietetic material to be used when composing functional foods were the leaves and the flowers of *S. officinalis* L., while the roots and the stalks were equally valuable plant materials.

Keywords: in vitro biological activity; bioactive compounds; morphological parts; medical plant

1. Introduction

The interest in alternative plants with a health-promoting potential has been growing in recent years not only in the pharmaceutical and cosmetic industries but also in the food industry where they are expected to contribute to the design of novel functional food. Therefore, it is believed that various morphological parts of *Sanguisorba officinalis* L. represent a good source of compounds exhibiting the aforementioned properties [1].

S. *officinalis* L. (great burnet or burnet bloodwort) is a species belonging to the Rosaceae family. It grows wild in Asia and Europe (except for the northern regions [1,2]. This melliferous, perennial plant usually occurs on arid and semi-arid grasslands and blooms from June till September. Its shoots can grow up to ca. 1.2–1.5 m. *S. officinalis* L. is resistant to frost as well as to diseases. It has been used for culinary purposes as an additive to salads and in animal feeding as an additive to feed mixtures due to its high nutritional value [3]. However, in folk medicine of both the Far East and Europe, *S. officinalis* L. was used as an herbal medicine in relieving inflammation, controlling external and internal bleeding, in the treatment of ulcers, burns, eczema, acne, as well as diarrhea [4,5]. In turn, the available experimental data prove a number of its biological properties, e.g., anti-inflammatory [3], anticancer [6], antiviral [7], antioxidant [1], prevention of the Alzheimer's disease [3], and anti-wrinkle effects. [8]. In addition, the above studies have shown that all the biological properties exhibited by this perennial plant are due to a broad range of its bioactive compounds such as phenolic acids, tannins, flavonoids, triterpenes, and polysaccharides [1,3–8]. The richness of these compounds is sought in alternative plant sources that could be used in the treatment and prevention of many diseases and even as a dietary component [9].

Considering a number of biological properties of *S. officinalis* L., this plant has a high nutraceutical potential. However, there are a few reports on the profile and content of secondary metabolites in all of its morphological parts, which may differ and therefore exhibit various properties. Thus, research was undertaken into the accurate characterization of flowers, leaves, stalks, and roots in terms of the profile and content of polyphenols using the highly sensitive LC-DAD-ESI-QTOF-MS/MS technique. Analyses were also conducted to determine the in vitro antioxidant, antiproliferative, and antidiabetic activity for the individual morphological parts of *S. officinalis* L. This study aims to provide valuable information about differences in contents of bioactive compounds and their biological properties in the flowers, leaves, stalks, and roots of *S. officinalis* L., which will be used to compose not only functional foods but also nutraceuticals in the future.

2. Results and Discussion

2.1. Identification of Polyphenolic Compounds

The present study involved a thorough identification of the profile of bioactive compounds in extracts from leaves, flowers, stalks, and roots of *Sanguisorba officinalis* L. plant with the use of an ultrasensitive LC-DAD-ESI-QTOF-MS/MS method in the negative and positive ion mode. In total, 130 compounds were identified in extracts from the selected morphological parts of *S. officinalis* L., including 77 hydrolyzable tannins, 9 sanguiins, 3 sanguisorbic acids, 13 phenolic acids, 6 anthocyanins, 12 catechins and proanthocyanidins, and 9 flavonols, as well as 1 triterpenoid saponins (Table 1; Figures S1–S4). In turn, 62 compounds were identified in *S. officinalis* L. for the first time ever, including 42 hydrolyzable tannins, 5 sanguiins, 8 phenolic acids, 2 anthocyanins, 1 proanthocyanidins, and 3 flavonols as well as 1 triterpenoid saponins. Peaks were identified based on the determined exact molecular weights, peak retention times, primary ions from MS fragmentation, and comparison of data obtained with commercial standards and literature findings (Table 1). However, the profile of the compounds examined was strongly dependent on the morphological part of the plant, since 70, 76, 66, and 62 compounds were identified in the flowers, leaves, roots, and stalks, respectively.

The prevailing group of polyphenolic compounds were hydrolyzable tannins belonging to the family of tannins and being hydrolyzed conjugates that contain one or more hexahydroxydiphenoyl (HHDP) groups, thus leading to the esterification of sugars, glucose in particular. During fragmentation of the primary ions, losses observed were typical of these compounds and involved losses of galloyl, hexahydroxydiphenoyl, gallic acid, HHDP glucose, galloyl-glucose, and galloyl-HHDP-glucose residues with 152, 302, 170, 482, 332, 634 Da, respectively. Additionally, fragments were noted at *m/z* 169 and at *m/z* 301 formed through lactonization of the characteristic hexahydroxydiphenoyl group to ellagic acid. These compounds comprise typical galloyl and HHDP groups, respectively, which have earlier been described in the available literature [1–3,9–11]. Furthermore, if ellagitannin or galloyl derivates are composed of one or a few galloyl groups taking part in sugar synthesis, the fragmentary ion first discards a molecule of gallic acid and then a galloyl group or groups during fragmentation [10]. Among the 77 compounds, only 36 had previously been identified in *S. officinalis* L., and they all were methyl-6-*O*-galloyl-β-ᴅ-glucopyranoside (peak 17, 64; *m/z* 345), pedunculagin1 (18, 23, 29; *m/z* 785), galloyl-HHDP-glucose otherwise called corilagin isomer (25, 44, 55; *m/z* 633), di-galloyl-glucoside (37; *m/z* 483), methyl-4,6-digalloyl-β-ᴅ-glucopyranoside (50, 62, 71, 88; *m/z* 497), HHDP-galloyl-glucose (53; *m/z* 633), ellagic acid pentoside (60, 99; *m/z* 433), ellagic acid hexoside (67, 68, 102; *m/z* 463), di-galloyl hexoside (72, 118; *m/z* 483), galloyl-bis-HHDP-glucose otherwise called potentilin/casuarictin isomer (84, 85, 95, 97, 104, 106; *m/z* 935), lambertianin C (86; *m/z* 1401), ellagic acid (108; *m/z* 300.99), trigalloyl-HHDP-glucose (92, 114; *m/z* 937), trigalloyl-β-D-methyl glucoside (115; *m/z* 649), 3,3′,4′-*O*-trimethyl ellagic acid (127, 128; *m/z* 343), and 3,4′-*O*-dimethyl ellagic acid (129, 130; *m/z* 329) [2,3,12]. In turn, 16 compounds had earlier been detected and identified in flowers and fruits of *Punica granatum* but in this study were for the first time detected in the morphological parts of *S. officinalis* L. These compounds were referred to as: 2,3-HHDP-(α/β)-glucose (1; *m/z* 481), HHDP-hexoside(2,3-(*S*)-Hexahydroxydiphenoyl-ᴅ-glucose) (2, 4; *m/z* 481), HHDP-hexoside(1-galloyl-2,3-hexahydroxydiphenoyl-α-glucose) (3; *m/z* 481), galloyl-hexoside(β-glucogallin) (5; *m/z* 331), galloyl-hexoside (7–10, 13; *m/z* 331), di-HHDP-glucoside (34; *m/z* 783), di-galloyl-HHDP-glucose (14, 56, 66; *m/z* 785), galloyl-HHDP-hexoside (77; *m/z* 633), and pentagalloyl-glucoside (111; *m/z* 939) [10,13]. Another 6 compounds belonging to the group of hydrolyzable tannins were detected during identification of *Duchesnea indica* and they were: di-HHDP-glucose also known as pedunculalagin isomer (15, 20, 24, 26, 27, 30; *m/z* 783) [14]. However, 12 subsequent compounds were identified and determined based on their main ion and MS/MS fragmentation as β-1-*O*-galloyl-2,3-(*S*)-HHDP-ᴅ-glucose (28; *m/z* 633), methyl ellagic acid-pentoside (35; *m/z* 477), HHDP-NHTP-glucose (47, 51; *m/z* 933), castalagin/vescalagin isomer (58, 70, 79, 81, 98, 110; *m/z* 933), HHDP-NHTP-glucose-galloyl-di-HHDP-glucose (cocciferind2) (82; *m/z* 933), and tetragalloyl-glucose (100; *m/z* 787). They had earlier been detected in various plant materials like *Castanea sativa* Miller, *Quercus suber* L., *Betula pubescens*, raspberry fruits, and oak [15–18]. However, 8 compounds were identified for the first time ever. Compound No. 6 was tentatively identified as galloyl-pentoside based on the primary ion at *m/z* 301 and the loss of the pentose group (132 Da) giving a peak at *m/z* 169. Compound No. 49 was tentatively identified as HHDP-glucose based the primary ion at *m/z* 481 and MS/MS fragment at *m/z* 301. In the case of compound No. 54, the primary peak was at *m/z* at 345 due to the loss of a 176 Da residue that resulted in a peak formed at *m/z* 169, which was tentatively identified as galloyl-glucoronide. Compounds No. 73 and 74 were tentatively identified as eucaglobulin based on the primary ion at *m/z* 497 and MS/MS fragmentary ions revealing peaks at *m/z* 345, 327, 313, 183, and 169. In turn, compounds No. 93 and 94 were tentatively described as ellagic acid-hexoside-pentoside based the primary ion at *m/z* 595 and its fragmentation ions at *m/z* 433 and 301 due to the loss of a hexose residue (162 Da) and a pentose residue (132 Da). Finally, compound No. 113 was tentatively identified as methyl galloyl-glucoside based on the primary peak at *m/z* 345 and the loss of a glucosyl residue (162 Da), yielding a base peak at *m/z* 183.

Another described class of polyphenolic compounds belonging to hydrolyzed tannins were sanguiins. Among the 9 identified compounds, only 4 had earlier been detected in *S. officinalis* L. as sanguiin H-6 (11, 89; *m/z* 1870), sanguiin H-4 (41; *m/z* 633), and sanguiin H-10 isomer (48; *m/z* 783) by Karkanis et al. [3] and Zhu et al. [2], whereas the other 5 were never identified, as shown by literature data. Therefore, based on the primary peak at *m/z* 785 and MS/MS fragmentation peaks at *m/z* 633 and 301, and due to the loss of 152 and 332 Da groups, compounds No. 65, 69, and 96 were tentatively identified as sanguiin H-1. In turn, compounds No. 119 and 122 were tentatively identified as sanguiin H-7 and sanguiin H-7 isomers considering their primary ion at *m/z* 801 and fragmentation peaks at *m/z* 649 and 301 resulting from the loss of 152, 332, and 16 Da.

Table 1. Characterization of polyphenolic compounds in *Sanguisorba officinalis* L. by LC-DAD-ESI-QTOF-MS/MS.

No	Compounds	Rt [min]	Δ [nm]	MS/MS	F‡	L	R	S
	Hydrolyzable Tannins							
1	2,3-HHDP-(α/β)-glucose	1.31	272	481/463/301			×	
2	HHDP-hex(2,3-(S)-Hexahydroxydiphenoyl-D-glucose)	1.34	314	481/332/301/182	×	×	×	×
3	HHDP-hexoside(1-galloyl-2,3-hexahydroxydiphenoyl-α-glucose)	1.41	218	481/301/275/257/229		×		
4	HHDP-hex(2,3-(S)-Hexahydroxydiphenoyl-D-glucose)	1.50	314	481/330/306/301/203/182	×	×	×	×
5	Galloyl-hexoside(β-glucogallin)	1.86	278	331/169			×	
6	Galloyl-pentoside	1.99	274	301/169			×	
7	Galloyl-hexoside	2.08	272	331/169			×	
8	Galloyl-hexoside	2.09	268	331/169		×		
10	Galloyl-hexoside	2.52	278	331/169		×		×
13	Galloyl-hexoside	3.08	273	331/169		×		
14	Di-galloyl-HHDP-glucose (tellimagrandin I)	3.16	236/322	785/633/615/483/301	×	×		×
15	Di-HHDP-glucose (pedunculagin isomer)	3.34	230, 275 sh	783/481/301/257	×	×	×	×
17	Methyl-6-O-galloyl-β-D-glucopyranoside	3.54	274	345/169/124.99				
18	Pedunculagin1	3.67	279	783/481/301	×			
20	Di-HHDP-glucose (pedunculagin isomer)	3.90	230, 275 sh	783/481/301/257	×			
23	Pedunculagin1	4.05	324	783/481/301	×			
24	Di-HHDP-glucose (pedunculagin isomer)	4.15	230, 275 sh	783/481/301/257	×			
25	Galloyl-HHDP-glucose (corilagin isomer)	4.18	235, 280 sh	633/300.99			×	
26	Di-HHDP-glucose (pedunculagin isomer)	4.24	326	783/481/301/257		×		
27	Di-HHDP-glucose (pedunculagin isomer)	4.24	230, 275 sh	783/481/301/257	×		×	
28	β-1-O-galloyl-2,3-(S)-HHDP-D-glucose	4.30	326	633/617/595/515/454/432/319/297/179	×	×		×
29	Pedunculagin1	4.30	279	783/481/301			×	
30	Di-HHDP-glucose (pedunculagin isomer)	4.40	313	783/613/447/423/274/211/196/169	×	×		×
34	Di-HHDP-glucoside	4.54	273	783/481/301	×		×	
35	Methylellagic acid-pentose	4.55	324	447/315/301	×	×		×
37	Di-galloyl-glucoside	4.59	273	463/313/169			×	
44	Galloyl-HHDP-glucose	4.98	219/276	633/463/301	×	×		×
47	HHDP-NHTP-glucose (castalagin/vescalagin)	5.08	219	933/915/889/871/631/613/587/569	×	×	×	×
49	HHDP-glucose	5.30	222	481/301	×	×	×	×
50	Methyl-4,6-digalloyl-β-D-glucopyranoside	5.39	212	497/345/169	×	×	×	×
51	HHDP-NHTP-glucose (castalagin/vescalagin)	5.44	282/343	933/915/889/871/631/613/587/569	×	×	×	
53	HHDP-galloyl-glucose	5.50	318	633/463/301/273/257/229/201/185	×			
54	Galloylglucoronide	5.52	276	345/169			×	
55	Galloyl-HHDP-glucose (corilagin isomer)	5.55	218	633/463/301		×		×
56	Di-galloyl-HHDP-glucose (tellimagrandin I)	5.63	230, 280 sh	785/633/615/483/301	×	×		×
58	Castalagin/vescalagin isomer	5.69	230, 285 sh	933/915/889/871/631/613/587/569	×	×		×

Table 1. Cont.

No	Compounds	Rt [min]	λ [nm]	MS/MS	F‡	L	R	S
60	Ellagic acid-pentoside	5.73	330	433/300.99	x	x		x
62	Methyl-4,6-digalloyl-β-D-glucopyranoside	5.90	216	497/345/169	x	x	x	x
64	Methyl-6-O-galloyl-β-D-glucopyranoside	5.97	374	345/169/124.99	x	x		x
66	Di-galloyl-HHDP-glucose (tellimagrandin I)	6.01	203/279	785/633/615/483/301			x	
67	Ellagic acid hexoside1	6.05	251/362	463/301	x	x	x	x
68	Ellagic acid hexoside	6.09	329	463/301				x
70	Castalagin/vescalagin isomer	6.15	230, 285 sh	933/915/889/871/631/613/587/569			x	
71	Methyl-4,6-digalloyl-β-D-glucopyranoside	6.19	213	497/345/169		x	x	x
72	Di-galloyl hexoside	6.22	203	483/301/169			x	
73	Eucaglobulin	6.23	276	497/345/327/313/183/169	x	x	x	x
75	Eucaglobulin	6.25	270	497/345/327/313/183/169	x	x	x	x
77	Galloyl-HHDP-hexoside	6.30	215	633/301				
79	Castalagin/vescalagin isomer	6.37	230, 285 sh	933/915/889/871/631/613/587/569	x	x	x	x
81	Castalagin/vescalagin isomer	6.41	222	933/915/889/871/631/613/587/569	x	x	x	x
82	HHDP-NHTP-glucose-galloyl-di-HHDP-glucose (cocciferind2)	6.46	224	933/915/633/631/301	x	x	x	x
84	Galloyl-bis-HHDP-glucose (potentilin/casuarictin isomer)	6.51	221	935/917/873//783/633/301	x	x	x	x
85	Galloyl-bis-HHDP-glucose (potentilin/casuarictin isomer)	6.55	225, 280 sh	935/917/873//783/633/301			x	
86	Lambertianin C	6.58	250	1401/1237/935/633303	x		x	x
88	Methyl-4,6-digalloyl-β-D-glucopyranoside	6.66	212	497/345/169			x	
92	Trigalloyl-HHDP-glucose	6.93	251 nm	937/767/635/465/301			x	
93	Ellagic acid-hexoside-pentoside	6.99	253/361	595/433/301	x	x	x	x
94	Ellagic acid-hexoside-pentoside	7.04	247/361	595/433/301		x		
95	Galloyl-bis-HHDP-glucose (potentilin/casuarictin isomer)	7.06	253/357	935/917/873//783/633/301				
97	Galloyl-bis-HHDP-glucose (potentilin/casuarictin isomer)	7.13	221	935/917/873//783/633/301	x			
98	Castalagin/vescalagin isomer	7.14	230, 285 sh	933/915/889/871/631/613/587/569				x
99	Ellagic acid pentoside	7.23	254/361	433/301	x	x	x	x
100	Tetragalloyl-glucose	7.27	227	787/635/617/573/465/403			x	
102	Ellagic acid hexoside	7.34	254/362	463/301	x	x	x	x
104	Galloyl-bis-HHDP-glucose (potentilin/casuarictin isomer)	7.41	218	935/917/873//783/633/301	x	x		
106	Galloyl-bis-HHDP-glucose (potentilin/casuarictin isomer)	7.43	219	935/917/873//783/633/301	x	x		
108	Ellagic acid ᵃ	7.50	255/365	300.99	x	x	x	x
110	Castalagin/vescalagin isomer	7.81	250/373	933/915/889/871/631/613/587/569		x	x	
111	Pentagalloylglucoside	8.04	280	939/769/617/465/313/169			x	
113	Methyl galloyl-glucoside	8.24	297/325	345/183		x		
114	Trigalloyl-HHDP- glucose	8.26	259/360	937/767/301				
115	Trigalloyl-β-D-methyl glucoside	8.35	263/356	649/497/479/345			x	
118	Di-galloyl hexoside	8.54	261/374	483/301	x	x	x	x
127	3,3',4'-O-trimethyl ellagic acid	9.66	352	343/328		x		
128	3,3',4'-O-trimethyl ellagic acid	9.79	353	343/328		x		
129	3,4'-O-dimethyl ellagic acid	10.55	249/359	329/314/298/285			x	

Table 1. *Cont.*

No	Compounds	Rt [min]	Λ [nm]	MS/MS	F‡	L	R	S
130	3,4'-O-dimethyl ellagic acid	11.11	247/362	329/314/298/285			x	
Sanguiin								
11	Sanguiin H-6	2.74	234/320	1870/1567/1265/933/631/301	x	x		x
41	Sanguiin H-4	4.84	235/280 sh	633/300.99	x			
48	Sanguiin H-10 isomer	5.23	313	1567/1265/1103/933/301	x	x		x
65	Sanguiin H-1	5.99	230/280 sh	785/633/465/301	x			
69	Sanguiin H-1	6.13	254/371	785/633/465/301		x	x	x
89	Sanguiin H-6	6.75	236	1870/1567/1265/933/631/301	x	x	x	x
96	Sanguiin H-1	7.12	221	785/633/465/301		x	x	
119	Sanguiin H-7	8.59	261/361	801/649/301			x	
122	Sanguiin H-7 isomer	9.05	334	801/649/301	x	x		x
Sanguisorbic acids								
9	Sanguisorbic acid dilactone	2.13	272	469/314/301/286		x	x	
12	Sanguisorbic acid dilactone	2.89	275	469/314/301/286		x	x	
52	Sanguisorbic acid glucoside	5.47	325	667/285	x	x		x
Phenolic acids								
16	Caffeoylquinic acid [a]	3.50	322	353/191/179/161	x	x		
19	3-O-caffeoylquinic acid [a]	3.72	323	353/191/179/135	x	x		x
32	3-O-p-coumaroylquinic acid [a]	4.50	311	337163	x	x		
33	Rosmarinic acid	4.54	325	359/191/179/173/163/152		x		x
42	5-O-caffeoylquinic acid [a]	4.87	324	353/191/179	x	x		x
78	3-O-feruloylquinic acid [a]	6.36	324	367/193/191	x	x		x
116	Disuccinoyl-caffeoylquinic acids	8.41	326	553/537/515/375/353/191/179/173	x	x		x
120	3,5-dicaffeoylquinic acid	8.83	326	515/353/191/179/173	x	x		x
121	3,5-dicaffeoylquinic acid	8.91	326	515/353/191/179/173	x	x		x
123	Caffeoyl dihexoside	9.27	325	503/341/179	x	x		x
124	Caffeoyl dihexoside	9.36	313	503/341/179	x	x		x
125	Caffeoyl dihexoside	9.50	326	503/341/179	x	x		x
126	Caffeoyl dihexoside	9.64	326	503/341/179	x	x	x	x
Anthocyanins								
21	Cyanidin 3,5-O-diglucoside	3.91	520	611/449/287	x			
46	Cyanidin 3-O-glucoside [a]	5.05	516	449/287	x			
76	Cyanidin 3-O-malonylglucoside	6.28	517	535/287	x			

Table 1. Cont.

No	Compounds	Rt [min]	λ [nm]	MS/MS	F‡	L	R	S
87	Cyanidin 3-O-rutinoside	6.60	518	595/449/287	x	x	x	x
90	Cyanidin 3-O-malonylglucoside	6.77	517	535/287	x	x		x
91	Cyanidin 3-(6-O-acetyl)-glucoside	6.91	518	491/317/303/287	x			x
Catechins and Proanthocyanidins								
31	(+)-Catechin [a]	4.43	281	289	x	x	x	x
36	B-type (epi)catechin dimmer [a]	4.58	276	577/289	x	x		x
38	B-type (epi)catechin dimmer [a]	4.67	279	577/289		x	x	x
39	B-type (epi)catechin dimmer [a]	4.69	279	577/289	x	x		x
40	(−)-Epicatechin [a]	4.83	279	289	x	x	x	x
43	B-type (epi)catechin trimmer	4.94	280	865/577/289		x	x	x
57	B-type (epi)catechin tetramer	5.63	278	1153/863/577/289	x	x	x	x
59	B-type (epi)catechin tetramer	5.70	278	1153/863/577/290	x	x	x	x
63	B-type (epi)catechin dimmer [a]	5.90	274	577/289	x	x	x	x
74	A-type procyanidins tetramer	6.23	221/273	1153/865/575/			x	x
80	B-type (epi)catechin tetramer	6.41	278	1153/863/577/289			x	x
83	B-type (epi)catechin dimmer [a]	6.46	276	577/289			x	x
Flavonols								
45	Quercetin 3-O-glucoside [a]	5.03	358	463/301		x		x
61	Kaempferol-di-O-rhamnoside	5.80	350	577/431/285	x	x		x
101	Quercetin 3-O-(6''-galloylglucose)	7.30	224	615/463/300.027		x		
103	Taxifolin 7-O-β-D-glucopyranoside	7.35	229	465/285			x	
105	Quercetin-glucoside-rhamnoside-rhamnoside	7.41	254/337	755/609/463/300.027	x	x		x
107	Quercetin rhamnosyl-rutinoside	7.47	368	755/609/301	x	x		x
109	Quercetin 3-O-glucuronide	7.68	255/353	477/300.027	x	x	x	x
112	Quercetin 3-O-acetyl glucoside	8.15	355	505/300.027	x	x		x
117	Kaempferol 3-O-glucuronide	8.49	347	461/285		x	x	x
Triterpenoid saponins								
22	Sanguisorbigenin	3.98	223/271	453/345/183/169	x	x		x

‡ F, flowers; L, leaves; R, roots; S, stalks; [a] identification confirmed by commercial standards.

In contrast, sanguisorbic acids, belonging to the hydrolyzed tannins, also have been previously defined for these plants by Zhu et al. [2] as sanguisorbic acid dilactone (9, 12; *m/z* 469) and sanguisorbic acid glucoside (52; *m/z* 667). These compounds were determined only in the leaves, stalks, and roots of *S. officinalis* L. Moreover, 1 sanguisorbigenin, belonging to the triterpenoid saponins, was detected during identification *P. granatum* [12].

UV detection at the characteristic absorption maximum between 310 and 330 nm [19] showed the presence of 13 hydroxycinnamic acids in flowers, leaves, and stalks in the case of which the esterification of their quinic acid residue occurs at positions 3, 4, and 5, but not at position 1 [19]. Of these, 5 were identified early in *S. officinalis* as caffeoylquinic acid (16, *m/z* 353), 3-*O*-caffeoylquinic acid (19; *m/z* 353), 3-*O*-*p*-coumaroylquinic acid (32; *m/z* 337), 5-*O*-caffeoylquinic acid (42; *m/z* 353), and 3-*O*-feruloylquinic acid (78; *m/z* 367) [12]. However, 4 more were previously identified in other botanical sources like *Eryngium alpinum* L. and *Chrysanthemum* as rosmarinic acid (33; *m/z* 359), disuccinoyl-caffeoylquinic acids (116; *m/z* 553), and 3,5-dicaffeoylquinic (120, 121; *m/z* 515), however, for the first time in *S. officinalis* L., compounds No. 123–125 were tentatively identified as caffeoyl dihexoside based on the highest peak at *m/z* 505 and its fragmentation yielding peaks at *m/z* 341 and 179 due to the loss of 2 hexose residues (162 + 162 Da). What is more, these compounds were also described for the first time ever in morphological parts of *S. officinalis* L.

Anthocyanins are natural plant pigments occurring in the plant kingdom. They were identified in the positive ion mode because they bear a positive charge and easily donate protons to free radicals under ESI conditions. In turn, their detection was carried out at the typical absorption maximum between 440 and 540 nm [10,20]. Among the tentatively identified 6 anthocyanins, that were detected only in the flowers, only 4 were earlier determined in *S. officinalis* L. as cyanidin 3,5-diglucoside (21; *m/z* 611), cyanidin 3-*O*-glucoside (46; *m/z* 449), and cyanidin 3-malonylglucoside (76, 90; *m/z* 535) [12]. The other 2 compounds were described based on previous information about fragmentation of pomegranate and grape berry skin [13,21] as cyanidin 3-*O*-rutinoside (87; *m/z* 595) and cyanidin 3-(6-*O*-acetyl)-glucoside (91; *m/z* 491).

Flavan-3-ols occur as monomers, oligomers, and polymers formed by linking to (epi)catechin monomers via interflavonoid bonds (C–C) [22]. Their fragmentation proceeds through the loss of a (epi)catechin unit with a molecular weight of 289 Da. The identified proanthocyanins occurred as catechin dimers, trimers, and tetramers and were identified as A and B procyanidins [22]. These 11 compounds were characterized based on available standards and the latest research works addressing *S. officinalis* L as (+)-catechin and (−)-epicatechin (31, 40; *m/z* 289), B-type (epi)catechin dimmer (36, 38, 39, 63, 83; *m/z* 577), B-type (epi)catechin trimmer (43; *m/z* 865), and B-type (epi)catechin tetramer (57, 59, 80; *m/z* 1153) [2,3]. In turn, compound No. 74 was tentatively identified as a A-type (epi)catechin tetramer at *m/z* 1153 and the base ion at *m/z* 289. Although it was earlier detected in black soybean [23], it was described in *S. officinalis* L. for the first time ever.

Flavonols were identified as derivatives of taxifolin, kaempferol, and quercetin based on the base fragments at *m/z* 300, 285, and 301. UV detection of flavonols revealed characteristic absorption maximum between 315 and 359 nm, and some of the identified compounds had additional peaks between 207 and 280 nm [24]. Besides, derivatives of these compounds are usually detected at positions C-7 and/or C-3. Fragmentation of the primary ions resulted in losses of hexose (162 Da), pentose (146 Da), and deoxyhexose (308 Da) [24]. Of the 9 flavonols initially suggested for *S. officinalis* L., only 6 have previously been described for this species as quercetin-3-*O*-glucoside (45; 463), quercetin-3-*O*-(6''-galloylglucose) (101; *m/z* 615), taxifolin-7-*O*-β-ᴅ-glucopyranoside (103; *m/z* 465), quercetin-3-*O*-glucuronide (109; *m/z* 477), quercetin-3-*O*-acetyl glucoside (112; *m/z* 505), and kaempferol-3-*O*-glucuronide (117; *m/z* 461) [2,3,12]. In turn, 3 compounds have not been previously described according to the available literature. Compound No. 61 was tentatively identified as kaempferol-di-*O*-rhamnoside based on the primary peak at *m/z* 577 and fragmentation peaks at *m/z* 431 and 285 due to the loss of two rhamnoside residues (146 + 146 Da). Another compound (103) was tentatively described as quercetin-glucoside-dirhamnoside based on the primary peak at *m/z* 755 and fragmentation peaks at *m/z* 609, 463, and 301 due to the loss of two rhamnose residues and one glycosyl residue. Finally, compound No. 107 was tentatively presented as quercetin rhamnosyl-rutinoside based on the primary peak at *m/z* 755 and fragmentation peaks at *m/z* 609 and 301.

2.2. Quantification of Polyphenolic Compounds

The content of polyphenols in the analyzed morphological parts of *S. officinalis* L. is shown in Table 2. The highest content of bioactive compounds was determined in the flowers, it reached 14,444.97 mg/100 g d.b. and was 1.5, 1.7, and 3.2 times higher than in the leaves, roots, and stalks, respectively. In turn, the content of polyphenols in the leaves + stalks of *Sanguisorba minor* Scop. was comparable to the content of these compounds in *S. officinalis* L., while the roots of *S. minor* Scop. were 4 times more abundant in the studied compounds than the roots of *S. officinalis* L. [3]. In turn, the sum of polyphenols analysed in the roots of the same species from Korea was 2 times lower than in the roots of plants grown in Poland. However, the extract from *S. officinalis* L. cultivated in China contained 3150 mg GAE/100 g dry weight polyphenols, which was 4.9, 3.2, 2.8, and 1.5 times lower compared to the flowers, leaves, roots, and stalks of the same species growing in Poland. The content of polyphenols in the leaves of green and white tea was 67.21 and 40.94 mg/g d.b. and was 1.5 and 2.4 times lower than in the leaves of the studied species, respectively [25]. Total content of polyphenols analyzed in the flowers, leaves, roots, and stalks of *S. officinalis* L. was 8.2, 8.4, 7.8, and 8.4 times higher, respectively, compared to edible flowers of *Allium schoenoprasum* (Liliaceae), *Salvia pratensis* (Lamiaceae), *Sambucus nigra* (Caprifoliaceae), *Taraxacum officinale* [26]. However, according to Zeng et al. [27] the contents of bioactive compounds in the flowers of green and black tea of *Camellia sinensis* were 2.4 and 5.4 times lower, respectively, compared to the flowers of *S. officinalis* L. Moreover, the content of bioactive compounds in the flowers and the leaves of *Punica granatum* L. was 2.2 and 6.7 times lower, respectively, than in the same morphological parts of *S. officinalis* L. [28]. In addition, the content of compounds tested in the leaves and the stalks of *Fallopia japonica* was 1.7 and 2.3 times lower, respectively, while their content in the roots of *F. japonica* was similar to *S. officinalis* L. [9]. The differences in the contents of polyphenolic compounds among individual species can be affected by various factors, such as the place of cultivation, climate, environmental conditions, and also the method of extraction and analysis [29]. Thus, the tested material is characterized by a high content of compounds exhibiting a number of biological properties and can be used to compose not only nutraceuticals in the pharmaceutical industry but also to produce functional food.

The profile and content of phenols present in various morphological parts of *S. officinalis* L. were quite diverse and strongly dependent on the morphological part tested. The flowers were dominated by hydrolyzed tannins (66.4% in all phenols) > flavan-3-ols (13.1%) > phenolic acids (9.9%) > flavonols (5%) > anthocyanins (3.8%) > triterpenoids (1.8%). In turn, in the leaves were dominated by hydrolyzed tannins (49.3%) > phenolic acids (20.5%) > flavonols (19.8%) > flavan-3-ols (7.4%) > triterpenoids (3%). However, in the roots, hydrolyzed tannins were also the dominant class (62.1%) > flavan-3-ols (37.3%) > phenolic acids and flavonols (<0.5%), whereas the stalks were dominated by hydrolyzed tannins (43.3%) > flavan-3-ols (26.2%) > flavonols (17.1%) > phenolic acids (7.8%) > triterpenes (5.5%). The analysis of phenols profile revealed flavonols to be the major group in leaf + stalks, whereas hydrolyzed tannins to be the major group in the roots of *S. minor* [3], similarly to the roots of *S. officinalis* L. and to the results presented in the work of Kim et al. [1].

Pharmaceuticals **2020**, *13*, 191

Table 2. Content of polyphenolic compounds in *Sanguisorba officinalis* [mg/100 g d.w.].

Compounds	Flower	Leaves	Roots	Stalk
Hydrolyzable tannins				
1 2,3-HHDP-(α/β)-glucose	nd‡	nd	12.33 ± 0.25a†	nd
2 HHDP-hex(2,3-(S)-Hexahydroxydiphenoyl-D-glucose)	141.89 ± 2.84a	102.71 ± 2.05b	13.28 ± 0.27c	11.49 ± 0.23c
3 HHDP-hexoside(1-galloyl-2,3-hexahydroxydiphenoyl-α-glucose)	nd	14.36 ± 0.29a	nd	nd
4 HHDP-hex(2,3-(S)-Hexahydroxydiphenoyl-D-glucose)	161.00 ± 3.22a	63.35 ± 1.27b	40.73 ± 0.81c	12.49 ± 0.25d
5 Galloyl-hexoside(β-glucogallin)	nd	nd	92.13±1.84a	nd
6 Galloyl-pentoside	nd	nd	38.51±0.77a	nd
7 Galloyl-hexoside	nd	nd	20.66±0.41a	nd
8 Galloyl-hexoside	nd	13.89 ± 0.28a	nd	nd
10 Galloyl-hexoside	nd	5.18 ± 0.10b	nd	9.52 ± 0.19a
13 Galloyl-hexoside	nd	4.41 ± 0.09a	nd	nd
14 Di-galloyl-HHDP-glucose (tellimagrandin I)	5.57 ± 0.11a	6.34 ± 0.13a	nd	1.35 ± 0.03b
15 Di-HHDP-glucose (pedunculagin isomer)	100.66 ± 2.01b	24.25 ± 0.49c	136.03 ± 2.72a	15.78 ± 0.32d
17 Methyl-6-O-galloyl-β-D-glucopyranoside	nd	nd	234.27 ± 4.69a	7.20 ± 0.14b
18 Pedunculagin1	2.55 ± 0.05a	nd	nd	nd
20 Di-HHDP-glucose (pedunculagin isomer)	2.23 ± 0.04a	nd	nd	nd
23 Pedunculagin1	9.08 ± 0.18a	nd	nd	nd
24 Di-HHDP-glucose (pedunculagin isomer)	20.00 ± 0.40a	nd	nd	nd
25 Galloyl-HHDP-glucose (corilagin isomer)	nd	nd	29.73 ± 0.59a	nd
26 Di-HHDP-glucose (pedunculagin isomer)	nd	17.21 ± 0.34a	nd	nd
27 Di-HHDP-glucose (pedunculagin isomer)	97.32 ± 1.95a	nd	42.58 ± 0.85b	nd
28 β-1-O-galloyl-2,3-(S)-HHDP-D-glucose	513.20 ± 10.26a	433.89±8.68b	nd	83.52 ± 1.67c
29 Pedunculagin1	nd	nd	24.37 ± 0.49a	nd
30 Di-HHDP-glucose (pedunculagin isomer)	9.66 ± 0.19b	11.96 ± 0.24a	nd	2.01 ± 0.04c
34 Di-HHDP-glucoside	nd	nd	19.51 ± 0.39a	0
35 Methylellagic acid-pentose	26.83 ± 0.54a	5.45 ± 0.11c	nd	8.17 ± 0.16b
37 Di-galloyl-glucoside	nd	nd	53.85 ± 1.08a	nd
44 Galloyl-HHDP-glucose	165.31 ± 3.31a	8.65 ± 0.17c	145.15 ± 2.90b	5.25 ± 0.11d
47 HHDP-NHTP-glucose (castalagin/vescalagin)	87.29 ± 1.75b	100.59 ± 2.01a	41.30 ± 0.83c	23.36 ± 0.47d
49 HHDP-glucose	97.26 ± 1.95a	45.3 ± 0.91b	11.32 ± 0.23c	11.44 ± 0.23c
50 Methyl-4,6-digalloyl-β-D-glucopyranoside	7.94 ± 0.16b	1.06 ± 0.02c	17.12 ± 0.34a	0.58 ± 0.01d

Pharmaceuticals **2020**, *13*, 191

Table 2. *Cont.*

	Compounds	Flower	Leaves	Roots	Stalk
51	HHDP-NHTP-glucose (castalagin/vescalagin)	nd	nd	24.08 ± 0.48a	nd
53	HHDP-galloyl-glucose	43.97 ± 0.88a	nd	nd	nd
54	Galloylglucoronide	nd	nd	93.44 ± 1.87a	nd
55	Galloyl-HHDP-glucose (corilagin isomer)	nd	22.90 ± 0.46a	nd	nd
56	Di-galloyl-HHDP-glucose (tellimagrandin I)	85.77 ± 1.72a	35.62 ± 0.71b	nd	nd
58	Castalagin/vescalagin isomer	37.38 ± 0.75a	70.71 ± 1.41b	nd	nd
60	Ellagic acid-pentoside	9.31 ± 0.19b	13.70 ± 0.27a	nd	3.96 ± 0.08c
62	Methyl-4,6-digalloyl-β-D-glucopyranoside	256.75 ± 5.14a	104.29 ± 2.09b	254.04 ± 5.08a	71.93 ± 1.44c
64	Methyl-6-O-galloyl-β-D-glucopyranoside	6.75 ± 0.14b	10.71 ± 0.21a	nd	3.47 ± 0.07c
66	Di-galloyl-HHDP-glucose (tellimagrandin I)	nd	nd	13.52 ± 0.27a	nd
67	Ellagic acid hexoside	5.76 ± 0.12b	7.16 ± 0.14a	4.05 ± 0.08b	2.61 ± 0.05c
68	Ellagic acid hexoside	nd	nd	nd	4.53 ± 0.09a
70	Castalagin/vescalagin isomer	nd	nd	68.46 ± 1.37a	nd
71	Methyl-4,6-digalloyl-β-D-glucopyranoside	nd	1.80 ± 0.04a	1.70 ± 0.03a	0.58 ± 0.01b
72	Di-galloyl hexoside	nd	nd	43.6±0.87a	nd
73	Eucaglobulin	51.84 ± 1.04b	102.83 ± 2.06a	nd	16.79 ± 0.34c
75	Eucaglobulin	71.19 ± 1.42a	71.72 ± 1.43a	nd	22.59 ± 0.45b
77	Galloyl-HHDP-hexoside	nd	nd	106.23 ± 2.12a	nd
79	Castalagin/vescalagin isomer	26.13 ± 0.52c	62.30 ± 1.25a	52.75 ± 1.06b	14.52 ± 0.29d
81	Castalagin/vescalagin isomer	nd	92.82 ± 1.86a	67.43 ± 1.35b	13.19 ± 0.26c
82	HHDP-NHTP-glucose-galloyl-di-HHDP-glucose (cocciferind2)	87.01 ± 1.74b	41.02 ± 0.82c	155.76 ± 3.12a	13.57 ± 0.27d
84	Galloyl-bis-HHDP-glucose (potentilin/casuarictin isomer)	38.45 ± 0.77b	132.33 ± 2.65a	32.87 ± 0.66c	30.56 ± 0.61c
85	Galloyl-bis-HHDP-glucose (potentilin/casuarictin isomer)	nd	nd	52.26 ± 1.05a	nd
86	Lambertianin C	3029.28 ± 60.59a	2232.84 ± 44.66b	898.98 ± 17.98d	1236.77 ± 24.74c
88	Methyl-4,6-digalloyl-β-D-glucopyranoside	nd	nd	4.82 ± 0.1a	nd
92	Trigalloyl-HHDP-glucose	nd	nd	86.34 ± 1.73a	nd
93	Ellagic acid-hexoside-pentoside	33.54 ± 0.67a	32.53 ± 0.65a	32.80 ± 0.66a	7.09 ± 0.14b
94	Ellagic acid-hexoside-pentoside	nd	51.34 ± 1.03a	nd	nd
95	Galloyl-bis-HHDP-glucose (potentilin/casuarictin isomer)	nd	nd	12.48 ± 0.25a	nd
97	Galloyl-bis-HHDP-glucose (potentilin/casuarictin isomer)	30.53 ± 0.61a	nd	nd	nd
98	Castalagin/vescalagin isomer	nd	nd	nd	43.38 ± 0.87a
99	Ellagic acid pentoside	14.50 ± 0.29b	15.22 ± 0.3b	18.07 ± 0.36a	3.47 ± 0.07c
100	Tetragalloyl-glucose	nd	nd	328.94 ± 6.58a	nd
102	Ellagic acid hexoside1	1.14 ± 0.02a	0.33 ± 0.01c	0.61 ± 0.01b	0.36 ± 0.01c

Table 2. *Cont.*

	Compounds	Flower	Leaves	Roots	Stalk
104	Galloyl-bis-HHDP-glucose (potentilin/casuarictin isomer)	nd	56.41 ± 1.13a	nd	nd
106	Galloyl-bis-HHDP-glucose (potentilin/casuarictin isomer)	202.46 ± 4.05a	nd	147.72 ± 2.95b	nd
108	Ellagic acid	17.69 ± 0.35c	26.90 ± 0.54a	13.49 ± 0.27b	5.20 ± 0.10d
110	Castalagin/vescalagin isomer	nd	nd	1.91 ± 0.04a	nd
111	Pentagalloylglucoside	nd	nd	36.57 ± 0.73a	nd
113	Methyl galloyl-glucoside	nd	13.75 ± 0.28a	nd	nd
114	Trigalloyl-HHDP- glucose	nd	nd	0.71 ± 0.01a	nd
115	Trigalloyl-β-*D*-methyl glucoside	nd	nd	35.65 ± 0.71a	nd
118	Di-galloyl hexoside	nd	nd	3.61 ± 0.07a	nd
127	3,3′,4′-*O*-trimethyl ellagic acid	nd	31.41 ± 0.63a	nd	nd
128	3,3′,4′-*O*-trimethyl ellagic acid	nd	1.47 ± 0.03a	nd	nd
129	3,4′-*O*-dimethyl ellagic acid	nd	nd	49.05 ± 0.98a	nd
130	3,4′-*O*-dimethyl ellagic acid	nd	nd	251.11 ± 5.02a	nd
	SUM	5497.24 ± 109.94a	4090.71 ± 81.81b	3865.92 ± 77.32c	1686.73 ± 33.73d
	Sanguiin				
11	Sanguiin H-6	2.57 ± 0.05b	10.13 ± 0.20a	nd	1.22 ± 0.02c
41	Sanguiin H-4	352.14 ± 7.04a	nd	nd	nd
48	Sanguiin H-10 isomer	130.92 ± 2.62a	5.33 ± 0.11b	nd	4.14 ± 0.08b
65	Sanguiin H-1	43.36 ± 0.87	nd	nd	nd
69	Sanguiin H-1	nd	1.01 ± 0.02b	2.95 ± 0.06a	0.15 ± 0.01c
89	Sanguiin H-6	3566.15 ± 71.32a	621.04 ± 12.42d	763.91 ± 15.28c	289.86 ± 5.80b
96	Sanguiin H-1	nd	61.95 ± 1.24b	730.22 ± 14.60a	nd
119	Sanguiin H-7	nd	nd	4.42 ± 0.09a	nd
122	Sanguiin H-7 isomer	1.89 ± 0.04a	2.24 ± 0.04a	nd	0.98 ± 0.02b
	SUM	4097.03 ± 81.94a	701.7 ± 14.03c	1501.5 ± 30.03b	296.35 ± 5.93d
	Sanguisorbic acids				
9	Sanguisorbic acid dilactone	nd	6.61 ± 0.13d	10.95 ± 0.22a	nd
12	Sanguisorbic acid dilactone	nd	nd	15.44 ± 0.31a	nd
52	Sanguisorbic acid glucoside	nd	109.18 ± 2.18a	nd	13.43 ± 0.27b
	SUM	nd	115.79 ± 2.32a	26.39 ± 0.53b	13.43 ± 0.27c
	Phenolic acids				
16	Caffeoylquinic acid	23.07 ± 0.46b	47.52 ± 0.95a	nd	nd

Table 2. Cont.

	Compounds	Flower	Leaves	Roots	Stalk
19	Caffeoylquinic acid	539.00 ± 10.78b	1363.67 ± 27.27a	nd	182.92 ± 3.66c
32	3-p-Coumaroylquinic acid	87.17 ± 1.74a	42.55 ± 0.85b	nd	nd
33	Rosmarinic acid	nd	8.39 ± 0.17a	nd	2.98 ± 0.06b
42	5-Caffeoylquinic acid	673.42 ± 13.47a	436.44 ± 8.73b	nd	129.09 ± 2.58c
78	3-Feruloylquinic acid	11.46 ± 0.23a	4.95 ± 0.10b	nd	3.17 ± 0.06c
116	Disuccinoyl-caffeoylquinic acids	69.02 ± 1.38b	89.00 ± 1.78a	nd	31.51 ± 0.63c
120	Di-caffeoylquinic	4.81 ± 0.10b	17.66 ± 0.35a	nd	2.79 ± 0.06c
121	Dicaffeoylquinic	4.12 ± 0.08c	12.78 ± 0.26a	nd	1.33 ± 0.03c
123	Caffeoyl dihexoside	2.72 ± 0.05b	6.68 ± 0.13a	nd	3.10 ± 0.06b
124	Caffeoyl dihexoside	13.38 ± 0.27a	8.47 ± 0.17b	nd	2.04 ± 0.04c
125	Caffeoyl dihexoside	3.51 ± 0.07b	6.26 ± 0.13a	nd	2.23 ± 0.04c
126	Caffeoyl dihexoside	nd	nd	6.64 ± 0.13a	nd
	SUM	1431.68 ± 28.63b	2044.37 ± 40.89a	6.64 ± 0.13d	361.16 ± 7.22c
	Anthocyanins				
21	Cyanidin 3,5-O-diglucoside	19.56 ± 0.39a	nd	nd	nd
46	Cyanidin 3-O-glucoside	339.87 ± 6.80a	nd	nd	nd
76	Cyanidin 3-O-malonylglucoside	154.35 ± 3.09a	nd	nd	nd
87	Cyanidin 3-O-rutinoside	4.83 ± 0.10a	nd	nd	nd
90	Cyanidin 3-O-malonylglucoside	14.40 ± 0.29a	nd	nd	nd
91	Cyanidin 3-(6-O-acetyl)glucoside	16.56 ± 0.33a	nd	nd	nd
	SUM	549.57 ± 10.99a			
	Catechins and Proanthocyanins				
31	(+)-Catechin	46.77 ± 0.94d	160.08 ± 3.20b	374.41 ± 7.49a	133.37 ± 2.67c
36	B-type (epi)catechin dimmer	111.05 ± 2.22a	33.03 ± 0.66b	nd	28.85 ± 0.58c
38	B-type (epi)catechin dimmer	nd	19.88 ± 0.40b	383.49 ± 7.67a	nd
39	B-type (epi)catechin dimmer	136.33 ± 2.73a	15.04 ± 0.30c	nd	125.77 ± 2.52b
40	(−)-Epicatechin	656.57 ± 13.13b	138.19 ± 2.76d	700.12 ± 14.00a	457.66 ± 9.15c
43	B-type (epi)catechin trimmer	nd	nd	nd	86.20 ± 1.72a
57	B-type (epi)catechin tetramer	120.62 ± 2.41c	45.32 ± 0.91d	448.56 ± 8.97a	142.85 ± 2.86b
59	B-type (epi)catechin tetramer	57.12 ± 1.14a	22.38 ± 0.45b	21.69 ± 0.43b	18.43 ± 0.37c

Table 2. *Cont.*

	Compounds	Flower	Leaves	Roots	Stalk
63	B-type (epi)catechin dimmer	760.26 ± 15.21b	305.55 ± 6.11c	796.86 ± 15.94a	214.39 ± 4.29d
74	A-type procyanidin tetramer	nd	nd	51.53 ± 1.03a	nd
80	B-type (epi)catechin tetramer	nd	nd	105.67 ± 2.11a	nd
83	B-type (epi)catechin dimmer	nd	nd	356.86 ± 7.14a	nd
	SUM	1888.72 ± 37.77b	739.47 ± 14.79d	3239.19 ± 64.78a	1207.52 ± 24.15c
	Flavonols				
45	Quercetin 3-O-glucoside	nd	15.00 ± 0.30a	nd	4.15 ± 0.08b
61	Kaempferol-di-O-rhamnoside	5.23±0.10a	0.59 ± 0.01b	nd	0.31 ± 0.01b
101	Quercetin 3-O-(6''-galloylglucose)	nd	77.72 ± 1.55a	nd	nd
103	Taxifolin 7-O-β-D-glucopyranoside	nd	nd	43.41 ± 0.87a	nd
105	Quercetin-glucoside-rhamnoside-rhamnoside	26.29 ± 0.53a	9.93 ± 0.20c	nd	13.33 ± 0.27b
107	Quercetin rhamnosyl-rutinoside	5.93 ± 0.12a	3.11 ± 0.06b	nd	2.54 ± 0.05b
109	Quercetin 3-O-glucuronide	494.97 ± 9.90c	1645.76 ± 32.92a	4.13 ± 0.08d	675.15 ± 13.50b
112	Quercetin 3-O-acetyl glucoside	47.89 ± 0.96b	54.56 ± 1.09a	nd	26.73 ± 0.53c
117	Kaempferol 3-O-glucuronide	137.89 ± 2.76b	163.18 ± 3.26a	nd	65.65 ± 1.31c
	SUM	718.2 ± 14.36c	1969.85 ± 39.40a	47.54 ± 0.95d	787.86 ± 15.76b
	Sanguisorbigenin	262.53 ± 5.25b	300.60 ± 6.01a	nd	253.28 ± 5.07c
	Total mg/100 g d.w.	14444.97 ± 288.90a	9962.55 ± 199.25b	8687.16 ± 173.74c	4606.33 ± 92.13d

[†] Values are expressed as the mean ($n = 3$) ± standard deviation and different letters (between morphological parts) within the same row indicates statistically significant differences ($p < 0.05$); [‡] nd, not identified.

Tannins are compounds that occur naturally in plants and also play a defensive role in them. They exhibit anti-inflammatory properties against inflammation of the mucous membranes and skin, as well as antiastringent, antioxidative, free radical-scavenging, and antiproliferative properties. In addition, they are also an important component of food because they affect its storage stability, taste, and color [30]. The highest content of these compounds was recorded in the flowers (9594.27 mg/100 g d.b.) and the lowest one in the stalks (1996.51 mg/100 g d.b.). According to Karkanis et al. [3], their content in *S. minor* was comparable in the leaves and stalks while 4 times higher in the roots compared to the morphological parts of *S. officinalis* L., respectively. In turn, the major compound in all morphological parts tested was Lambertian C, with its content ranging from 62% in the roots to 17% in the stalks, and similar observations were made in *S. minor* [3].

Phenolic acids are another naturally occurring class of polyphenolic compounds that have a number of biological properties, including antioxidative ones, or are used in the prevention of cardiovascular diseases. They also affect the sour and bitter taste of food of plant origin, imparting them astringent flavones [31]. They dominated in the leaves of *S. officinalis* L. and their content amounted to 2044.37 mg/100 g d.b., while their poorest presence was in the roots (only 6.64 mg/100 g d.b.). Their content in the leaves was 5.3 times higher compared to their total content in leaves and stalks of *S. minor*, but similar while comparing to the stalks of *S. officinalis* L. and *S. minor* [3]. In turn, chlorogenic acid turned out to be the major compound in the flowers, neochlorogenic acid prevailed in the stalks and leaves, while ellagic acid was found in the leaves and stalks of *S. minor* [3].

Anthocyanins occurred only in flowers, giving them an intense red color. They belong to the group of polyphenols which show a number of health-promoting properties [9,32]. Their content was 549.57 mg/100 g d.b., and the dominant compounds were cyanidin 3-*O*-glucoside and cyanidin 3-*O*-malonylglucoside and they constituted of 62% and 28% of all anthocyanins, respectively.

Catechins and proanthocyanidins are compounds that also play an important role in the prevention of many diseases [9,32]. Their content ranged from 739.47 to 3239.19 mg/100 g d.b. in the leaves and roots of *S. officinalis* L, respectively, and was 5.6 and 20 times higher compared to the leaves and roots of *Fallopia japonica*, respectively [9]. The dominant compounds were: B-type (epi)catechin dimmer constituting 41% in the leaves to 18% in the stalks of all flavan-3-ols, and (−)-epicatechin constituting from 37% in the stalks to 19% in the leaves. Although in *F. japonica*, the major compound was procyanidin dimer B [9].

Flavonols are also a valuable class of natural secondary metabolites due to their anti-inflammatory and antioxidative properties [9]. The highest content of these compounds was noted in the leaves and reached 1969.85 mg/100 g d.b. It was 2.7, 2.5, and 41 times higher compared to the flowers, stalks, and roots, respectively. This difference results from the fact that these compounds are mainly located in the top layer of plants, protecting them from harmful UV radiation [32]. In turn, quercetin-*O*-glucuronide was the dominant compound in the flowers, leaves, and stalks, constituting 69%, 83%, and 85% of all flavonols, respectively, whereas taxifolin 7-*O*-β-D-glucopyranoside prevailed in the roots, constituting 91%. These observations have also been confirmed by Kim et al. [1].

2.3. Pro-Health Properties

The average antioxidative activity determined for *S. officinalis* L. was 4.45 mmol Troloxu (TE)/g dry basis (d.b.) in the ABTS test and 0.18 mmol TE/g d.b. in the FRAP assay (Table 3). The highest activity was determined in the leaves and was 6.63 and 0.30 mmol TE/g d.b. in the ABTS and FRAP tests, respectively. It was 1.2 and 1.6 times higher than in the stalks, 12.0 and 2.1 times higher than in the roots, and comparable to that found in the flowers for the ABTS radicals and for Fe^{3+} reduction to Fe^{2+}, respectively (Table 3). Similar results of the antioxidative activity assays were obtained for the roots of *S. officinalis* gathered in China [5]. In turn, previous research shows that the antiradical activity of the leaves, stalks, and roots of *S. officinalis* L. was 6.2, 1.7, and 10.6 times higher compared to the same parts of *F. japonica* as well as 7.9, 1.8, and 9.3 times higher compared to the same parts of *F. sachalinensis*, respectively [9]. Antiradical activity for the roots was comparable to that obtained for the medical plant—*Ruta montana* [33]. Moreover, the average reducing activity of the tested parts of *S. officinalis* L. was comparable to the antioxidant potential determined for *Melissae* folium and about 6 times higher than for *Spiraea herba*, *Uvae ursi* folium, *Rubi fructose* folium, or *Fragariae herba* folium [34]. Thus, the results obtained indicate that the roots, flowers, and leaves of *S. officinalis* L. have a high ability to scavenge free radicals, which may be due to the high content of bioactive compounds determined for these morphological parts of the plant. What's more, the results presented a strong Pearson's correlation with the sum content of phenolic acids and anthocyanins and with the antioxidative activity as $r^2 = 0.734$ and 0.539 for ABTS assay and $r^2 = 0.746$ and 0.869 for FRAP, whereas the correlation between the reducing activity and sum of hydrolysable tannins and polyphenols was also strong $r^2 = 0.769$ and 0.823.

Table 3. The antioxidant activity and the biological activity in vitro.

Components	α-Amylase [EC$_{50}$ MG/ML]	α-Glucosidase [EC$_{50}$ MG/ML]	Pancreatic Lipase [EC$_{50}$ MG/ML]	ABTS [mmol/g d.b.]	FRAP [mmol/g d.b.]
Leaves	9.48 ± 0.24b ‡	11.86 ± 0.24b	18.75 ± 0.38a	6.63 ± 0.1a3	0.30 ± 0.01a
Flowers	6.03 ± 0.19a	9.60 ± 0.19a	21.40 ± 0.43b	5.56 ± 0.11b	0.20 ± 0.01b
Stalks	23.91 ± 0.63c	31.74 ± 0.63d	56.47 ± 1.13c	0.52 ± 0.01d	0.09 ± 0.01d
Roots	10.44 ± 0.39b	19.54 ± 0.39c	72.68 ± 1.45d	5.08 ± 0.10c	0.13 ± 0.01c

‡ Values are expressed as the mean ($n = 3$) ± standard deviation and different letters (between morphological parts) within the same row indicates statistically significant differences ($p < 0.05$).

The leaves, flowers, stalks, and roots of *S. officinalis* L. were also tested for their ability of inhibition of α-amylase (αA) and α-glucosidase (αG) activity, and their ability of inhibition of pancreatic lipase (LP) activity (Table 3). αA and αG are carbohydrate-degrading enzymes, but the mechanisms of their action differ; αA accelerates the hydrolysis of bonds inside a compound, whereas αG hydrolyzes α-1,4-glucosidic bonds, leading to the release of glucose absorbed by the body [35]. In turn, LP is an enzyme responsible for the degradation of triglycerides to simple lipids and fatty acids absorbable by the human body. However, it has been proved that excess fatty acids can lead to the formation of free radicals and insulin resistance [36]. Therefore, the inhibition of the above enzymes may be used in the treatment of diabetes type II or obesity [35]. The obtained results show that the highest ability to inhibit αA and αG activity was recorded for flowers of *S. officinalis* L. and reached EC$_{50}$ 6.03 and 9.60 mg/mL, respectively. Therefore, the flowers were 1.6 and 1.3 times more active than the leaves, 4.0 and 3.3 times more active than the stalks, and 1.7 and 2.0 times more active than the roots, respectively. In turn, the highest ability to inhibit pancreatic lipase was found for the leaves of *S. officinalis* L. (EC$_{50}$ = 18.75 mg/mL) which were 1.2, 3.0, and 3.9 times more active compared to the flowers, stalks, and roots of the tested plant, respectively. As far as the results showed that the ability to inhibit αA, αG, and LP strongly depended on the sum of flavan-3-ols and the correlations were $r^2 = 0.944$, 0.836, and 0.593, respectively. However, in the case of phenolic acids and flavonols, the correlations were strongly negative: $r^2 = 0.813$, 0.921, and 0.872 and $r^2 = 0.842$, 0.825, and 0.857, respectively.

The antiproliferative potency of the flowers, leaves, roots, and stems of *S. officinalis* L. were tested against four different cancer cell lines as BxPC3 (pancreatic ductal adenocarcinoma), DLD-1 (colorectal adenocarcinoma), HCV29T (bladder cancer), and Jurkat (T-cell leukemia). This is the first report on these cancer cell lines. The effect against the used cell lines was clearly noted (Figure 1). The extract from *S. officinalis* L. leaves significantly reduces the viability of all tested cell lines, especially DLD-1 colon cancer cells (to 19%) and Jurkat leukemia cells (to 22%). The flower extract reduced the viability of Jurkat cells to 32% and the remaining cells by 39–50%. Extract from the root showed similar results. In contrast, the extract from the stem acted the weakest on all cell lines, reducing cell viability to 85–97%. What's more, the results presented a strong Pearson's correlation between the sum of flavan-3-ols and with the viability of Jurkat leukemia cells and DLD-1 colon cancer cells—$r^2 = 0.731$ and 0.545, while lower the viability of HCV29T cells strongly depended on anthocyanins and the correlation was $r^2 = 0.705$. Liu et al. [37] noted that aqueous root extracts of *S. officinalis* L. showed synergic effect on inhibition of activity against HCT-116 and CPR cell lines (colon cancer) with 5-fluorouracil. Shin et al. [38] observed that the extract of *S. officinalis* L. inhibited cell growth against HSC4 and HN22 cell line (oral cancer) and induced death. According to Liu et al. [39], aqueous plant extracts of *S. officinalis* L. decreased the target Wnt and β-catenin genes by inhibiting the signal pathway of Wnt/β-catenin in cells of colorectal cancer. Moreover, Karkanis et al. [3] noted that the highest ability to inhibit of cervical carcinoma (HeLa), breast adenocarcinoma (MCF-7), and nonsmall cell lung cancer (NCl-H460) cell line was recorded for extract of roots of *S. minor*, whereas the extract of leaves + stalks of *S. minor* showed high ability to inhibit of hepatocellular carcinoma (HepG2) cell line. Thus, our own results and other authors presented that the highest cytotoxicity for the examined tumor cell lines covered depends on the analyzed morphological parts of *S. officinalis* L. and their bioactive substances. Moreover, the leaves, flowers, and roots showed high and differed antiproliferative potency to inhibit activity of various tumor cell lines.

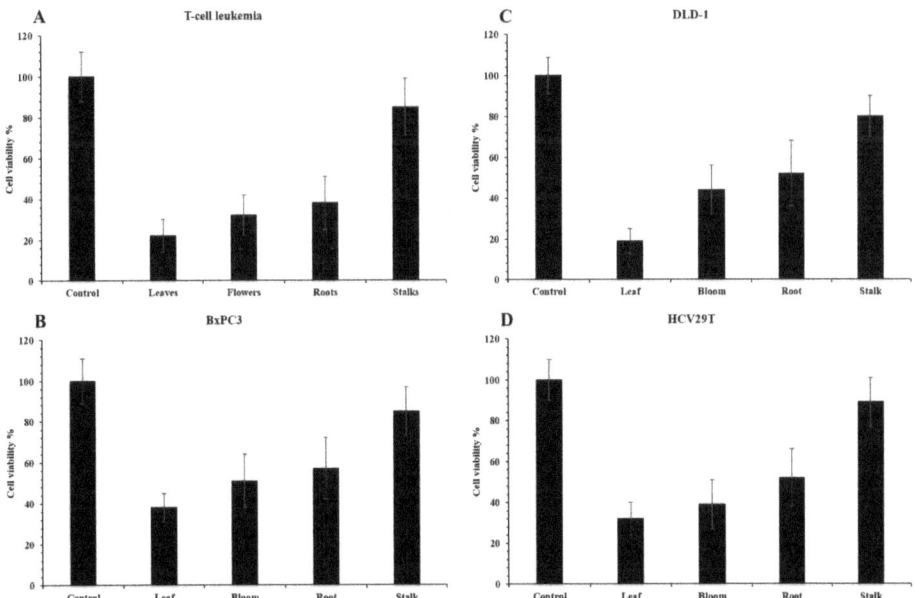

Figure 1. Cell viability of Jurkat (**A**), BxPC3 (**B**), DLD-1 (**C**), and HCV29T (**D**) cell lines after treatment with plant extracts for 48 h. Data are presented as means SD normalized to untreated control (1% ethanol).

3. Materials and Methods

3.1. Material, Reagents, and Instruments

Materials: *Sanguisorba officinalis* L. flowers, stalks, roots, and leaves (~5 kg) were obtained from a private garden in Szczytna (53°33′46″ N 20°59′07″ E), Lower Silesia, Poland. The plant was collected randomly in August 2019 from different parts of field (total area of cultivation is 1 ha). Then, material was washed and dried in a freeze dryer Alpha 1-4 LSC (Christ, Osterode, Germany).

Reagents: acetonitrile, formic acid, methanol, ABTS (2,2′-azinobis(3-ethylbenzothiazoline-6-sulfonic acid), 6-hydroxy-2,5,7,8-tetramethylchroman-2-carboxylic acid (Trolox), 2,4,6-tri(2-pyridyl)-s-triazine (TPTZ), methanol, acetic acid, α-amylase from porcine pancreas, α-glucoamylase from *Rhizopus* sp., lipase from porcine pancreas, Antibiotic-Antimycotic Solution, and RPMI 1640 culture medium were purchased from Sigma-Aldrich (Steinheim, Germany). (−)-Epicatechin, (+)-catechin, procyanidin B2, *p*-coumaric acid, ferulic acid, 5-caffeoylquinic acid, procyanidin A2, caffeic acid, quercetin 3-*O*-rutinoside, quercetin-3-*O*-galactoside, quercetin-3-*O*-glucoside, kaempferol 3-*O*-galactoside, ellagic acid, and cyanidin-3-*O*-glucoside were purchased from Extrasynthese (Lyon, France). DMEM culture medium with 10% FBS were purchased from Gibco (Thermo Fisher Scientific, Waltham, MA, USA), and MTS solution was purchased from Promega (Madison, WI, USA).

Instruments: UV-2401 PC spectrophotometer (Shimadzu, Kyoto, Japan) for antioxidant activity; Sonic 6D, Polsonic, Warsaw, Poland, for extraction; LC-DAD-ESI-QTOF-MS/MS (ultraperformance liquid chromatography equipped with a binary solvent manager and a Q-Tof Micro Mass Spectrometer (Waters, Manchester, UK) with an ESI source operating in negative and positive modes (Waters Corporation, Milford, MA, USA) for polyphenolic compounds; and Wallac 1420 VICTOR2 Plate Reader (PerkinElmer, Waltham, MA, USA) for antiproliferative activity.

3.2. Determination of Polyphenols

For the extraction and determination of phenolic compounds, a protocol described before by Lachowicz et al. [9] was followed. Briefly, samples (0.1 g) were mixed with 5 mL of 30% of UPLC-grade methanol. The extracts were sonicated for 20 min and centrifuged (at 19,000× g/10 min). Finally, the extracts were filtered by hydrophilic PTFE 0.20 μm membrane (Millex Samplicity Filter, Darmstadt, Germany) and used for testing.

The runs were monitored at the following wavelengths: phenolic acids at 320 nm, flavonols at 360 nm, anthocyanins at 520 nm, flavan-3-ols at 280 nm, and hydrolysable tannins at 240 nm. Separations of individual polyphenols were carried out using a UPLC BEH C18 column (1.7 μm, 2.1 mm × 100 mm) at 30 °C. The samples (10 μL) were injected, and the elution was completed in 15 min with a sequence of linear gradients and isocratic flow rates of 0.45 mL/min. The mobile phase consisted of solvent A (0.1% formic acid, v/v) and solvent B (100% acetonitrile). The program began with isocratic elution with 99% solvent A (0–1 min), and then, a linear gradient was used until 12 min, lowering solvent A to 0%; from 12.5 to 13.5 min, the gradient returned to the initial composition (99% A), and then, it was held constant to re-equilibrate the column. The analysis was carried out using full-scan, data-dependent MS scanning from m/z 100 to 1500. Leucine enkephalin was used as the reference compound at a concentration of 500 pg/μL, at a flow rate of 2 μL/min, and the $[M - H]^-$ ion at 554.2615 Da was detected. The $[M - H]^-$ ion was detected during 15 min analysis performed within ESI–MS accurate mass experiments, which were permanently introduced via the LockSpray channel using a Hamilton pump. The lock mass correction was ±1.000 for the mass window. The mass spectrometer was operated in negative- and positive-ion mode, set to the base peak intensity (BPI) chromatograms, and scaled to 12,400 counts per second (cps) (100%). The optimized MS conditions were as follows: capillary voltage of 2500 V, cone voltage of 30 V, source temperature of 100 °C, desolvation temperature of 300 °C, and desolvation gas (nitrogen) flow rate of 300 L/h. Collision-induced fragmentation experiments were performed using argon as the collision gas, with voltage ramping cycles from 0.3 to 2 V. Characterization of the single components was carried out via the retention time and the accurate molecular masses. Each compound was optimized to its estimated molecular mass [M − H]$^-$/[M + H]$^+$ in the negative and positive mode before and after fragmentation. The data obtained from UPLC-MS were subsequently entered into the MassLynx 4.0ChromaLynx Application Manager software. On the basis of these data, the software is able to scan different samples for the characterized substances. The PDA spectra were measured over the wavelength range of 200–800 nm in steps of 2 nm. The calibration curves were prepared for the standard: gallic acid (y = 1222.5x − 1972.7; r^2 = 0.9999), procyanidin B2 (y = 6566.2x − 15,957; r^2 = 0.9999), (+)-catechin (y = 1565.9x + 2243; r^2 = 0.9999), *p*-coumaric acid (y = 68.109x + 49.224; r^2 = 0.9996), ferulic acid (y = 50,215x + 36,206; r^2 = 0.9997), 5-caffeoylquinic acid (y = 14,332x + 1315.1; r^2 = 0.9999), procyanidin A2 (y = 9484.1x − 6770.5; r^2 = 0.9997), caffeic acid (y = 17,431x + 40,114; r^2 = 0.9999), quercetin 3-*O*-rutinoside (y = 13,362x − 1795; r^2 = 0.9997), qercetin-3-*O*-galactoside (y = 20,926x − 18,309; r^2 = 0.9991), qercetin-3-*O*-glucoside (y = 11,923x + 8188; r^2 = 0.9999), kaempferol 3-*O*-galactoside (y = 12,057x − 1922.4; r^2 = 0.9997), ellagic acid (y = 26754x + 172359; r^2 = 0.9995), cyanidin-3-*O*-glucoside (y = 30,726x + 190,297; r^2 =

0.9976), and (−)-epicatechin (y = 39,233x − 360,853; r^2 = 0.9994) at concentrations ranging between 0.05 and 0.5 mg/mL. All data were obtained in triplicate. The results were expressed as mg/100 g of dry basis (d.b.).

3.3. Pro-Health Properties

3.3.1. Antiradical Capacity

Samples (1 g) were mixed with methanol (80%; 10 mL) and then with hydrochloric acid (1%). This process was performed twice by incubating the above slurry for 20 min under sonication. Next, the slurry was centrifuged at 19,000× *g* for 10 min, and the supernatant was filtered through a hydrophilic PTFE 0.20 μm membrane (Merck, Darmstadt, Germany) and used for analysis.

The ABTS method was carried out with the method described by Re et al. [40]. For this, 0.03 mL of sample was mixed with 3 mL of ABTS + solution, and after 6 min of reaction, the absorbance was measured at 734 nm using the spectrophotometer. All data were obtained in triplicate. The activity was expressed in mmol Trolox/g d.b.

3.3.2. Reducing Potential

The FRAP method was carried out with the method described by Benzie et al. [41]. The reagent was prepared by mixing 10 mmol 2,4,6-Tris(2-pyridyl)-s-triazine (TPTZ)/L reagent with 20 mmol/L ferric chloride in acetate buffer (pH 3.6). Precisely, 0.1 mL of sample was mixed with 0.9 mL of distilled water and 3 mL of ferric complex. After 10 min of reaction, the absorbance was measured at 593 nm using the spectrophotometer. All data were obtained in triplicate. The activity was expressed in mmol Trolox/g d.b.

3.3.3. Determination of Enzyme Inhibition Potency

Anti-diabetic activity, α-amylase, α-glucosidase inhibitory, and lipase activity effect of the materials were described previously by Nakai et al. [42], Podsędek et al. [43], and Nickavar et al. [44]. The extraction of mixed material was done with 70% acetone (or water) at room temperature for 60 min with constant stirring. After centrifuging at 4000 rpm for 10 min, and filtration, the supernatants were concentrated at 40 °C (vacuum evaporator) to remove the acetone and the aqueous phase was diluted with water. For further analytical and biological activity assays, a gradient of concentrations was prepared via serial dilution of the fruit extracts in pure water. The amount of the inhibitor (expressed as mg of fruit per 1 mL of reaction mixture under assay conditions) required to inhibit 50% of the enzyme activity was defined as the IC_{50} value. The IC_{50} of the fruits tested was obtained from the line of the plot of the fruit concentration in 1 mL of reaction mixture versus the % inhibition. All samples were assayed in triplicate.

3.3.4. Antiproliferative Potency

Cell Lines and Cell Culture

The human cancer cell lines BxPC3 (pancreatic ductal adenocarcinoma), DLD-1 (colorectal adenocarcinoma), and HCV29T (bladder cancer) were cultured in DMEM culture medium with 10% FBS and Antibiotic-Antimycotic Solution. Jurkat cell line (T-cell leukemia) was maintained in RPMI 1640 culture medium supplemented with 2 mM L-glutamine, 100 U/mL penicillin, 100 μg/mL streptomycin, and 10% fetal bovine serum (FBS). All cell lines were cultured at 37 °C in a humidified atmosphere of 5% CO_2. The cells were seeded at densities of 5×10^3 cells/0.1 mL (0.32 cm^2) for cell viability assay. All cell lines were obtained from the collection of the Institute of Immunology and Experimental Therapy, Polish Academy of Sciences, Wroclaw, Poland.

Determination of Cell Viability

For determination of cell viability, cells were seeded in 96-well-plate (NUNC, Roskilde, Denmark). The plant extract was prepared by suspending 100 mg of dry plant material in 1 mL of 30% ethanol. The suspension was heated at 50 °C for 30 min and then centrifuged at 10,000× *g* for 15 min. The clear supernatant was diluted 30-fold in cell culture medium. As a control, 1% ethanol in the cell medium was used. The cells were incubated in 200 μL of the above culture medium for 48 h. Following the incubation, 20 μL of MTS solution was added to each well for 4 h; next, absorbance at 490 nm was recorded by a plate reader. Each treatment within a single experiment was performed in triplicate. Data were normalized to control medium containing 1% ethanol.

3.4. Statistical Analysis

Statistical analysis such as one-way ANOVA ($p < 0.05$) was analyzed using Statistica 12.5 (StatSoft, Kraków, Poland).

4. Conclusions

It needs to be noted that the flowers and leaves of *S. officinalis* L. are a good source of polyphenols, including hydrolyzable tannins, phenolic acids, flavonols, and anthocyanins, and exhibit a significant antiradical and reducing potential. In turn, the roots and stalks are a valuable source of flavan-3-ols. The most effective the inhibition of α-amylase, α-glucosidase, and pancreatic lipase and antiproliferative activities, reflected in the inhibition of viability of pancreatic ductal adenocarcinoma, colorectal adenocarcinoma, and bladder cancer as well as T-cell leukemia cell, were shown by the flowers and leaves of *S. officinalis* L. Thus, the data provided in this work indicate the possibility of using its individual morphological parts in the prevention of selected disease entities. In addition, this plant material can be used not only in the food industry as a functional additive to food, increasing its health value, but also in the cosmetic and pharmaceutical industries as a nutraceutical. The data obtained justify the need for further research on the morphological parts of *S. officinalis* L. with special emphasis put on leaves and flowers, to identify mechanisms potentially responsible for the antiproliferative activity.

Supplementary Materials: The following are available online at http://www.mdpi.com/1424-8247/13/8/191/s1. Figure S1: LC-DAD-ESI-QTOF-MS/MS chromatogram fragile of the *Sanguisorba officinalis* L. flowers extract at 320 and 360 nm; Figure S2: LC–DAD-ESI–QTOF–MS/MS chromatogram fragile of the *Sanguisorba officinalis* L. leaves extract at 320 and 360 nm; Figure S3: LC-DAD-ESI-QTOF-MS/MS chromatogram fragile of the *Sanguisorba officinalis* L. roots extract at 320 and 360 nm; Figure S4: LC–DAD-ESI–QTOF–MS/MS chromatogram fragile of the *Sanguisorba officinalis* L. stalks extract at 320 and 360 nm.

Author Contributions: Conceptualization, S.L. and J.O.; methodology, S.L., J.O., A.R. and I.O.; validation, S.L. and J.O.; formal analysis, S.L. and J.O.; investigation, S.L. and J.O.; resources, S.L. and J.O.; data curation, S.L. and J.O.; writing—original draft preparation, S.L. and J.O.; writing—review and editing, S.L. and J.O.; visualization, S.L. and J.O.; project administration, S.L. and J.O.; and funding acquisition, S.L. and J.O. All authors have read and agreed to the published version of the manuscript.

Funding: This research received no external funding.

Acknowledgments: The work was created in a leading research team "Food&Health".

Conflicts of Interest: The authors declare no conflicts of interest.

References

1. Kim, S.; Oh, S.; Noh, H.B.; Ji, S.; Lee, S.H.; Koo, J.M.; Choi, C.W.; Jhun, H.P. In vitro antioxidant and anti-propionibacterium acnes activities of cold water, hot water, and methanol extracts, and their respective ethyl acetate fractions, from Sanguisorba officinalis L. Roots. *Molecules* **2018**, *23*, 3001. [CrossRef]
2. Zhu, H.-L.; Chen, G.; Chen, S.-N.; Wang, Q.-R.; Wan, L.; Jian, S.-P. Characterization of polyphenolic constituents from Sanguisorba officinalis L. and its antibacterial activity. *Eur. Food Res. Technol.* **2019**, *245*, 1487–1498. [CrossRef]

3. Karkanis, A.C.; Fernandes, A.; Vaz, J.; Petropoulos, S.A.; Georgiou, E.; Ćirić, A.; Sokovic, M.D.; Oludemi, T.; Barros, L.; Ferreira, I.C. Chemical composition and bioactive properties of Sanguisorba minor Scop. under Mediterranean growing conditions. *Food Funct.* **2019**, *10*, 1340–1351. [CrossRef]

4. Nguyen, T.T.H.; Cho, S.O.; Ban, J.Y.; Kim, J.Y.; Ju, H.S.; Koh, S.B.; Song, K.-S.; Seong, Y.H. Neuroprotective effect of Sanguisorbae radix against oxidative stress-induced brain damage: In vitro and in vivo. *Boil. Pharm. Bull.* **2008**, *31*, 2028–2035. [CrossRef]

5. Zhang, L.; Koyyalamudi, S.R.; Jeong, S.C.; Reddy, N.; Smith, P.T.; Rajendran, A.; Longvah, T. Antioxidant and immunomodulatory activities of polysaccharides from the roots of Sanguisorba officinalis. *Int. J. Boil. Macromol.* **2012**, *51*, 1057–1062. [CrossRef]

6. Wang, Z.; Loo, W.T.; Wang, N.; Chow, L.W.; Wang, N.; Han, F.; Zheng, X.; Chen, J.-P. Effect of Sanguisorba officinalis L on breast cancer growth and angiogenesis. *Expert Opin. Ther. Targets* **2012**, *16*, S79–S89. [CrossRef] [PubMed]

7. Liang, J.; Chen, J.; Tan, Z.; Peng, J.; Zheng, X.; Nishiura, K.; Ng, J.; Wang, Z.; Wang, D.; Chen, Z.; et al. Extracts of the medicinal herb Sanguisorba officinalis inhibit the entry of human immunodeficiency virus-1. *J. Food Drug Anal.* **2013**, *21*, S52–S58. [CrossRef] [PubMed]

8. Kim, Y.H.; Chung, C.B.; Kim, J.G.; Ko, K.I.; Park, S.H.; Kim, J.-H.; Eom, S.-Y.; Kim, Y.S.; Hwang, Y.-I.; Kim, K.-H. Anti-Wrinkle Activity of Ziyuglycoside I Isolated from a Sanguisorba officinalis Root Extract and Its Application as a Cosmeceutical Ingredient. *Biosci. Biotechnol. Biochem.* **2008**, *72*, 303–311. [CrossRef]

9. Lachowicz, S.; Oszmiański, J.; Wojdyło, A.; Cebulak, T.; Hirnle, L.; Siewiński, M. UPLC-PDA-Q/TOF-MS identification of bioactive compounds and on-line UPLC-ABTS assay in Fallopia japonica Houtt and Fallopia sachalinensis (F.Schmidt) leaves and rhizomes grown in Poland. *Eur. Food Res. Technol.* **2018**, *245*, 691–706. [CrossRef]

10. Yisimayili, Z.; Abdulla, R.; Tian, Q.; Wang, Y.; Chen, M.; Sun, Z.; Li, Z.; Liu, F.; Aisa, H.A.; Huang, C. A comprehensive study of pomegranate flowers polyphenols and metabolites in rat biological samples by high-performance liquid chromatography quadrupole time-of-flight mass spectrometry. *J. Chromatogr. A* **2019**, *1604*, 460472. [CrossRef] [PubMed]

11. Nawrot-Hadzik, I.; Ślusarczyk, S.; Granica, S.; Hadzik, J.; Matkowski, A. Phytochemical Diversity in Rhizomes of Three Reynoutria Species and their Antioxidant Activity Correlations Elucidated by LC-ESI-MS/MS Analysis. *Molecules* **2019**, *24*, 1136. [CrossRef] [PubMed]

12. Bunse, M.; Lorenz, P.; Stintzing, F.C.; Kammerer, D.R. Characterization of Secondary Metabolites in Flowers of Sanguisorba officinalis L. by HPLC-DAD-MS n and GC/MS. *Chem. Biodivers.* **2020**, *17*, 1900724. [CrossRef] [PubMed]

13. Sentandreu, E.; Cerdán-Calero, M.; Sendra, J.M. Phenolic profile characterization of pomegranate (Punica granatum) juice by high-performance liquid chromatography with diode array detection coupled to an electrospray ion trap mass analyzer. *J. Food Compos. Anal.* **2013**, *30*, 32–40. [CrossRef]

14. Zhu, M.-Z.; Dong, X.; Guo, M. Phenolic Profiling of Duchesnea indica Combining Macroporous Resin Chromatography (MRC) with HPLC-ESI-MS/MS and ESI-IT-MS. *Molecules* **2015**, *20*, 22463–22475. [CrossRef] [PubMed]

15. Esposito, T.; Celano, R.; Pane, C.; Piccinelli, A.L.; Sansone, F.; Picerno, P.; Zaccardelli, M.; Aquino, R.P.; Mencherini, T. Chestnut (Castanea sativa Miller.) burs extracts and functional compounds: UHPLC-UV-HRMS profiling, antioxidant activity, and inhibitory effects on Phytopathogenic Fungi. *Molecules* **2019**, *24*, 302. [CrossRef] [PubMed]

16. Fernandes, A.; Sousa, A.; Mateus, N.; Cabral, M.; De Freitas, V. Analysis of phenolic compounds in cork from Quercus suber L. by HPLC-DAD/ESI-MS. *Food Chem.* **2011**, *125*, 1398–1405. [CrossRef]

17. Mämmelä, P.; Savolainen, H.; Lindroos, L.; Kangas, J.; Vartiainen, T. Analysis of oak tannins by liquid chromatography-electrospray ionisation mass spectrometry. *J. Chromatogr. A* **2000**, *891*, 75–83. [CrossRef]

18. Mullen, W.; Yokota, T.; Lean, M.E.; Crozier, A. Analysis of ellagitannins and conjugates of ellagic acid and quercetin in raspberry fruits by LC-MSn. *Phytochemistry* **2003**, *64*, 617–624. [CrossRef]

19. Clifford, M.N.; Johnston, K.L.; Knight, S.; Kuhnert, N. Hierarchical Scheme for LC-MSnIdentification of Chlorogenic Acids. *J. Agric. Food Chem.* **2003**, *51*, 2900–2911. [CrossRef]

20. Sun, J.; Lin, L.-Z.; Chen, P. Study of the mass spectrometric behaviors of anthocyanins in negative ionization mode and its applications for characterization of anthocyanins and non-anthocyanin polyphenols. *Rapid Commun. Mass Spectrom.* **2012**, *26*, 1123–1133. [CrossRef]

21. Brar, H.S.; Singh, Z.; Swinny, E. Dynamics of anthocyanin and flavonol profiles in the 'Crimson Seedless' grape berry skin during development and ripening. *Sci. Hortic.* **2008**, *117*, 349–356. [CrossRef]
22. Rockenbach, I.I.; Jungfer, E.; Ritter, C.; Santiago-Schübel, B.; Thiele, B.; Fett, R.; Galensa, R. Characterization of flavan-3-ols in seeds of grape pomace by CE, HPLC-DAD-MSn and LC-ESI-FTICR-MS. *Food Res. Int.* **2012**, *48*, 848–855. [CrossRef]
23. Ito, C.; Oki, T.; Yoshida, T.; Nanba, F.; Yamada, K.; Toda, T. Characterisation of proanthocyanidins from black soybeans: Isolation and characterisation of proanthocyanidin oligomers from black soybean seed coats. *Food Chem.* **2013**, *141*, 2507–2512. [CrossRef] [PubMed]
24. Abad-García, B.; Garmón-Lobato, S.; Berrueta, L.; Gallo, B.; Vicente, F. Practical guidelines for characterization ofO-diglycosyl flavonoid isomers by triple quadrupole MS and their applications for identification of some fruit juices flavonoids. *J. Mass Spectrom.* **2009**, *44*, 1017–1025. [CrossRef] [PubMed]
25. Lin, Y.-S.; Tsai, Y.-J.; Tsay, J.-S.; Lin, J.-K. Factors Affecting the Levels of Tea Polyphenols and Caffeine in Tea Leaves. *J. Agric. Food Chem.* **2003**, *51*, 1864–1873. [CrossRef]
26. López-García, J.; Kucekova, Z.; Humpolíček, P.; Mlček, J.; Saha, P. Polyphenolic Extracts of Edible Flowers Incorporated onto Atelocollagen Matrices and Their Effect on Cell Viability. *Molecules* **2013**, *18*, 13435–13445. [CrossRef]
27. Zeng, Y.; Deng, M.; Lv, Z.; Peng, Y. Evaluation of antioxidant activities of extracts from 19 Chinese edible flowers. *SpringerPlus* **2014**, *3*, 315. [CrossRef]
28. Elfalleh, W. Total phenolic contents and antioxidant activities of pomegranate peel, seed, leaf and flower. *J. Med. Plants Res.* **2012**, *6*, 4724–4730. [CrossRef]
29. Loza-Mejía, M.A.; Salazar, J.R. Sterols and triterpenoids as potential anti-inflammatories: Molecular docking studies for binding to some enzymes involved in inflammatory pathways. *J. Mol. Graph. Model.* **2015**, *62*, 18–25. [CrossRef]
30. Arapitsas, P. Hydrolyzable tannin analysis in food. *Food Chem.* **2012**, *135*, 1708–1717. [CrossRef]
31. Parus, A. Antioxidant and pharmacological properties of phenolic acids. *Postępy Fitoter.* **2012**, *1*, 48–53.
32. Lachowicz, S.; Oszmiański, J. Profile of Bioactive Compounds in the Morphological Parts of Wild Fallopia japonica (Houtt) and Fallopia sachalinensis (F. Schmidt) and Their Antioxidative Activity. *Molecules* **2019**, *24*, 1436. [CrossRef] [PubMed]
33. Djeridane, A.; Yousfi, M.; Nadjemi, B.; Boutassouna, D.; Stocker, P.; Vidal, N. Antioxidant activity of some algerian medicinal plants extracts containing phenolic compounds. *Food Chem.* **2006**, *97*, 654–660. [CrossRef]
34. Katalinic, V.; Milos, M.; Kulisic, T.; Jukić, M. Screening of 70 medicinal plant extracts for antioxidant capacity and total phenols. *Food Chem.* **2006**, *94*, 550–557. [CrossRef]
35. Kunyanga, C.N.; Imungi, J.K.; Okoth, M.W.; Biesalski, H.K.; Vadivel, V. Total phenolic content, antioxidant and antidiabetic properties of methanolic extract of raw and traditionally processed Kenyan indigenous food ingredients. *LWT* **2012**, *45*, 269–276. [CrossRef]
36. Koska, J.; Yassine, H.; Trenchevska, O.; Sinari, S.; Schwenke, D.C.; Yen, F.T.; Billheimer, D.; Nelson, R.W.; Nedelkov, B.; Reaven, P.D. Disialylated apolipoprotein C-III proteoform is associated with improved lipids in prediabetes and type 2 diabetes1[S]. *J. Lipid Res.* **2016**, *57*, 894–905. [CrossRef]
37. Liu, M.-P.; Liao, M.; Dai, C.; Chen, J.-F.; Yang, C.-J.; Liu, M.; Chen, Z.-G.; Yao, M.-C. Sanguisorba officinalis L synergistically enhanced 5-fluorouracil cytotoxicity in colorectal cancer cells by promoting a reactive oxygen species-mediated, mitochondria-caspase-dependent apoptotic pathway. *Sci. Rep.* **2016**, *6*, 34245. [CrossRef]
38. Shin, J.-A.; Kim, J.-S.; Kwon, K.-H.; Nam, J.-S.; Jung, J.-Y.; Cho, N.-P.; Cho, S.-D. Apoptotic effect of hot water extract of Sanguisorba officinalis L. in human oral cancer cells. *Oncol. Lett.* **2012**, *4*, 489–494. [CrossRef]
39. Liu, M.-P.; Li, W.; Dai, C.; Lam, C.W.K.; Li, Z.; Chen, J.-F.; Chen, Z.-G.; Zhang, W.; Yao, M. Aqueous extract of Sanguisorba officinalis blocks the Wnt/β-catenin signaling pathway in colorectal cancer cells. *RSC Adv.* **2018**, *8*, 10197–10206. [CrossRef]
40. Re, R.; Pellegrini, N.; Proteggente, A.; Pannala, A.; Yang, M.; Rice-Evans, C. Antioxidant activity applying an improved ABTS radical cation decolorization assay. *Free. Radic. Boil. Med.* **1999**, *26*, 1231–1237. [CrossRef]
41. Benzie, I.F.; Strain, J. The Ferric Reducing Ability of Plasma (FRAP) as a Measure of "Antioxidant Power": The FRAP Assay. *Anal. Biochem.* **1996**, *239*, 70–76. [CrossRef] [PubMed]
42. Nakai, M.; Fukui, Y.; Asami, S.; Toyoda-Ono, Y.; Iwashita, T.; Shibata, H.; Mitsunaga, T.; Hashimoto, A.F.; Kiso, Y. Inhibitory effects of oolong tea polyphenols on pancreatic lipase in vitro. *J. Agric. Food Chem.* **2005**, *53*, 4593–4598. [CrossRef] [PubMed]

Pharmaceuticals **2020**, *13*, 191

43. Podsędek, A.; Majewska, I.; Redzynia, M.; Sosnowska, D.; Koziolkiewicz, M. In vitro inhibitory effect on digestive enzymes and antioxidant potential of commonly consumed fruits. *J. Agric. Food Chem.* **2014**, *62*, 4610–4617. [CrossRef] [PubMed]

44. Nickavar, B.; Yousefian, N. Evaluation of α-amylase inhibitory activities of selected antidiabetic medicinal plants. *J. Consum. Prot. Food Saf.* **2010**, *6*, 191–195. [CrossRef]

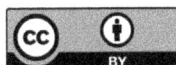

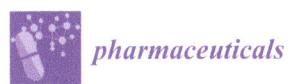

pharmaceuticals

Article

Development, Characterization, and Stability Evaluation of the Anti-Cellulite Emgel Containing Herbal Extracts and Essential Oils

Ngamrayu Ngamdokmai [1], Kornkanok Ingkaninan [1,*], Nattiya Chaichamnong [2], Krongkarn Chootip [3], Nitra Neungchamnong [4] and Neti Waranuch [5,6,*]

1 Centre of Excellence in Cannabis Research, Department of Pharmaceutical Chemistry and Pharmacognosy, Faculty of Pharmaceutical Sciences and Center of Excellence for Innovation in Chemistry, Naresuan University, Phitsanulok 65000, Thailand; ngamrayun59@nu.ac.th
2 Division of Applied Thai Traditional Medicine, Faculty of Public Health, Naresuan University, Phitsanulok 65000, Thailand; nattiyach@nu.ac.th
3 Department of Physiology, Faculty of Medical Sciences, Naresuan University, Phitsanulok 65000, Thailand; krongkarnc@nu.ac.th
4 Science Laboratory Centre, Faculty of Science, Naresuan University, Mueang, Phitsanulok 65000, Thailand; nitran@nu.ac.th
5 Department of Pharmaceutical Technology, Faculty of Pharmaceutical Sciences and Center of Excellence for Innovation in Chemistry, Naresuan University, Phitsanulok 65000, Thailand
6 Cosmetics and Natural Products Research Center, Faculty of Pharmaceutical Sciences, Naresuan University, Phitsanulok 65000, Thailand
* Correspondence: k_ingkaninan@yahoo.com (K.I.); netiw@nu.ac.th (N.W.); Tel.: +66-814817350 (K.I.); +66-97482792 (N.W.)

Citation: Ngamdokmai, N.; Ingkaninan, K.; Chaichamnong, N.; Chootip, K.; Neungchamnong, N.; Waranuch, N. Development, Characterization, and Stability Evaluation of the Anti-Cellulite Emgel Containing Herbal Extracts and Essential Oils. *Pharmaceuticals* **2021**, *14*, 842. https://doi.org/10.3390/ph14090842

Academic Editors: Jan Oszmianski and Sabina Lachowicz

Received: 5 August 2021
Accepted: 23 August 2021
Published: 25 August 2021

Publisher's Note: MDPI stays neutral with regard to jurisdictional claims in published maps and institutional affiliations.

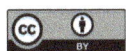
Abstract: Recently, the herbal compress was successfully developed and applied for cellulite treatment. The aim of this study was to formulate a more convenient dosage form of herbal application from the original formula. In addition, we aimed to characterize and evaluate the stability of the developed dosage form. A gelled emulsion, or an "emgel," incorporated with 0.1 wt% tea and coffee extracts (1:1 ratio) plus 5 wt% essential oils (mixed oil) was prepared. The caffeine content in the finished product obtained from tea and coffee extracts analyzed by HPLC was 48.1 ± 2.3 µg/g. The bio-active marker monoterpenes of mixed oil characterized by headspace GCMS were camphene 50.8 ± 1.8 µg/mg, camphor 251.0 ± 3.2 µg/mg, 3-carene 46.7 ± 1.8 µg/mg, α-citral 75.0 ± 2.1 µg/mg, β-citral 65.6 ± 1.3 µg/mg, limonene 36.8 ± 6.7 µg/mg, myrcene 53.3 ± 4.5 µg/mg, α-pinene 85.2 ± 0.6 µg/mg, β-pinene 88.4 ± 1.1 µg/mg, and terpinene-4-ol 104.3 ± 2.6 µg/mg. The stability study was carried out over a period of 3 months at 4, 25, and 50 °C. The caffeine content showed no significant changes and passed the acceptance criteria of ≥80% at all tested temperatures. However, monoterpenes showed their stability for only 2 months at 50 °C. Therefore, the shelf-life of the emgel was, consequently, calculated to be 31 months using the Q10 method. Thus, the anti-cellulite emgel was successfully formulated. The characterization methods and stability evaluation for caffeine and monoterpenes in an emgel matrix were also successfully developed and validated.

Keywords: topical formulation; anti-cellulite; cosmetic; monoterpenoids; accelerated stability

1. Introduction

Cellulite, popularly called orange peel skin, affects mostly women and is found in more than 80% of women of post-pubertal age, which can be treated either medically or cosmetically to enhance the appearance of this issue [1]. Natural ingredients are preferable in cosmetic treatment due to their safety image [2]. Several studies have shown that various natural components are clinically effective [3–6]. These indicate that plants are a particularly rich source of providing components for cellulite treatment. Previously, anti-cellulite treatment by applying a warmed traditional herbal compress comprising aromatic herbs, i.e., ginger (*Zingiber officinale* Roscoe), black pepper (*Piper nigrum* L.), java long pepper (*Piper retrofractum* Vahl.), plai (*Zingiber montanum* (J. Koenig) Link ex A.Dietr.), turmeric (*Curcuma longa* L.), lemon grass (*Cymbopogon citratus* DC. Stapf.), and kaffir lime (*Citrus hystrix* DC.), and herbs containing xanthine alkaloids, i.e., tea (*Camellia sinensis* (L.) Kuntze) and coffee (*Coffea arabica* L.), on the cellulite area was proven to be effective [7,8]. The anti-cellulite ingredients were considered for their prospective complementarities in combating the cellulite problem. Caffeine [9] (in tea and coffee), limonene [10] (in ginger, black pepper, java long pepper, lemon grass, and kaffir lime), citral [11] (in black pepper, java long pepper, lemon grass, and kaffir lime), and terpinene-4-ol [12] (in plai) among others are cosmetic agents with well-documented anti-adipogenesis action.

The anti-cellulite mechanisms of the essential oils, including monoterpenoids, constituents of aromatic herbs as well as extracts of tea and coffee, have also been elucidated in vitro as a reduction in lipid accumulation and vasorelaxation [13]. Therefore, the active formulation of a smooth-texture gelled emulsion, or an "emgel," with a pH range of 5.5–7.0 included a combination of essential oil and extract actives, considered for their way of treating all the major mechanisms related to the development of cellulite. Recently, the more convenient dosage form, anti-cellulite emgel, was freshly prepared and clinically tested. Its effectiveness was already proved and reported [14].

The aim of this study was to demonstrate headspace gas chromatography/mass spectrometry (HS-GCMS) and high-performance liquid chromatography (HPLC) methods for monoterpenoid and caffeine determination for the main constituents in the anti-cellulite emgel matrix and evaluate product stability after storage over a period of 12 weeks at 4, 25, and 50 °C.

2. Results and Discussion

2.1. Anti-Cellulite Emgel Formulation

Many active ingredients from medicinal plants, primarily in the form of standardized botanical extracts, can act synergistically on various biological targets and improve unwanted signs and symptoms [15]. The main ingredients of this formulation were mixed essential oils from well-documented anti-inflammatory and anti-lipogenesis or lipolysis herbs used in our herbal compress, such as ginger [16,17], black pepper [18,19], java long pepper [20,21], and lemon grass [22,23], and water extracts of tea [24,25] and coffee [26,27].

Anti-cellulite emgels were formulated by using a carbomer (Carbopol 940) combined with an emulsion to create a delivery base for hydrophobic substances. The carbomer-to-emulsion ratio was optimized to accommodate the hydrophobic actives. A mixture of seven essential oils of herbal ingredients in the compress (mixed oil) and tea and coffee extracts were chosen as active ingredients of the anti-cellulite formulation. The problem of water insolubility, high volatility, and instability of the short-chain hydrocarbon molecules of the essential oils (e.g., α-pinene, camphene, myrcene, and terpinen-4-ol), being incompatible with the emulsion droplets in the formulation [28], was resolved by introducing a carrier oil with a long lipid tail into the emulsion system as a diluent for the essential oils. The carrier oil also enhanced the viscosity of the oil combination and promoted the development of the emulsion. The carrier oil for this emulsion system was virgin cold-pressed rice bran oil. This mixed oil and two extracts were successfully incorporated into the preliminary developed stable emgel base. The formulation is shown in Table 1.

Texture, color, odor, pH (at 25 °C), and viscosity (spindle no. 5, 20 rpm, 25 °C) of the formulation were observed during the stability tests. Measurements were taken before and after 24 days of storage at 4 °C, followed by six cycles of heating and cooling at 4 and 45 °C for 48 h per cycle. A formulation kept at 25 °C was used as a control.

Table 1. Anti-cellulite emgel formula.

Ingredient	Formula (wt%)
Deionized water	66.00
Carbopol 940	0.80
Disodium EDTA	0.10
Propylene glycol	2.00
Glycerin	6.00
Phenoxyethanol and chlorphenesin	1.00
Triethanolamine (TEA)	1.00
PEG-40 hydrogenated castor oil	5.00
Rice bran oil	8.00
Tea extract	0.05
Coffee extract	0.05
Mixed oil	5.00
Camphor	5.00

2.2. Chemical Characterization of the Anti-Cellulite Emgel

HS-GCMS was used for qualitative and quantitative analyses of volatile substances in the anti-cellulite emgel. The advantage of headspace analysis over standard GC methods is the ability to determine only volatile analytes, without concern for other matrix components. Headspace sampling is therefore suitable to determine volatile compounds in our emgel or other semisolid cosmetic products. Moreover, the headspace GCMS method provides several advantages, including no use of organic solvents, potential automation, and the ease of sample preparation [29,30]. Twenty-nine constituents of the anti-cellulite emgel were characterized by HS-GCMS (Table 2). The monoterpenes from the essential oil constituents were detected as major constituents. The rank by %peak area was camphor (100.0%), δ-Curcumene (21.6%), limonene (8.8%), β-sesquiphellandrene (8.6%), α-curcumene (6.6%), β-bisabolene (6.4%), sabinene (6.3), tumerone (5.8%), α-citral (5.2%), and β-citral (4.6%).

Table 2. The volatile composition of the anti-cellulite emgel analyzed by using HS-GCMS.

Peak No.	RT (min)	RI [1]	Identified Compounds	Relative Area (%)
1	1.66	562	Trimethoxyborane	2.57
2	3.67	939	α-Pinene	2.06
3	3.86	955	Camphene	2.81
4	4.14	978	Sabinene	6.31
5	4.21	984	β-Pinene	4.38
6	4.31	992	Myrcene	2.03
7	4.57	1009	α-Phellandrene	1.14
8	4.67	1014	3-Carene	3.93
9	4.75	1019	α-Terpinene	1.22
10	4.95	1029	Limonene	8.84
11	5.03	1033	Eucalyptol	1.39
12	5.49	1058	γ-Terpinene	1.64
13	6.13	1092	α-Terpinolene	1.55
14	7.71	1152	Camphor	100.00
15	8.49	1180	(Internal standard) menthol	31.01
16	8.63	1185	γ-Terpinene	4.29

Table 2. *Cont.*

Peak No.	RT (min)	RI [1]	Identified Compounds	Relative Area (%)
17	8.92	1195	α-Terpineol	1.83
18	9.45	1227	(Preservative) phenoxyethanol	7.95
19	9.73	1250	β-Citral	4.60
20	10.19	1277	α-Citral	5.22
21	11.75	1373	Caryophyllene	2.26
22	12.15	1395	α-Curcumene	6.66
23	12.20	1400	Germacrene D	1.87
24	12.23	1404	delta-Curcumene	20.43
25	12.28	1409	β-Selinene	3.15
26	12.32	1413	β-Bisabolene	6.41
27	12.43	1424	β-Sesquiphellandrene	8.46
28	13.25	1511	Tumerone	5.81
29	13.42	1530	Curlone	1.26

[1] Comparison with Kováts retention index (RI), the NIST library (version 2.2) comparison using GCMS (SCAN) analysis.

2.3. HS-GCMS Method Validation

2.3.1. Selectivity

These values demonstrate that no interfering peaks occurred in the corresponding retention time of each analyte (Figure 1). The selected ion mode (SIM) and retention time (RT) for compounds of interest in HS-GCMS analysis were (1) α-pinene (specific m/z ratios: 91, 92, 93), RT 3.611; (2) camphene (specific m/z ratios: 79, 93, 121), RT 3.810; (3) β-pinene (specific m/z ratios: 69, 91, 93), RT 4.166; (4) myrcene (specific m/z ratios: 69, 91, 93), RT 4.257; (5) 3-carene (specific m/z ratios: 79, 91, 93), RT 4.605; (6) D-limonene (specific m/z ratios: 91, 136), RT 4.895; (7) camphor (specific m/z ratios: 69, 81, 95), RT 7.588; (7) menthol (specific m/z ratios: 71, 81, 95), RT 8.420; (8) terpinen-4-ol (specific m/z ratios: 43, 71, 111), RT 8.560; (9) β-citral (specific m/z ratios: 41, 69, 94), RT 9.747; and (10) α-citral (specific m/z ratios: 69, 84, 94), RT 10.16.

2.3.2. Linearity

The range of linearity of the 10 constituents with their LOD and LOQ are shown in Table 3. The r^2 for the calibration curves for all compounds was >0.990. For all substances, the signals were linear over concentration ranges, suggesting that the method was appropriate for analyzing these compounds in the same sample.

Table 3. Correlation coefficient (r^2), linear range, LOD, and LOQ of 10 monoterpenoids in the anti-cellulite emgel analyzed by HS-GCMS.

Analytes	RT	(r^2)	Linear Range (µg/mL)	LOD (µg/mL)	LOQ (µg/mL)
α-Pinene	3.611	0.9997	39.1–1250	13.0	39.1
Camphene	3.810	0.9989	62.5–2000	20.8	62.5
β-Pinene	4.166	0.9982	39.1–1250	13.0	39.1
Myrcene	4.257	0.9978	62.5–2000	20.8	62.5
3-Carene	4.605	0.9987	39.1–1250	13.0	39.1
Limonene	4.895	0.9974	39.1–1250	13.0	39.1
Camphor	7.588	0.9989	62.5–2000	20.8	62.5
Terpinene	8.420	0.9964	39.1–1250	13.0	39.1
β-Citral	8.560	0.9988	62.5–2000	20.8	62.5
α-Citral	9.747	0.9976	62.5–2000	20.8	62.5

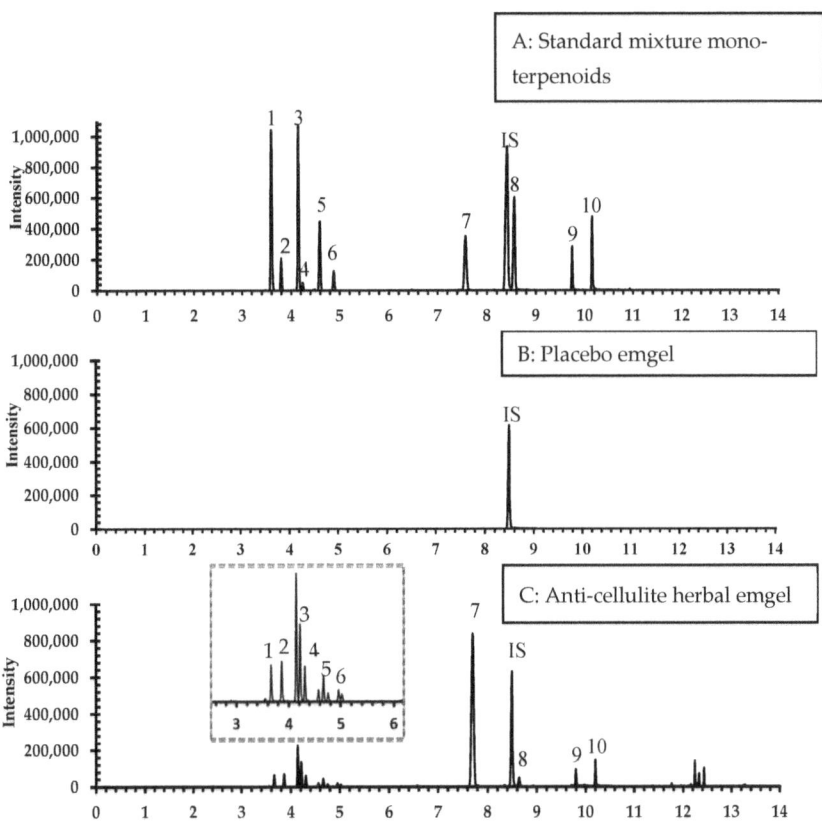

Figure 1. HS-GCMS (SIM) total ion chromatograms of (**A**) standard monoterpenoid mixture (2.5 µg/mL), (**B**) placebo emgel (20 mg), and (**C**) anti-cellulite herbal emgel. The peaks of 10 constituents were identified by comparison with standard references as (1) α-pinene (RT 3.61), (2) camphene (RT 3.81), (3) β-pinene (RT 4.16), (4) myrcene (RT 4.25), (5) 3-carene (RT 4.61), (6) D-limonene (RT 4.89), (7) camphor (RT 7.59), (8) terpinene-4-ol (RT 8.55), (9) β-citral (RT 9.75), and (10) α-citral (RT 10.16).

2.3.3. Precision and Accuracy

Intra-day and inter-day precision and accuracy at three concentrations were studied. Both precision and accuracy were within reasonable limits (%RSD was less than 15%, and percentage accuracy was between 85 and 110%) [31] (Table 4).

Table 4. Intra-day and inter-day precision and accuracy of the HS-GCMS method for determination of 10 monoterpenoid standards assessed at three different concentration levels (*n* = 3) on three consecutive days. Accuracy was expressed as the percentage recovery of 10 monoterpenoid standards in three different concentrations in the placebo emgel.

Analytes	Concentration Levels/Spiked Mount (µg/mL)	Intra-Day (*n* = 3)		Inter-Day (*n* = 9)		Accuracy (*n* = 9)
		Measured Concentration (µg/mL) ± SD	Precision (%RSD)	Measured Concentration (µg/mL)	Precision (%RSD)	Recovery (%)
α-Pinene	120	126.62 ± 4.07	3.21	124.45 ± 3.54	2.85	105.5
	190	190.75 ± 1.38	0.73	190.90 ± 1.03	0.54	98.6
	1000	1013.42 ± 5.56	0.54	1004.97 ± 10.63	1.06	98.8
Camphene	125	131.09 ± 2.41	1.84	128.40 ± 3.88	3.02	97.4
	300	284.46 ± 6.33	2.23	277.07 ± 11.66	4.21	101.8
	1600	1561.43 ± 7.74	0.49	1568.28 ± 9.42	0.60	99.4

Table 4. Cont.

Analytes	Concentration Levels/Spiked Mount (µg/mL)	Intra-Day (*n* = 3)		Inter-Day (*n* = 9)		Accuracy (*n* = 9)
		Measured Concentration (µg/mL) ± SD	Precision (%RSD)	Measured Concentration (µg/mL)	Precision (%RSD)	Recovery (%)
β-Pinene	120	109.23 ± 3.17	2.91	107.70 ± 2.83	2.63	100.5
	190	192.64 ± 4.88	2.53	193.65 ± 4.11	2.12	100.4
	1000	1013.34 ± 9.99	0.98	1012.33 ± 9.53	0.94	100.0
Myrcene	125	112.72 ± 4.11	3.64	113.48 ± 2.846	2.50	100.6
	300	273.69 ± 3.84	1.40	272.10 ± 8.16	2.99	101.1
	1600	1436.74 ± 4.31	0.30	1442.68 ± 11.36	0.78	106.7
3-Carene	120	124.26 ± 4.42	3.56	122.61 ± 4.22	3.44	94.4
	190	189.28 ± 3.96	2.09	186.85 ± 3.96	2.45	102.0
	1000	924.90 ± 6.15	0.66	927.38 ± 5.33	0.57	102.6
Limonene	120	130.95 ± 3.20	2.44	129.40 ± 2.91	2.91	105.5
	190	194.62 ± 5.02	5.02	191.83 ± 5.34	2.78	102.1
	1000	1025.84 ± 9.62	0.94	1025.34 ± 13.53	1.32	98.3
Camphor	125	134.15 ± 5.09	3.79	134.26 ± 5.09	3.79	98.2
	300	286.33 ± 8.94	3.12	291.26 ±9.32	3.20	96.7
	1600	1718.85 ± 2.75	0.16	1718.85 ± 11.69	0.68	97.8
Terpinene-4-ol	120	114.58 ± 2.17	1.89	112.78 ± 4.19	3.71	100.4
	190	177.21 ± 4.89	2.76	176.40 ± 3.47	1.97	107.5
	1000	942.44 ± 7.19	0.76	934.46 ± 10.47	1.12	101.6
β-Citral	125	107.75 ± 0.95	0.89	108.02 ± 2.31	2.14	98.3
	300	314.81 ± 9.63	3.06	311.76 ± 8.18	2.62	96.2
	1600	1649.47 ± 13.03	0.79	1663.07 ± 14.08	0.85	99.0
α-Citral	125	128.02 ± 4.96	3.88	127.39 ± 4.07	3.19	99.5
	300	329.87 ± 7.54	2.28	329.24 ± 5.74	1.74	99.0
	1600	1642.30 ± 12.91	0.79	1645.17 ± 11.29	0.69	99.0

The accuracy was determined by spiking the three different concentrations of 10 monoterpenoid standards. Recovery in the range of 94–107 (%RSD ≤ 4.21%) was obtained (Table 4).

2.4. HPLC Method Validation

The HPLC method for determination of caffeine was developed and validated according to ICH guidelines.

2.4.1. Selectivity

Separation was done on a C18 column with isocratic elution of 40% methanol in water. The tailing factor and resolution of the caffeine standard met ICH guidelines. The identification of caffeine in the sample was confirmed with the retention time of the caffeine standard (Figure 2).

2.4.2. Linearity

The calibration equations, linearity, limit of detection (LOD), and limit of quantitation (LOQ) values are presented in Table 5. The HPLC chromatograms of the caffeine standard, placebo, and anti-cellulite emgel are shown in Figure 2A–C.

Table 5. Correlation coefficient (r^2), linear range, LOD, and LOQ of the caffeine standard in the anti-cellulite emgel analyzed by HPLC.

Analyte	RT (min)	(r^2)	Linear Range (µg/mL)	LOD (ng/mL)	LOQ (ng/mL)
Caffeine	4.015	1.00	0.3125–20	156.250	15.625

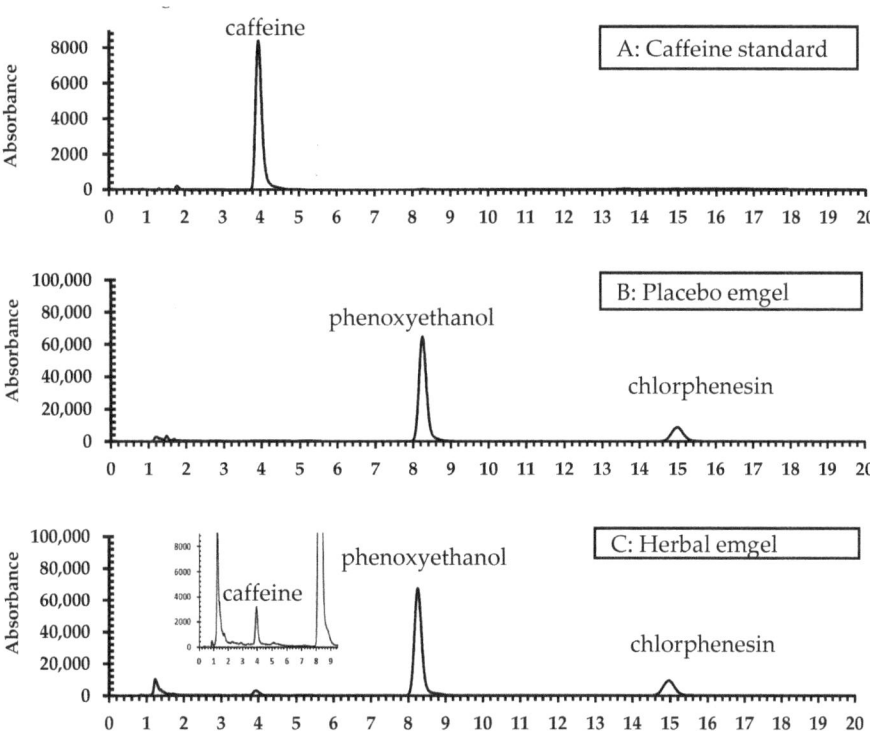

Figure 2. HPLC chromatograms of (**A**) caffeine standard (2.5 μg/mL) (RT 4.015), (**B**) placebo emgel (20 mg/mL), and (**C**) anti-cellulite emgel (20 mg/mL).

2.4.3. Precision and Accuracy

Intra-day and inter-day precision and accuracy at three concentrations were determined. Both precision and accuracy were within reasonable limits (% RSD was less than 15%, and percentage accuracy was between 85 and 110%) (AOAC, 2012). (Table 6. The %RSD, which reflected the intra-day and inter-day precision of the caffeine standard, was not more than 2.5%.

Table 6. Intra-day and inter-day precision and accuracy of the HPLC method for determination of the caffeine standard assessed at two different concentration levels ($n = 3$) on three consecutive days. Accuracy was expressed as the percentage recovery of the caffeine standard at two different concentrations in the coffee extract.

Standard	Concentration Levels/Spiked Mount (μg/mL)	Intra-Day Precision ($n = 6$)		Inter-Day Precision ($n = 9$)		Accuracy ($n = 9$)
		Measured Concentration (μg/mL) ± SD	Precision (%RSD)	Measured Concentration (μg/mL) ± SD	Precision (%RSD)	Recovery (%)
Caffeine	1.88	1.86 ± 0.03	1.70	1.81 ± 0.05	2.51	101.0
	7.50	7.49 ± 0.19	2.52	7.32 ± 0.18	2.51	100.6

The accuracy was determined by spiking the two different concentrations of caffeine standard (1.8 and 7.5 ppm) at 0.1 mg/mL of coffee extract. Recovery in the range of 98–103 (%RSD ≤ 6.32%) was obtained. All data are shown in Table 6.

2.5. Quantitation of Constituents of Interest in the Anti-Cellulite Emgel Using HS-GCMS

The 10 constituents of interest were analyzed in the anti-cellulite emgel by HS-GCMS (SIM) (Table 7). The major monoterpene in the formula was camphor (251.0 µg/mg).

Table 7. The contents of 10 monoterpenoid constituents in the anti-cellulite emgel analyzed by HS-GCMS (n = 3).

Anti-Cellulite Emgel	Monoterpenoids Presented in the Formulation (µg/mg) Average ± S.D.
α-Pinene	85.2 ± 0.6
Camphene	50.8 ± 1.8
β-Pinene	88.4 ± 1.1
Myrcene	53.3 ± 4.5
3-Carene	46.7 ± 1.8
Limonene	36.8 ± 6.7
Camphor	251.0 ± 3.2
Terpinene-4-ol	104.3 ± 2.6
β-Citral	65.6 ± 1.3
α-Citral	75.0 ± 2.1

2.6. Determination of Caffeine Content in Tea, Coffee Material, and the Anti-Cellulite Emgel by HPLC

The caffeine concentrations of coffee, tea, and anti-cellulite emgel were analyzed by HPLC. For the anti-cellulite emgel, a content of 0.05% of each tea and coffee extract in the formulation contained approximately 1% of caffeine (Table 8).

Table 8. The content of caffeine in the anti-cellulite emgel was analyzed by HPLC (n = 3).

Sample	Caffeine Content Ave ± S.D. (µg/g)
Coffee extract (freeze-dried)	45.0 ± 0.4
Tea extract (freeze-dried)	64.2 ± 1.1
Anti-cellulite emgel with tea and coffee extracts in this formulation	48.1 ± 2.3

2.7. Physical Stability of the Anti-Cellulite Emgel

Physical stability is important to consider while maintaining lipophilic chemicals in emulsion formulae and subsequently in cosmetic products to prevent or mitigate deterioration during storage. The anti-cellulite emgel was evaluated for qualities such as color, odor, pH, viscosity, and phase separation. The anti-cellulite emgel had a homogeneous texture with a buttermilk color and a characteristic odor of herbal essential oils. After storage for 12 weeks (Table 9), the physical properties of the anti-cellulite emgel remained similar to baseline, while after a heating-cooling stability study and after storage at 50 °C for 3 months, there was only a minor change in the appearance of the anti-cellulite emgel.

Table 9. The physical stability of the anti-cellulite emgel at initiation day and after being stored at 4 °C, 25 °C, and 50 °C for 3 months and after 6 heating-cooling cycles.

Conditions	Physical Examination	pH	Viscosity (Cp)	Separation
Initiation	Smooth texture, pale brown	6.89 ± 0.02	1715 ± 5.29	No phase separation
4 °C	Smooth texture, pale brown	6.61 ± 0.04	1681 ± 6.81	No phase separation
25 °C	Smooth texture, pale brown	6.68 ± 0.05	1632 ± 5.50	No phase separation
50 °C	Smooth texture, pale brown (darker, slightly stronger smell)	6.63 ± 0.02	1616 ± 5.03	No phase separation
Heating-cooling 6 cycles 45 °C/4 °C	Smooth texture, pale brown (slightly darker, slightly stronger smell)	6.65 ± 0.03	1654 ± 3.21	No phase separation

2.8. Chemical Stability Evaluation Using GCMS and HPLC

The active monoterpenoids and caffeine in the anti-cellulite emgel were determined using our validated HS-GCMS and HPLC methods. The anti-cellulite emgel was stored for 12 weeks at 4 °C, room temperature, 50 °C.

After 8 weeks storage at 50 °C, the active monoterpenoids in the emgel formulation retained more than 80% of the initiation concentration (Figure 3), whereas caffeine retained more than 80% after 12 weeks (Figure 3).

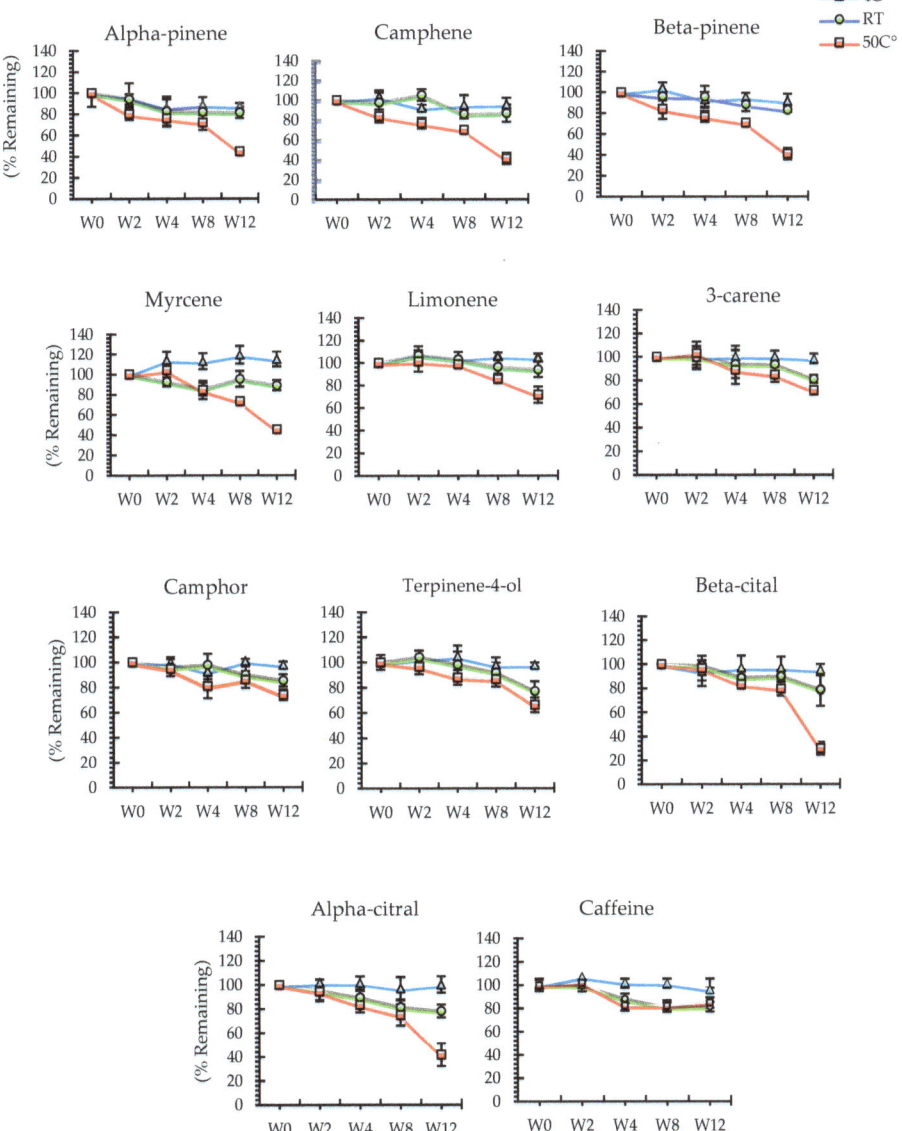

Figure 3. The percentages of the relationship between the time of storage and temperature under room temperature (25 °C), refrigerator (4 °C), and oven (50 °C) conditions. Change in the percentage of constituents of interest, camphor, camphene, citral, 3-carene, limonene, myrcene, α-pinene, β-pinenen, terpinene-4-ol, and caffeine, for 12 weeks.

2.9. Microbiological Stability Evaluation

The durability of preservatives is a critical element in ensuring microbial efficiency. To demonstrate microbiological stability, we conducted a preservation challenge test. Our results, shown in Table 10, indicate the acceptance criteria required by the method for acceptability in each time (day 0, day 7, day 14, and day 28). The anti-cellulite emgel was resistant to microbial proliferation, which could pose a risk if used improperly.

Table 10. Preservation efficacy of the anti-cellulite emgel.

Microbes	Log_{10} CFU/g			
	Day 0	Day 7	Day 14	Day 28
Staphylococcus aureus	6.0	3.3	<2.0	<2.0
Pseudomonas aeruginosa	5.9	3.0	<2.0	<2.0
Escherichia coli	6.0	<2.0	<2.0	<2.0
Candida albicans	4.4	<2.0	<2.0	<2.0
Aspergillus niger	4.6	<2.0	<2.0	<2.0

2.10. Calculation of Monoterpenoids and Caffeine Accelerated Shelf Life by the Q10 Method

The accelerated stability test, which predicts the potential behavior of the anti-cellulite emgel, was quite informative. The shelf life of the anti-cellulite emgel was calculated using the Q10 equation [32,33], which is considered a cornerstone in estimating the storage life of monoterpenoids with heat-sensitive degradation. The storage life of the monoterpenoids in the anti-cellulite emgel was estimated to be 31 months, while that of caffeine was 46 months in the same concentration of the anti-cellulite herbal emgel.

3. Materials and Methods

3.1. Chemicals and Standards

Methanol and water were of LC-MS grade and purchased from RCI Labscan Ltd., (Bangkok, Thailand). Reference standards, camphor (purity $\geq$ 95%), camphene (purity $\geq$ 95%), caffeine anhydrous (purity > 99%), citral (purity $\geq$ 98%), 3-carene (purity $\geq$ 90%), limonene (purity $\geq$ 97%), myrcene (purity $\geq$ 90%), α-pinene (purity $\geq$ 98%), β-pinene (purity $\geq$ 99%), and terpinen-4-ol (purity $\geq$95%), were products from Sigma-Aldrich (St. Louis, MO, USA). The internal standard, menthol (purity $\geq$ 98%), was from TCI (Shanghai, China). The standard homologous series of n-alkanes (C8-C40) was obtained from Sigma-Aldrich (St. Louis, MO, USA). Camphor (cosmetic grade) was purchased from Chemipan (Bangkok, Thailand).

3.2. Essential Oils and Extracts

Essential oils of ginger, black pepper, java long pepper, plai, turmeric, lemon grass, and kaffir lime were purchased from Thai-China Flavours and Fragrances Industry Co., Ltd. (Ayutthaya, Thailand). They were mixed in a ratio equivalent to the composition of the herbs used in the herbal compress formula [13] and called a "mixed oil." Tea of the Three Horses brand and roasted coffee of the Arabica 100% Coffman brand were purchased in Phitsanulok, Thailand. Ground tea leaves and coffee beans were separately extracted with boiling water for 20 min. After filtration and 5 min of centrifuging, the aqueous solutions were lyophilized to obtain tea and coffee extracts, which were then stored at -20 °C until use.

3.3. Preparation of the Anti-Cellulite Emgel

The anti-cellulite emgel was composed of 5% mixed oil, 5% camphor, 0.05% tea extract, and 0.05% coffee extract. The other ingredients and their functions are listed in Table 11. Camphor was dissolved in the mixed oil, while tea and coffee extracts were added to the carbopol gel and mixed with other ingredients, resulting in the formation of an emgel.

The base sample (without the mixed oil) was prepared with similar materials and under identical conditions for formulation.

Table 11. Anti-cellulite emgel ingredients.

Anti-Cellulite Emgel	Function
Deionized water	Diluent
Carbopol 940	Gelling agent
Disodium EDTA	Chelating agent
Propylene glycol	Moisturizing agent
Glycerin	Moisturizing agent
Phenoxyethanol and chlorphenesin	Preservatives
Triethanolamine (TEA)	pH adjuster
PEG-40 hydrogenated castor oil	Solubilizer
Rice bran oil	Emollient
Tea extract	Active ingredient
Coffee extract	Active ingredient
Mixed oil	Active ingredient
Camphor	Active ingredient

3.4. Headspace Gas Chromatography/Mass Spectrometry (HS-GCMS) and High-Performance Liquid Chromatography (HPLC) Analyses

The HS-GCMS and HPLC methods for determination of chemical ingredients in the anti-cellulite emgel were developed and validated in terms of the limit of detection (LOD), limit of quantitation (LOQ), linearity, accuracy, and precision [31]. A placebo emgel was used as a blank sample.

3.4.1. HS-GCMS Instruments and Chromatographic Conditions

HS analysis was performed using the Agilent G4556-64000 network. The HS auto sampler Agilent PN 7697A was used to directly introduce samples automatically into the Agilent 7890B Gas Chromatography System-5977B MSD model mass spectrometer. After the vials were pressurized with carrier gas, the emgel HS samples were injected into an HP-5 capillary column (5% phenyl methyl silox) (30 m × 250 μm × 0.25 μm; Agilent 19091S-433). The carrier gas was helium (He) with a constant flow rate of 1.3 mL/min. The GC oven temperature was initially set at 70 °C for 3 min, then increased to 100 °C at a rate of 3 °C/min and held for 3 min, and then increased to 250 °C at a rate of 20 °C/min and held for 1 min, with a total run time of 22 min. Mass spectrometry analysis was carried out using an Agilent mass selective detector model 5977B MSD coupled with the gas chromatograph in selected ion mode (SIM) of specific *m/z* ratios for each of the 10 compounds and one internal standard. The mass spectrometer was operated in electron impact ionization mode (70 eV) with a scan range of 50 to 550 amu.

3.4.2. HS-GCMS Method Validation

The method was validated according to ICH guidelines by determining linearity, LOD, LOQ, precision, and accuracy. The calibration curves were obtained with the average of peak area ratios of three replicates. To find the correlation coefficient (r^2) value, six concentration levels of standard solutions were analyzed. Precision was determined using the repeatability between 6 replicate samples of the placebo emgel and spiked with the concentrations of QC1, QC2, and QC3 of the calibration curve and reported as a coefficient of variation (percentage). The accuracy was calculated as the percentage recovery from three replicates of samples spiked with the same concentration that was used for the determination of precision. Intra-day and inter-day precision and accuracy were performed at three concentrations.

3.4.3. Sample Preparation for HS-GCMS

Mixture standard solutions in methanol at concentrations of 500, 250, 125, 62.5, 31.2, and 15.6 µg/mL (camphene, myrcene) and 2500, 1250, 625, 312.5, 156.2, and 78.1 mg/mL (camphor, α-citral, β-citral, 3-carene, limonene, α-pinene, β-pinene, and terpinen-4-ol) were prepared for generating the calibration curve. Menthol in methanol (2 mg/mL) was used as the internal standard.

For preparing the validation samples, 1 mg of a blank matrix (placebo emgel) and a blank sample (blank vial) were spiked with the internal standard and prepared in a headspace vial of 20 mL and then injected into each batch of samples to demonstrate that there was no cross-contamination and interference during the analysis.

3.4.4. Qualitative Analyses of Constituents in the Anti-Cellulite Emgel Using the HS-GCMS Method

Volatile compounds of the anti-cellulite emgel were analyzed by using the HS-GCMS method, stated above, and identified by comparing their spectra and retention times to those of the standard compounds or to those of the NIST MS search 2.2 library, in addition to comparison with their GC Kováts retention indices (RIs) from the literature. The linear RIs for all components were determined by co-injecting the samples with a solution containing the homologous series of n-alkanes (C8-C20). Caffeine was identified by the retention time of the standard compound.

3.4.5. HPLC Instruments and Chromatographic Conditions

Chromatographic analysis was performed using a Shimadzu SCL-10A HPLC system equipped with a Shimadzu SPD-10A UV/Vis detector, an LC-10AT pump, SIL-20AC HT auto-samplers, and a CTO-10ASVP column oven. Chromatographic separation was performed on a Phenomenex Synergi 4u Hydro-RP 80A column (150 × 4.60 mm, 4 µm particle size) connected to a Phenomenex C18 (10 × 4.6 mm, 5 µm) guard column that maintained the temperature at 35 °C. The isocratic mobile phase was methanol and water (40:60 *v/v*) at a flow rate of 1.0 mL/min. The injection volume was 10 µL, and the eluates were monitored at 275 nm. The total run time was 8 min.

3.4.6. HPLC Method Validation

The method was validated according to ICH guidelines by determining linearity, LOD, LOQ, precision, and accuracy. The linearity range of the standards was determined on seven concentration levels that ranged from 0.3125 to 20 µg/mL. Calibration curves were measured on every analysis day, and each sample was determined in triplicate. The standard curves were plotted by areas under the curve of the caffeine standard. The linearity of the calibration curve was assessed by calculating the coefficient of determination (r^2). The LOD and LOQ under the present chromatographic conditions were determined by injecting the standard solutions until the signal-to-noise ratio of each compound was 3 for LOD and 10 for LOQ. The intra-day precision of the method was analyzed from the measurement of two concentration levels of caffeine for six times within 1 day. Precision is represented by the relative standard deviation (%RSD) calculated by standard deviation/mean × 100. Inter-day precision was validated by measuring the %RSD for three consecutive days at two concentration levels, 1.875 and 7.5 µg/mL ($n = 3$, each level). The accuracy and recovery were determined by spiking the known concentration of the standard solution with the coffee extract to obtain two different concentrations (1.875 and 7.5 µg/mL). These experiments were done in triplicate. The accuracy is presented as percentage recovery of the spiked concentration, which was calculated as [(measured standard concentration – standard concentration in the non-spiked sample)/standard concentration spiked] × 100.

3.4.7. Caffeine Standard Solutions for the HPLC Method

The stock solution of the caffeine standard was freshly prepared by dissolving it in methanol to obtain a concentration of 10 mg/mL. This solution was further diluted with water to create standard calibration curves, LOD, and LOQ. The solutions were then filtered through nylon syringe filters with a 0.45 μm pore size.

3.5. Determination of Marker Compounds in the Anti-Cellulite Emgel by HS-GCMS and HPLC

Ten monoterpenoids in the anti-cellulite emgel were quantitatively determined by HS-GCMS, and caffeine was analyzed by HPLC analysis.

3.5.1. Sample Preparation for HS-GCMS

A 1 mg sample of the anti-cellulite emgel was weighed in an HS vial of 20 mL and covered with an aluminum crimp cap with a silicon septum. Next, 10 μL of the internal standard was added to each sample vial.

3.5.2. Sample Preparation for HPLC

A 20 mg sample of the anti-cellulite emgel was weighed in a vial of 1.5 mL, dissolved in methanol, and then vortexed for 1 min. The sample solution was filtered through nylon syringe filters with a 0.45 μm pore size.

3.6. Accelerated Stability Study of the Anti-Cellulite Emgel

The anti-cellulite emgel was stored at ambient temperature, 4 °C ($\pm$2 °C), and 50 °C ($\pm$2 °C). The physical properties, including color, odor, pH, viscosity, and phase separation, as well as chemical markers were determined every 2 weeks for 12 weeks. The heating-cooling cycle test was performed by alternating conditions between 4 °C ($\pm$2 °C) for 48 h and 45 °C ($\pm$2 °C) for 48 h of each cycle for 6 cycles. The studies were conducted in triplicate.

3.7. Shelf Life Prediction by the Q10 Method

The Q10 approach is a tool for forecasting the product shelf life. It is assumed that the ratio of times to equal harm at two temperatures, which are usually 10 °C apart, is constant [32–34]. The shelf life of the anti-cellulite emgel at 25 °C was calculated using the following equation:

$$t_{80}(\mathrm{T}_2) = \frac{t_{80}(\mathrm{T}_1)}{\mathrm{Q}^{(\Delta T/10)}}$$

where t_{80} (T2) denotes the shelf life at 25 °C and t_{80} (T1) denotes the shelf life at 50 °C.

3.8. Microbial Stability Studies

Microbial testing of the anti-cellulite emgel was carried out using a preservation test with the plate method. Five types of microorganisms, i.e., *Staphylococcus aureus* TISTR 1466, *Pseudomonas aeruginosa* ATCC 25783, *Escherichia coli* ATCC 25922, *Candida albicans* ATCC 10231, and *Aspergillus niger*, were added to the anti-cellulite emgel formulation. The criteria of acceptance and the consideration of preservative stability were measured according to USP 29 Chapter 51 Antimicrobial Effectiveness [35].

3.9. Statistical Analysis for Quality Control Studies

Data were expressed as the average $\pm$ standard deviation (SD). Statistical analysis was conducted using analysis of variance (ANOVA) and Student's *t*-test using GraphPad.

4. Conclusions

An anti-cellulite herbal emgel of smooth texture with pH 6.89 $\pm$ 0.02 was successfully formulated. HS-GCMS and HPLC methods were developed and validated to quantitatively determine the monoterpenoid and caffeine constituents in the formulation, respectively. The emgel was physically stable up to 3-month storage at 4 °C, room temperature, and 50 °C. The caffeine content showed no significant changes and passed the acceptance criteria of $\geq$80% at all temperature tests, while monoterpenes showed some degree of degradation at

50 °C after 2 months. The shelf life of the emgel was, consequently, calculated as 31 months by using the Q10 method.

5. Patents

The petit patent for the anti-cellulite herbal emgel product was obtained from the Department of Intellectual Property (DIP), Thailand (no. 17425, date 11 March 2021).

Author Contributions: Conceptualization, N.N. (Ngamrayu Ngamdokmai), K.I., K.C. and N.W.; methodology and experimental design, N.N. (Ngamrayu Ngamdokmai), N.C., K.C., N.N. (Nitra Neungchamnong), K.I. and N.W.; software, N.N. (Ngamrayu Ngamdokmai); validation, N.N. (Ngamrayu Ngamdokmai), N.C., K.I. and N.W.; formal analysis, N.N. (Ngamrayu Ngamdokmai), N.C., N.N. (Nitra Neungchamnong), and N.W.; investigation, N.N. (Ngamrayu Ngamdokmai), N.C. and K.I.; resources, N.W., K.C. and K.I.; data curation and interpretation, N.N. (Ngamrayu Ngamdokmai), N.N. (Nitra Neungchamnong), K.I. and N.W.; writing—original draft preparation, N.N. (Ngamrayu Ngamdokmai), K.I. and N.W.; writing—review and editing, N.N. (Ngamrayu Ngamdokmai), K.I. and N.W.; visualization, N.N. (Ngamrayu Ngamdokmai), K.C., N.C., N.N. (Nitra Neungchamnong), and N.W.; supervision, K.I., K.C. and N.W.; project administration, K.I.; funding acquisition, K.I. and N.W. All authors have read and agreed to the published version of the manuscript.

Funding: This research was funded by (i) the Royal Golden Jubilee Program (RGJ-PhD) (0008/2560) for the scholarship of NN, (ii) the Thailand Center of Excellence for Life Sciences (TCEL) (TC-A2/62), (iii) the National Research Council of Thailand (NRCT) (DBG6080005, IRN61W0005) and (iv) the Center of Excellence for Innovation in Chemistry (PERCH-CIC), Ministry of Higher Education, Science, Research and Innovation.

Institutional Review Board Statement: Not applicable.

Informed Consent Statement: Not applicable.

Data Availability Statement: Data are contained within the article.

Acknowledgments: We would like to acknowledge the Royal Golden Jubilee Program, PERCH-CIC, NRCT, TCELs, and the Cosmetics and Natural Products Research Center (COSNAT).

Conflicts of Interest: All authors completed the ICMJE disclosure form and reported the following: KI is the PI for the funding listed above and has received an honorarium from the university, and K.I., N.N. (Ngamrayu Ngamdokmai), K.C., and N.W. are named in the petit patent (Thailand) lodged by TCEL (no. 12872).

References

1. Rawlings, A.V. Cellulite and its treatment. *Int. J. Cosmet. Sci.* **2006**, *28*, 175–190. [CrossRef]
2. Morganti, P.; Morganti, G.; Gagliardini, A.; Lohani, A. From cosmetics to innovative cosmeceuticals—non-woven tissues as new biodegradable carriers. *Cosmetics* **2021**, *8*, 65. [CrossRef]
3. Puviani, M.; Tovecci, F.; Milani, M. A two-center, assessor-blinded, prospective trial evaluating the efficacy of a novel hypertonic draining cream for cellulite reduction: A clinical and instrumental (Antera 3D CS) assessment. *J. Cosmet. Dermatol.* **2018**, *17*, 448–453. [CrossRef]
4. Roure, R.; Oddos, T.; Rossi, A.; Vial, F.; Bertin, C. Evaluation of the efficacy of a topical cosmetic slimming product combining tetrahydroxypropyl ethylenediamine, caffeine, carnitine, forskolin and retinol, In vitro, ex vivo and in vivo studies. *Int. J. Cosmet. Sci.* **2011**, *33*, 519–526. [CrossRef]
5. Al-Bader, T.; Byrne, A.; Gillbro, J.; Mitarotonda, A.; Metois, A.; Vial, F.; Rawlings, A.V.; Laloeuf, A. Effect of cosmetic ingredients as anticellulite agents: Synergistic action of actives with in vitro and in vivo efficacy. *J. Cosmet. Dermatol.* **2012**, *11*, 17–26. [CrossRef] [PubMed]
6. Yimam, M.; Lee, Y.-C.; Jiao, P.; Hong, M.; Brownell, L.; Jia, Q. A randomized, active comparator-controlled clinical trial of a topical botanical cream for skin hydration, elasticity, firmness, and cellulite. *J. Clin. Aesthet. Dermatol.* **2018**, *11*, 51–57. [PubMed]
7. Ngamdokmai, N.; Waranuch, N.; Chootip, K.; Neungchamnong, N.; Ingkaninan, K. HPLC-QTOF-MS method for quantitative determination of active compounds in an anti-cellulite herbal compress. *Songklanakarin J. Sci. Technol.* **2017**, *39*, 463–470.
8. Ngamdokmai, N.; Waranuch, N.; Chootip, K.; Jampachaisri, K.; Scholfield, C.N.; Ingkaninan, K. Cellulite reduction by modified Thai herbal compresses; A randomized double-blind trial. *J. Evid.-Based Integr. Med.* **2018**, *23*, 2515690X18794158. [CrossRef]
9. Zapata, F.J.; Rebollo-Hernanz, M.; Novakofski, J.E.; Nakamura, M.T.; Gonzalez de Mejia, E. Caffeine, but not other phytochemicals, in mate tea (Ilex paraguariensis St. Hilaire) attenuates high-fat-high-sucrose-diet-driven lipogenesis and body fat accumulation. *J. Funct. Foods* **2020**, *64*, 103646. [CrossRef]

10. Lone, J.; Yun, J.W. Monoterpene limonene induces brown fat-like phenotype in 3T3-L1 white adipocytes. *Life Sci.* **2016**, *153*, 198–206. [CrossRef]
11. Sri Devi, S.; Ashokkumar, N. Citral, a monoterpene inhibits adipogenesis through modulation of adipogenic transcription factors in 3T3-L1 cells. *Indian J. Clin. Biochem.* **2018**, *33*, 414–421. [CrossRef]
12. Wong-a-nan, N.; Inthanon, K.; Saiai, A.; Inta, A.; Nimlamool, W.; Chomdej, S.; Kittakoop, P.; Wongkham, W. Lipogenesis inhibition and adipogenesis regulation via PPARγ pathway in 3T3-L1 cells by *Zingiber cassumunar* Roxb. rhizome extracts. *Egypt. J. Basic Appl. Sci.* **2018**, *5*, 289–297. [CrossRef]
13. Ngamdokmai, N.; Paracha, T.U.; Waranuch, N.; Chootip, K.; Wisuitiprot, W.; Suphrom, N.; Insumrong, K.; Ingkaninan, K. Effects of essential oils and some constituents from ingredients of anti-cellulite herbal compress on 3T3-L1 adipocytes and rat aortae. *Pharmaceuticals* **2021**, *14*, 253. [CrossRef]
14. Ngamdokmai, N.; Waranuch, N.; Chootip, K.; Jampachaisri, K.; Scholfield, C.N.; Ingkaninan, K. Efficacy of an anti-cellulite herbal emgel: A randomized clinical trial. *Pharmaceuticals* **2021**, *14*, 683. [CrossRef] [PubMed]
15. Sparavigna, A.; Guglielmini, G.; Togni, S.; Cristoni, A.; Maramaldi, G. Evaluation of anti-cellulite efficacy: A topical cosmetic treatment for cellulite blemishes—A multifunctional formulation. *J. Cosmet. Sci.* **2011**, *62*, 305. [PubMed]
16. Aafreen, M.M.; Anitha, R.; Preethi, R.C.; Rajeshkumar, S.; Lakshmi, T. Anti-Inflammatory activity of silver nanoparticles prepared from ginger oil-an invitro approach. *Indian J. Public Health Res. Dev.* **2019**, *10*, 145–149. [CrossRef]
17. Funk, J.L.; Frye, J.B.; Oyarzo, J.N.; Chen, J.; Zhang, H.; Timmermann, B.N. Anti-inflammatory effects of the essential oils of ginger (Zingiber officinale Roscoe) in experimental rheumatoid arthritis. *PharmaNutrition* **2016**, *4*, 123–131. [CrossRef] [PubMed]
18. Eren, H.; Turkmen, A.S.; Aslan, A. Effect of topical application of black pepper essential oil on peripheral intravenous catheter insertion: A randomized controlled study. *Explore* **2021**. [CrossRef] [PubMed]
19. Jeena, K.; Liju, V.B.; Umadevi, N.P.; Kuttan, R. Antioxidant, anti-inflammatory and antinociceptive properties of black pepper essential oil (piper nigrum linn). *J. Essent. Oil Bear. Plants* **2014**, *17*, 1–12. [CrossRef]
20. Zhang, Y.; Wang, X.; Ma, L.; Dong, L.; Zhang, X.; Chen, J.; Fu, X. Anti-inflammatory, antinociceptive activity of an essential oil recipe consisting of the supercritical fluid CO_2 extract of white pepper, long pepper, cinnamon, saffron and myrrh in vivo. *J. Oleo Sci.* **2014**, ess14061. [CrossRef]
21. Wang, B.; Zhang, Y.; Huang, J.; Dong, L.; Li, T.; Fu, X. Anti-inflammatory activity and chemical composition of dichloromethane extract from Piper nigrum and P. longum on permanent focal cerebral ischemia injury in rats. *Rev. Bras. Farmacogn.* **2017**, *27*, 369–374. [CrossRef]
22. Han, X.; Parker, T.L. Lemongrass (*Cymbopogon flexuosus*) essential oil demonstrated anti-inflammatory effect in pre-inflamed human dermal fibroblasts. *Biochim. Open* **2017**, *4*, 107–111. [CrossRef] [PubMed]
23. Katsukawa, M.; Nakata, R.; Takizawa, Y.; Hori, K.; Takahashi, S.; Inoue, H. Citral, a component of lemongrass oil, activates PPARα and γ and suppresses COX-2 expression. *Biochim. Biophys. Acta (BBA)-Mol. Cell Biol. Lipids* **2010**, *1801*, 1214–1220. [CrossRef]
24. Koch, W.; Zagórska, J.; Marzec, Z.; Kukula-Koch, W. Applications of Tea (*Camellia sinensis*) and its active constituents in cosmetics. *Molecules* **2019**, *24*, 4277. [CrossRef] [PubMed]
25. Susanto, H.; Kharisma, V.D.; Listyorini, D.; Taufiq, A. Effectivity of black tea polyphenol in adipogenesis related IGF-1 and its receptor pathway through in silico based study. In *Journal of Physics: Conference Series*; IOP Publishing: Bristol, UK, 2018.
26. Farias-Pereira, R.; Park, C.S.; Park, Y. Mechanisms of action of coffee bioactive components on lipid metabolism. *Food Sci. Biotechnol.* **2019**, *28*, 1287–1296. [CrossRef]
27. Duangjai, A.; Nuengchamnong, N.; Suphrom, N.; Trisat, K.; Limpeanchob, N.; Saokaew, S. Potential of coffee fruit extract and quinic acid on adipogenesis and lipolysis in 3T3-L1 adipocytes. *Kobe J. Med. Sci.* **2018**, *64*, E84–E92. [PubMed]
28. Pavoni, L.; Benelli, G.; Maggi, F.; Bonacucina, G. Green nanoemulsion interventions for biopesticide formulations. In *Nano-Biopesticides Today and Future Perspectives*; Academic Press: Cambridge, MA, USA, 2019; pp. 133–160. ISBN 978-0-12-815829-6.
29. Ferreiro-González, M.; Ayuso, J.; Álvarez, J.A.; Palma, M.; Barroso, C.G. Application of an HS–MS for the detection of ignitable liquids from fire debris. *Talanta* **2015**, *142*, 150–156. [CrossRef]
30. Zhang, C.Y.; Lin, N.B.; Chai, X.S.; Barnes, D.G. A rapid method for simultaneously determining ethanol and methanol content in wines by full evaporation headspace gas chromatography. *Food Chem.* **2015**, *183*, 169–172. [CrossRef]
31. AOAC International; Guideline Working Group. AOAC International guidelines for validation of botanical identification methods. *J. AOAC Int.* **2012**, *95*, 268–272.
32. Charde, M.; Shinde, M.; Welankiwar, A.; Jitendra, K. Development of analytical and stability testing method for vitamin-A palmitate formulation. *Int. J. PharmaceutChem.* **2014**, *4*, 39–51.
33. Moussa, N.; Haushey, L. The shelf life of Vitamin C in aw/o emulsion according to the Q10 Method. *Int. J. Pharm. Sci. Rev. Res.* **2015**, *30*, 33–39.
34. Khathir, R.; Agustina, R.; Nurba, D.; Syafriandi; Putra, D. Shelf-life estimation of cauliflower based on total soluble solids by using the arrhenius and Q10 approach. In Proceedings of the IOP conference Series: Earth and Environmental Science, Banda Aceh, Indonesia, 21–22 August 2019; Volume 365, p. 012006.
35. Sutton, S.V.; Porter, D. Development of the antimicrobial effectiveness test as USP chapter 51. *PDA J. Pharm. Sci. Technol.* **2002**, *56*, 300–311. [PubMed]

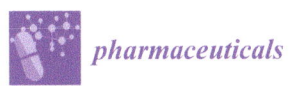 *pharmaceuticals*

Article

RP-18 TLC Chromatographic and Computational Study of Skin Permeability of Steroids

Anna W. Weronika Sobanska [1,*](iD), Jeremy Robertson [2] and Elżbieta Brzezińska [1]

1   Department of Analytical Chemistry, Faculty of Pharmacy, Medical University of Lodz, ul. Muszyńskiego 1, 90-151 Łódź, Poland; elzbieta.brzezinska@umed.lodz.pl
2   Chemistry Research Laboratory, Department of Chemistry, University of Oxford, Mansfield Road, Oxford OX1 3TA, UK; jeremy.robertson@chem.ox.ac.uk
*   Correspondence: anna.sobanska@umed.lodz.pl

Abstract: The skin permeability of steroids, as investigated in this study, is important because some of these compounds are, or could, be used in preparations applied topically. Several models of skin permeability, involving thin layer chromatographic and calculated descriptors, were generated and validated using K_p reference values obtained in silico and then tested on a group of solutes whose experimental K_p values could be found (log K_p^{exp}). The study established that the most applicable log K_p model is based on RP-18 thin layer chromatographic data (R_M) and the calculated descriptors V_M (molar volume) and PSA (polar surface area). Two less efficient, yet simple, equations based on PSA or V_M combined with HD (H-donor count) can be used with caution for rapid, rough estimations of compounds' skin permeability prior to their chemical synthesis.

Keywords: steroids; skin permeability; thin layer chromatography; calculated physicochemical descriptors

Citation: Sobanska, A.W.W.; Robertson, J.; Brzezińska, E. RP-18 TLC Chromatographic and Computational Study of Skin Permeability of Steroids. *Pharmaceuticals* **2021**, *14*, 600. https://doi.org/10.3390/ph14070600

Academic Editors: Jan Oszmianski and Sabina Lachowicz

Received: 30 May 2021
Accepted: 16 June 2021
Published: 22 June 2021

Publisher's Note: MDPI stays neutral with regard to jurisdictional claims in published maps and institutional affiliations.

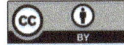
1. Introduction

Steroids are an important class of pharmaceutical actives which may be administered by different routes, including transdermal delivery [1]. Their skin permeation has been a subject of interest for a relatively long time [2–4]. In addition to experimental studies of steroids' ability to cross the skin barrier, attempts have been made to predict this property in silico. However, due to their polyfunctionality and relatively large molecular volumes, steroids are significantly different from many substances whose skin permeability has been studied, and not all the known algorithms of skin permeability are suitable for this group of solutes [4].

The rate of a molecule's permeation through skin is expressed as the flux (J), which is the amount of substance permeated per unit area and unit time. The flux depends on the permeability of the skin to the permeant (K_p) and the gradient of permeant concentration across the skin (Δc):

$$J = K_p \cdot \Delta c$$

For passive diffusion, the permeability coefficient K_p depends, in turn, on the partition coefficient P, the diffusion coefficient D and the diffusional path length h:

$$K_p = \frac{P \cdot D}{h}$$

Transdermal permeation of drugs may be studied using many techniques, including in vitro permeation experiments on excised human skin [5], animal skin, cultured human skin cells or synthetic membranes [5,6]. It is also known that skin permeation correlates with some easily obtained physicochemical parameters of a molecule, including log P_{ow}, which is the partition coefficient between octanol and water and a well-established predictor of a compound's lipophilicity and biological activity [7]. However, it has been demonstrated that log P_{ow} is not applicable as a single measure of log K_p across a very wide range of chemical families, so molecular weight (M_w) or volume (V_M), hydrogen bond donor and acceptor activity (H_d and H_a, respectively), and melting point (M_{Pt}) values are incorporated as additional descriptors [8–14]. Different computational skin permeability models have been reviewed and compared by several authors [3,15–20].

Liquid chromatography is frequently used to investigate physicochemical properties and biological activity of solutes, including their skin permeability. The chromatographic techniques used to predict the ability of molecules to cross the skin barrier include normal and reversed-phase thin layer chromatography [21,22], immobilized artificial membrane (IAM) column chromatography [23–26], RP-18 column chromatography [24,25], column chromatography on a unique stationary phase based on immobilized keratin [27], and biopartitioning micellar chromatography (BMC) [28–30]. The skin permeability coefficient K_p is connected with the chromatographic retention parameters log k or R_M^0 (obtained for column and thin layer chromatography, respectively) via linear or reverse parabolic relationships [22,26]. Chromatographic retention parameters are used either as sole skin permeability predictors, or they are combined with additional descriptors (log P_{ow}, V_M, M_w or M_{Pt}) [23,24,28,30].

Transdermal drug delivery is an important strategy employed to improve the bioavailability of drugs whose administration by other routes suffers from limitations such as poor drug stability in the gastrointestinal tract, poor permeability through the intestinal membrane or problems caused by first pass metabolism [31]. Although oral delivery remains to date the preferred method of drug administration, transdermal drug delivery systems are gaining in popularity [18,32]. Skin permeability, expressed by the coefficient K_p, is an important parameter affecting the systemic uptake of drugs after transdermal delivery. The objective of this study was to examine the relationships between the skin permeability coefficient K_p and calculated and RP-18 TLC-chromatographic descriptors for a group of steroid drugs acting upon different therapeutic targets. Descriptors derived from the RP-18 thin layer chromatographic system used in this study have appeared in previous works on blood-brain barrier (BBB) permeability [33–35] and skin permeation [36] and, according to [37], in some instances the RP-18 TLC retention parameters are better predictors of biological activity than the RP-18 HPLC data.

2. Results and Discussion

The skin permeability coefficient (K_p) is an important parameter that helps in the assessment of a compound's epidermal permeability; however, the experimentally determined values of K_p are available for only some of the drugs within the studied group. For this reason, it was decided that models of skin permeability based on thin layer chromatographic and calculated descriptors should be generated and validated using K_p values obtained in silico, then tested on a group of solutes whose experimental K_p values could be found (log K_p^{exp}). The estimation methodology used in this study is based on the approaches A to C (Table 1).

Table 1. Calculated and experimental log K_p values for compounds **1** to **46**.

	$\log K_p^{EPI}$	$\log K_p^{pre}$	$\log K_p^{exp}$	$\log K_p^{(1)}$	$\log K_p^{(3)}$	$\log K_p^{(4)}$	$\log K_p^{(5)}$	$\log K_p^{(6)}$	$\log K_p^{(7)}$	$\log K_p^{(8)}$	$\log K_p^{(9)}$	$\log K_p^{(10)}$
1	−3.72	−3.88	−4.19	−3.55	−3.75	−3.57	−4.06	−3.57	−3.47	−3.30	−3.46	−3.56
2	−3.77	−4.71	−4.79	−3.62	−3.65	−3.45	−4.22	−3.39	−3.35	−3.10	−3.46	−3.44
3	−2.00	−2.15	−1.36	−1.47	−1.87	−1.48	−2.04	−1.57	−1.48	−1.51	−1.33	−1.68
4	−3.75	−4.24	−4.35	−3.25	−3.63	−3.41	−4.29	−3.33	−3.31	−3.03	−3.46	−3.39
5	−2.24	−2.49	−2.44	−1.75	−2.49	−1.80	−2.64	−1.94	−1.73	−1.82	−1.44	−1.84
6	−4.11	−4.42	−4.41	−3.54							−3.07	−2.76
7	−3.46	−4.23	−3.26	−2.98							−2.75	−2.86
8	−1.78	−2.35	−2.82	−1.62							−1.44	−2.30
9	−2.55	−2.97	−3.22	−2.23							−2.04	−2.26
10	−2.20	−3.42	−3.22	−2.38							−2.15	−2.88
11	−2.74	−3.42	−3.34	−2.15							−2.04	−2.27
12	−2.22	−2.54	−2.65	−1.78							−1.44	−2.03
13	−2.70	−3.90	−4.12	−3.29							−2.75	−4.07
14	−1.67	−2.72	−2.21	−1.91							−1.56	−2.45
15	−2.80	−4.05	−4.39	−2.68							−2.26	−3.04
16	−3.85	−4.54	−5.00	−3.38							−3.35	−2.83
17	−4.44	−4.42	−4.59	−4.90							−5.18	−4.61
18	−4.20	−4.24	−4.17	−4.35							−4.38	−3.67
19	−3.75	−3.53	−3.68	−4.27							−4.59	−3.54
20	−4.00	−3.63	−3.20	−4.59							−4.98	−3.95
21	−3.47	−2.45	−2.74	−4.43							−4.98	−4.33
22	−4.10	−3.43	−3.05	−4.26							−4.38	−4.05
23	−3.63	−3.11	−3.04	−4.13							−4.38	−4.23
24	−3.29	−3.26	−2.47	−3.49							−3.67	−3.26
25	−3.26	−2.35	−2.27	−4.12							−4.59	−3.92
26	−2.41	−1.82	−1.74	−3.24							−3.67	−3.64
27	−1.90	−1.35	−1.21	−3.08							−3.67	−3.90
28	−1.28	−2.33		−1.71	−1.25	−1.63	−2.07	−1.58	−1.51	−1.28	−1.77	−2.51
29	−3.62	−4.13		−3.57	−3.69	−3.42	−4.24	−3.30	−3.46	−3.15	−3.67	−3.14
30	−2.85	−2.81		−2.10	−2.67	−2.19	−2.79	−2.21	−2.30	−2.25	−2.25	−1.96
31	−3.67	−3.35		−3.34	−3.89	−3.24	−4.30	−3.11	−3.40	−3.14	−3.56	−2.52
32	−1.58	−2.03		−1.69	−1.56	−1.48	−2.19	−1.44	−1.49	−1.32	−1.66	−1.85
33	−2.27	−2.19		−1.70	−1.99	−1.74	−2.18	−1.87	−1.63	−1.68	−1.44	−2.16
34	−0.58	−1.28		−1.36	−0.72	−1.36	−1.46	−1.30	−1.31	−1.07	−1.66	−2.36
35	−3.64	−3.68		−2.31	−3.53	−2.81	−3.76	−2.73	−3.05	−2.86	−3.14	−2.05
36	−4.10	−4.19		−3.34	−4.09	−2.96	−3.70	−3.04	−3.20	−3.27	−2.90	−1.89
37	−6.35	−4.98		−7.56	−6.34	−7.54	−5.15	−7.68	−7.44	−7.35	−7.25	−7.57
38	−1.95	−1.32		−1.70	−2.16	−1.83	−2.17	−2.01	−1.73	−1.85	−1.44	−2.17
39			−1.44		−2.39	−1.60	−2.99	−1.64	−1.54	−1.48	−1.44	−1.59
40			−4.05		−4.69	−3.73	−5.31	−3.55	−3.86	−3.53	−4.05	−2.71
41			−2.14		−3.63	−2.08	−4.80	−1.88	−2.18	−1.86	−2.37	−1.11
42			−2.04		−3.20	−1.71	−4.23	−1.60	−1.73	−1.53	−1.77	−0.99
43			−2.84		−2.91	−1.77	−4.79	−1.47	−1.70	−1.19	−2.15	−1.41
44			−3.67		−3.29	−2.56	−3.62	−2.55	−2.62	−2.51	−2.58	−2.13
45			−3.81		−3.13	−2.68	−5.72	−2.04	−2.76	−1.75	−3.92	−2.29
46			−2.54		−2.94	−1.89	−3.48	−1.90	−1.88	−1.82	−1.77	−1.52

A.   Equation (1), developed and validated in our earlier research [36]:

$$\log K_p^{(1)} = -1.39\ (\pm 0.18) - 0.35\ (\pm 0.03)\ (N + O) + 0.15\ (\pm 0.04)\ \log D - 0.23\ (\pm 0.06)\ HD$$

$$(n = 60, R^2 = 0.83, R^2_{adj.} = 0.82, F = 92.3, p < 0.01, s_e = 0.44) \tag{1}$$

B. EpiSuite software (DERMWIN v. 2 module) (log K_p^{EPI}), recommended by the US Environmental Protection Agency and related to the widely recognized Potts' model of skin permeability [10]:

$$\log K_p = -2.80 + 0.66 \log P_{ow} - 0.0056 M_w \ (R^2 = 0.66) \qquad (2)$$

C. PreADMET 2.0 software [38] (log K_p^{pre})

Initially, attention was turned to partition phenomena in the human stratum corneum. It was noted that Equation (1) may be a source of valuable information on solute partitioning between water and the stratum corneum. The process of skin absorption of topically applied compounds is relatively complex and consists of three steps: (i) penetration of the stratum corneum (SC), either by polar or lipid transport pathways; (ii) permeation through deeper skin layers and (iii) resorption, i.e., the uptake of a substance into the vascular system [39]. The SC is the rate-limiting skin layer [39,40] and good partition between water and the SC is an important prerequisite for effective skin absorption. Skin permeability coefficients calculated according to Equation (1) were correlated with experimental values of SC/water partition coefficients for lipid and protein domains (log $K_{sc/w}^{lip}$ and log $K_{sc/w}^{prot}$, respectively) determined by Anderson et al. [40]. The correlations obtained for a group of hydrocortisone esters (compounds **17** to **27**) were moderate (R^2 = 0.70 for lipid and 0.41 for protein domain, respectively). A group of 14 other steroid compounds (**2**, **3**, **5** to **16**), whose SC/water and lipid/water partition parameters were studied by other authors [2,41], showed good correlations between log $K_{sc/w}$ and log $K_p^{(1)}$ (R^2 = 0.80, n = 14). For compounds **3**, **6**, **7**, **12** and **14**, the correlation between log $K_{sc/w}^{lip}$ and log $K_p^{(1)}$ was also linear (R^2 = 0.85, n = 5).

Equation (1) was applied to a group of 27 steroid drugs whose experimental skin permeability coefficients are available (Table 1). It was discovered that these drugs formed two subgroups (Figure 1): compounds **1** to **16** (log K_p^{exp} taken from Refs. [2,4,42–44]) and **17** to **27** (log K_p^{exp} given by Anderson et al. [40]). The skin permeability coefficients calculated for these compounds according to Equation (1) (log $K_p^{(1)}$) were in good agreement with the experimental values (log K_p^{exp}) (linear relationships within the subgroups, R^2 = 0.81 for compounds **1** to **16** and 0.74 for compounds **17** to **27**, respectively). The correlation between calculated (Equation (1)) and experimental values of log K_p for compounds **17** to **27** was even better (R^2 = 0.84) once two ionic molecules that contain free carboxyl groups (**20** and **21**) were removed as outliers.

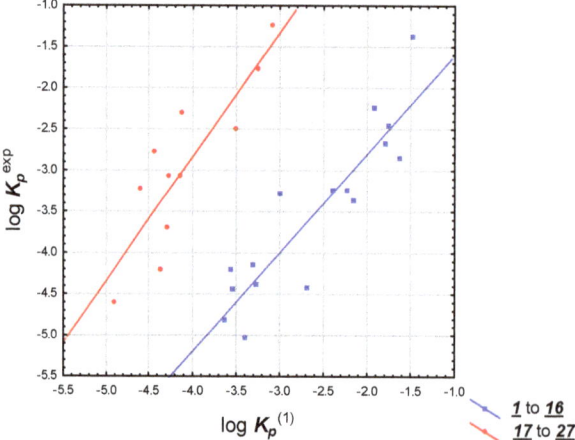

Figure 1. log K_p experimental values vs. Equation (1), compounds **1** to **27**.

A similar situation arose when log K_p^{EPI} values were considered; thus, compounds **1** to **27** again formed two subgroups (**1** to **16** and **17** to **27**) whose experimental log K_p values gave reasonable correlations with log K_p^{EPI} ($R^2 = 0.69$ and 0.86, respectively), although the subgroups partially overlapped (Figure 2). The reasons for discrepancies between experimental log K_p^{exp} values for compounds **1** to **16** and **17** to **27** are unclear. However, because the log K_p^{exp} values for compounds **17** to **27** were taken from a single source [40], the differences in experimental methodology may have had more influence on log K_p^{exp} values obtained by different authors than the physicochemical properties of the studied compounds. Related problems with the "Anderson's dataset" (with a similar explanation) were described by Abraham et al. [4].

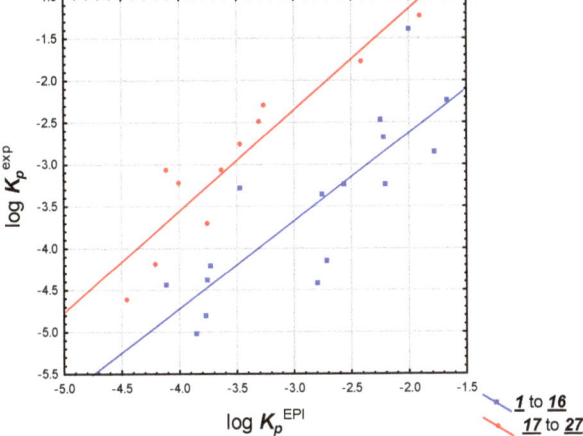

Figure 2. log K_p experimental values vs. EpiSuite, compounds **1** to **27**.

The results of log K_p calculations using preADMET software seemed more consistent (Figure 3); compounds **1** to **27** gave a single group whose calculated (log K_p^{pre}) and experimental (log K_p^{exp}) values were in good agreement ($R^2 = 0.87$, $n = 27$). However, since there was no reason to suspect that, for studied compounds, the predicted values of log K_p^{pre} were more (or less) reliable than the values calculated by other methods, the decision was made to consider also log K_p^{EPI} and log $K_p^{(1)}$ as reference values in further investigations.

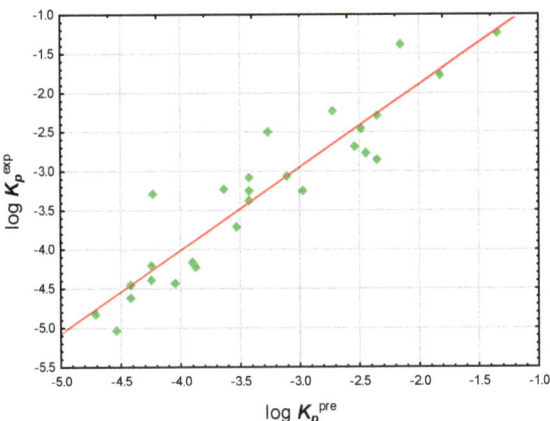

Figure 3. log K_p experimental values vs. preADMET, compounds **1** to **27**.

One of the key properties responsible for skin permeability of solutes is lipophilicity. Some earlier chromatographic studies of lipophilicity of steroids and steroid analogues [45,46] were based on the linear extrapolation approach. Chromatographic parameters for a single-solvent mobile phase were obtained by using a series of chromatographic experiments with mobile phases containing different concentrations φ of a modifier. Plots of R_M or $\log k$ (for TLC and HPLC, respectively) vs. φ were extrapolated to zero concentration of the modifier to furnish $R_M{}^0$ ($\log k_0$). The most common method to do so is by using the linear Soczewiński-Wachmeister equation: $R_M = R_M{}^0 + S\varphi$ [47]. Apart from the $R_M{}^0$ value, other useful chromatographic descriptors derived from the linear extrapolation method are the slope S and $C_0 = -R_M{}^0/S$. The extrapolation method, although commonly used and recognized, has certain drawbacks. Several chromatographic experiments are required and the extrapolated $R_M{}^0$ values depend on a modifier and its concentration range used to generate $R_M = f(\varphi)$ plots. In this study, therefore, the single chromatographic run approach was used. It was established that for the 16 steroids analyzed chromatographically, R_M values collected using a single concentration of an organic modifier in a mobile phase were very closely related to their lipophilicity. For example, for lipophilicity calculated using ACDLabs v. 8.0 software, the relationship between $\log P$ and R_M was linear ($R^2 = 0.92$, Figure 4).

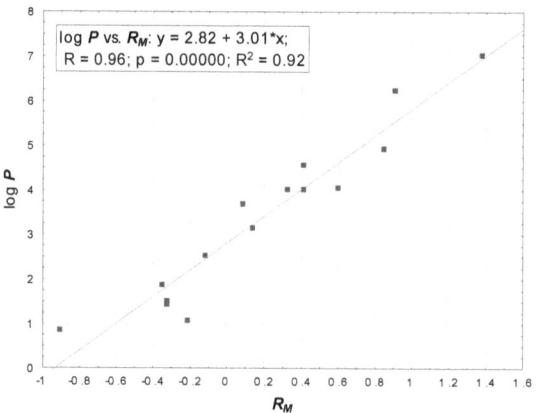

Figure 4. Correlation between calculated $\log P$ and R_M.

Based on $\log K_p$ reference values obtained by methods A to C, Equations (3)–(5) were developed for compounds **1** to **5** and **28** to **38**, whose RP-18 thin layer chromatographic retention data are available: (Figure 5)

$$\log K_p{}^{EPI} = -1.66\ (\pm 0.24) - 0.011\ (\pm 0.005)\ \textbf{PSA} + 0.24\ (\pm 0.05)\ \textbf{HD} - 0.0036\ (\pm 0.0017)\ \textbf{V}_M + 2.01\ (\pm 0.24)\ \textbf{R}_M$$
$$(n = 16, R^2 = 0.99, R^2{}_{adj} = 0.98, RMSECV = 0.21, F = 229.0, p < 0.01, s_e = 0.18) \tag{3}$$

$$\log K_p{}^{(1)} = 0.17\ (\pm 0.31) - 0.011\ (\pm 0.006)\ \textbf{PSA} - 0.14\ (\pm 0.06)\ \textbf{HD} - 0.0065\ (\pm 0.0022)\ \textbf{V}_M + 1.01\ (\pm 0.30)\ \textbf{R}_M$$
$$(n = 16, R^2 = 0.99, R^2{}_{adj.} = 0.78, RMSECV = 0.31, F = 174.8, p < 0.01, s_e = 0.22) \tag{4}$$

$$\log K_p{}^{pre} = -3.77\ (\pm 0.61) - 0.043\ (\pm 0.012)\ \textbf{PSA} + 0.18\ (\pm 0.13)\ \textbf{HD} + 0.011\ (\pm 0.004)\ \textbf{V}_M + 0.027\ (\pm 0.600)\ \textbf{R}_M$$
$$(n = 16, R^2 = 0.90, R^2{}_{adj.} = 0.86, RMSECV = 0.60, F = 23.6, p < 0.01, s_e = 0.45) \tag{5}$$

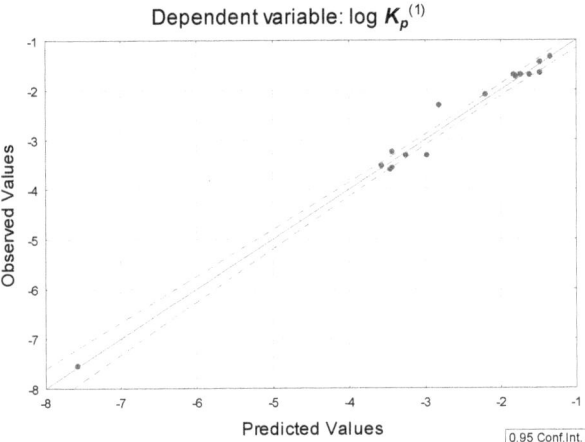

Figure 5. Equation (4) predicted vs. observed values.

The selection of independent variables in Equations (3)–(5) is a logical consequence of the influence on skin permeability of molecules of lipophilicity, polarity, molecular size and ability to form hydrogen bonds. For example, in Equation (3) the variables were selected by stepwise regression in the following order: R_M (which accounts for 89% of total variability), V_M, HD and PSA. Equations (3) to (5) were also tested on a subgroup of five compounds analyzed in this study whose chromatographic data and log K_p^{exp} values were available. The resulting dependences between the calculated and experimental log K_p values were linear, with $R^2 = 0.97$, 0.94 and 0.98, respectively. However, when eight additional, nonsteroid compounds (mainly drugs of low to medium lipophilicity, not particularly bulky molecules, with moderate ability to form H-bonds) **39** to **46** (ibuprofen, salicylic acid, indomethacin, naproxen, methylparaben, aspirin, piroxicam, and ranitidine) were incorporated in a test set, the correlations between the calculated and experimental log K_p values remained linear only for Equation (4), with $R^2 = 0.85$ (for Equation (3) and Equation (5) $R^2 = 0.53$ and 0.30, respectively).

The result obtained for Equation (4) (as compared to Equations (3) and (5)) confirms the versatility of Equation (4) which was tested on a set of compounds of different physicochemical properties. It is stressed here that the coefficients for PSA, HD and V_M in Equation (4) are negative (as opposite to Equations (3) and (5)) which (as already observed, e.g., by Lien and Gaot [48]) suggests that excessive hydrogen bonding, polar surface area and molecular size are obstacles to epidermal permeability.

Equation (4), efficient as it may be, seems somewhat over-parameterized. In search for a simpler, yet efficient model, Equations (6)–(10) were considered: (Figure 6)

$$\log K_p^{(1)} = 0.43 \ (\pm 0.30) - 0.17 \ (\pm 0.07) \ HD - 0.010 \ (\pm 0.001) \ V_M + 1.48 \ (\pm 0.17) \ R_M$$

$$(n = 16, R^2 = 0.98, R^2_{adj.} = 0.97, RMSECV = 0.42, F = 195.2, p < 0.01, s_e = 0.24) \qquad (6)$$

$$\log K_p^{(1)} = 0.20 \ (\pm 0.35) + 1.09 \ (\pm 0.34) \ R_M - 0.0063 \ (\pm 0.0025) \ V_M - 0.015 \ (\pm 0.007) \ PSA$$

$$(n = 16, R^2 = 0.98, R^2_{adj.} = 0.97, RMSECV = 0.41, F = 176.0, p < 0.01, s_e = 0.26) \qquad (7)$$

$$\log K_p^{(1)} = 0.58 \ (\pm 0.35) + 1.80 \ (\pm 0.14) \ R_M - 0.011 \ (\pm 0.001) \ V_M$$

$$(n = 16, R^2 = 0.97, R^2_{adj.} = 0.96, RMSECV = 0.31, F = 201.5, p < 0.01, s_e = 0.29) \qquad (8)$$

$$\log K_p^{(1)} = -0.14 \ (\pm 0.16) - 0.035 \ (\pm 0.002) \ PSA.$$

$$(n = 16, R^2 = 0.96, R^2_{adj.} = 0.96, RMSECV = 0.40, F = 327.3, p < 0.01, s_e = 0.32) \qquad (9)$$

$$\log K_p^{(1)} = 0.60 \ (\pm 0.78) - 0.61 \ (\pm 0.12) \ \mathit{HD} - 0.0079 \ (\pm 0.0026) \ V_M$$

$$(n = 16, \text{R}^2 = 0.85, \text{R}^2_{adj.} = 0.83, \text{RMSECV} = 0.69, \text{F} = 37.5, p < 0.01, s_e = 0.64) \qquad (10)$$

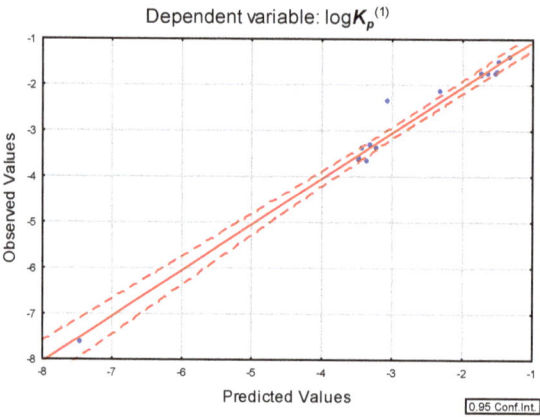

Figure 6. Equation (7) predicted vs. observed values.

Equations (6)–(10) were tested on a set of 13 compounds whose $\log K_p^{exp}$ values were available (compounds **1** to **5** and **39** to **46**), giving correlations of different quality ($\text{R}^2 = 0.75$, 0.83, 0.67, 0.79 and 0.74, respectively). Equation (7), which is a simplified version of Equation (4) (with one independent variable (**HD**) omitted), gave the best fit with experimental $\log K_p$ data. However, Equations (9) and (10), unlike other equations developed in this study, do not require access to compound samples, so they have the benefit of applicability, e.g., to new drugs at the design stage. Equation (9), which contains only one independent variable (**PSA**), is somewhat similar to the blood and brain barrier (BBB) permeability and human intestinal absorption (HIA) models developed by Clark [49,50], which strengthens the notion that physicochemical properties associated with good penetration of different biological barriers are interrelated.

Equations (9) and (10) were tested on a group of all compounds (steroids and nonsteroids) whose $\log K_p^{exp}$ values were available, including solutes that had not been used for validation of other equations because of the lack of chromatographic data. It was established that $\log K_p$ values calculated according to these equations ($\log K_p^{(9)}$ and $\log K_p^{(10)}$) were in moderate agreement with experimental data for a dataset containing 24 compounds (**1** to **16** and **39** to **46**) ($\text{R}^2 = 0.65$ and 0.62), but correlations were poorer for the group of hydrocortisone esters **17** to **27** studied by Anderson [40]. It was, therefore, concluded that Equations (9) and (10) should be used with caution for rapid, rough estimations of skin permeability of compounds before they are synthesized. In other situations, predictions based on more sophisticated models (e.g., Equations (1) or (7)) are recommended.

3. Materials and Methods

3.1. Chemicals

The 16 steroid drugs analyzed experimentally during these investigations (**1** to **16**: cortisol, hydrocortisone acetate, methyltestosterone, progesterone, testosterone propionate, testosterone heptanoate, cortisone acetate, prednisolone, estrone, estradiol benzoate, desoxycorticosterone acetate, tibolone, spironolactone, eplerenone, digoxin and dexamethasone) were donated as free samples by Polfa-Pabianice or isolated from pharmaceutical preparations. Nonsteroid compounds **39** to **46** (ibuprofen, salicylic acid, indomethacin, naproxen, methylparaben, aspirin, piroxicam, and ranitidine) were also donated as free samples by Polfa-Pabianice or isolated from pharmaceutical preparations. The purity of solutes isolated from pharmaceutical preparations was assessed by thin layer chromatography and densitometry. All isolated compounds gave single chromatographic spots (densitometric peaks) and were used without further purification. Compounds obtained from Polfa-Pabianice were of analytical or pharmacopeial grade. Distilled water used for chromatography was obtained from an in-house distillation apparatus. Analytical grade acetonitrile and methanol were obtained from Avantor Performance Materials (formerly Polskie Odczynniki Chemiczne, Gliwice, Poland). pH 7.4 phosphate buffered saline was obtained from Sigma-Aldrich.

3.2. Thin Layer Chromatography

Thin layer chromatography was performed according to [33] on 10×20 cm glass-backed RP-18 F_{254s} TLC plates from Merck, Germany (layer thickness 0.25 mm). Before use, the plates were prewashed with methanol-dichloromethane 1:1 (v/v) and dried overnight in ambient conditions. Solutions of compounds **1** to **16** in methanol (1 μg·μL^{-1}, spotting volume 1 μL), were spotted with a Hamilton microsyringe 15 mm from the plate bottom edge, starting 10 mm from the plate edge, at 8 mm intervals. The chromatographic plates were developed in a vertical chromatographic chamber lined with filter paper and previously saturated with the mobile phase vapor for 20 min. The mobile phase consisted of acetonitrile/pH 7.4 phosphate buffered saline 70:30 (v/v). The development distance was 95 mm from the plate bottom edge. After development, the plates were dried at room temperature and examined under UV light (254 nm) and with the Desaga CD60 densitometer (Multiwavelength Scan, 200–300 nm at 20 nm intervals). All chromatograms were repeated in duplicate, and the mean R_f values were used in further investigations. The chromatographic parameter R_M considered in these investigations was defined by Bate-Smith and Westall: $R_M = \log (1/R_{f-1})$ [51]. The chromatographic data are presented in Table 2.

3.3. Calculated Molecular Descriptors

The molecular descriptors for compounds investigated during this study (octanol water partition coefficient log P_{ow}; molecular weight M_W; distribution coefficient log$D$; polar surface area *PSA*; H-bond donors count *HD*; H-bond acceptors count *HA*; freely rotatable bonds count *FRB*; molar volume V_M; polarizability α; molar refractivity *R*) were calculated using ACD/Labs 8.0 software. Total oxygen and nitrogen atom count ($N + O$) was calculated from molecular formulae. The calculated molecular descriptors are given in Table 2. Statistical analysis was done using Statistica v.13 or StatistiXL v. 2. Equations (3)–(10) were tested using leave-one-out methodology.

Table 2. Physicochemical and chromatographic descriptors for compounds **1** to **46**.

		log P	M_W	PSA	FRB	HD	HA	R	V_M	α	$N+O$	log$D$	R_M
1	Dexamethasone	1.87	392.5	94.8	5	3	5	100.2	296.2	39.7	5	1.87	−0.35
2	Hydrocortisone (HC)	1.43	362.5	94.8	5	3	4	95.6	281.4	37.9	5	1.43	−0.33
3	Progesterone	4.04	314.5	34.1	1	0	2	91.0	289.0	36.6	2	4.04	0.60
4	Prednisolone	1.49	360.4	94.8	5	3	5	95.5	274.7	37.9	4	1.49	−0.33
5	Estrone	3.69	270.4	37.3	1	1	2	78.1	232.2	30.9	2	3.69	0.09
6	Aldosterone	0.46	360.4	83.8	4	2	5	93.7	272.1	37.1	5	0.46	
7	Corticosterone	1.76	346.5	74.6	4	2	4	94.0	284.3	37.3	4	1.76	
8	Pregnenolone	4.52	316.5	37.3	2	1	2	92.4	290.0	36.6	2	4.52	
9	17-α-Hydroxyprogesterone	2.89	330.5	54.4	2	1	3	92.6	286.1	36.7	3	2.89	
10	17-α-Hydroxypregnenolone	3.38	332.5	57.5	3	2	3	93.9	287.2	37.2	3	3.38	
11	Deoxycorticosterone	3.41	330.5	54.4	3	1	3	92.5	286.3	36.7	3	3.41	
12	Testosterone	3.48	288.4	37.3	1	1	2	83.1	257.0	33.0	2	3.48	
13	Cortexolone	1.74	346.5	74.6	2	4	2	94.1	283.4	37.3	4	2.74	
14	Estradiol	4.13	272.4	40.5	2	2	2	79.5	232.6	31.5	2	4.13	
15	Estriol	2.94	288.4	60.7	3	3	3	81.1	229.6	32.2	3	2.94	
16	Cortisone	1.44	360.4	91.7	4	2	5	94.2	280.3	37.3	5	1.44	
17	HC succinamate	1.45	461.6	144.0	9	4	8	118.2	351.8	46.8	8	1.45	
18	HC N,N-dimethylsuccinate	2.05	489.6	121.2	9	2	8	127.7	386.8	50.6	8	2.05	
19	HC methylsuccinate	2.53	476.6	127.2	10	2	8	120.9	370.4	47.9	8	2.53	
20	HC hemisuccinate	2.13	462.5	138.2	9	3	8	116.1	345.6	46.0	8	1.95	
21	HC pimelate	3.07	504.6	138.2	12	3	8	130.0	393.9	51.5	8	2.99	
22	HC pimelamate	2.61	531.7	121.2	12	2	8	141.6	435.0	56.1	8	2.61	
23	HC 6-hydroxyhexanoate	2.63	476.6	121.1	12	3	7	125.2	381.0	49.6	7	2.63	
24	HC propionate	3.05	418.5	100.9	7	2	6	109.8	335.4	43.5	6	3.04	
25	HC methylpimelate	3.53	518.6	127.2	13	2	8	134.8	418.7	53.4	8	3.53	
26	HC hexanoate	4.64	460.6	100.9	10	2	6	123.7	383.7	49.0	6	4.64	
27	HC octanoate	5.70	488.7	100.9	12	2	6	132.9	415.9	52.7	6	5.70	
28	Estradiol benzoate	6.24	376.5	46.53	4	1	3	109.3	317.6	43.3	3	6.24	0.91
29	HC acetate	2.51	404.5	100.9	6	2	6	105.2	319.3	41.7	6	2.51	−0.12
30	Deoxycortisone acetate	4.53	372.5	60.4	4	0	4	102.1	324.3	40.5	4	4.53	0.41
31	Cortisone acetate	2.53	402.5	97.7	5	1	6	103.8	318.2	41.1	6	2.53	−0.12
32	Testosterone propionate	4.90	344.5	43.4	3	0	3	97.3	311.2	38.6	3	4.90	0.85
33	Methyltestosterone	4.02	302.5	37.3	1	1	2	87.8	273.0	34.8	2	4.02	0.41
34	Testosterone enanthate	7.03	400.6	43.4	7	0	3	115.9	375.9	45.9	3	7.03	1.38
35	Spironolactone	3.12	416.6	85.7	2	0	4	112.7	335.8	44.7	4	3.12	0.14
36	Eplerenone	1.05	414.5	78.9	2	0	6	106.1	315.7	42.1	6	1.05	−0.21
37	Digoxin	0.85	780.9	203.1	13	6	14	196.4	572.3	77.9	14	0.85	−0.91
38	Tibolone	4.02	312.5	37.3	1	1	2	90.0	274.2	35.7	2	4.02	0.33
39	Ibuprofen			37.3		1			200.3				0.08
40	Ranitidine			111.6		2			265.5				−0.66
41	Aspirin			63.6		1			139.6				−0.50
42	Methylparaben			46.5		1			124.8				−0.41
43	Salicylic acid			57.5		2			100.4				−0.37
44	Indomethacin			69.6		1			269.6				−0.07
45	Piroxicam			108		2			212.0				0.00
46	Naproxen			46.5		1			192.3				−0.16

4. Conclusions

The skin permeability of steroids, as investigated in this study, is important because some of these compounds are, or could be used in preparations applied topically. Predicting skin permeability of steroids is a difficult task because steroid drugs have very different physicochemical properties and may cross the skin barrier by a variety of mechanisms [4]. Experimental skin permeability data exist only for a part of the studied group and they form three mutually incompatible steroid datasets [1,4], with experimental values given by Anderson et al. [40] distinctively higher than expected, as already reported by Abraham et al. [4]. Due to the limited availability of consistent experimental data for the studied solutes, the reference skin permeability coefficients log K_p were calculated using three methods: log $K_p{}^{\mathrm{EPI}}$ based on log P_{ow} and M_w as proposed by Potts and Guy [10]; Equation (1) developed earlier [36] and based on $(N + O)$, HD and log D; and by preADMET software [38]. It was established that Equation (1), proposed for structurally unrelated, nonsteroid drugs was also applicable to the group of studied steroids, as shown using a subset of compounds whose experimental log K_p data were available. It is also a useful tool to study the partition between the stratum corneum (especially the lipid domain) and water. However, the solutes from the so-called "Anderson dataset" [40] form a separate subgroup, parallel to the correlation line obtained for compounds studied by other authors [1,2] (Figures 1 and 2). Skin permeability models developed earlier (Equation (1) [36]) or in this study (Equations (4), (7), (9) and (10)) were found to predict log K_p of steroids fairly well (especially Equations (1) and (7)) and have the benefit of being based only on calculated descriptors (Equations (1), (9) and (10)). It was established that the applicability of equations proposed in this study ((7), (9) and (10)) extend beyond steroid compounds.

Author Contributions: Conceptualization, A.W.W.S.; methodology, A.W.W.S. and E.B.; investigation, A.W.W.S.; writing—original draft preparation, A.W.W.S. and J.R. All authors have read and agreed to the published version of the manuscript.

Funding: This research was supported by an internal grant of the Medical University of Łódź no. 503/3-016-03/503-31-001.

Institutional Review Board Statement: Not applicable.

Informed Consent Statement: Not applicable.

Data Availability Statement: The data presented in this study are available in this manuscript.

Conflicts of Interest: The authors declare no conflict of interest. The funders had no role in the design of the study; in the collection, analyses, or interpretation of data; in the writing of the manuscript, or in the decision to publish the results.

References

1. Johnson, M.E.; Blankschtein, D.; Langer, R. Permeation of steroids through human skin. *J. Pharm. Sci.* **1995**, *84*, 1144–1146. [CrossRef]
2. Scheuplein, R.J.; Blank, I.H.; Brauner, G.J.; MacFarlane, D.J. Percutaneous Absorption of Steroids. *J. Investig. Derm.* **1969**, *52*, 63–70. [CrossRef] [PubMed]
3. Lian, G.; Chen, L.; Han, L. An Evaluation of Mathematical Models for Predicting Skin Permeability. *J. Pharm. Sci.* **2008**, *97*, 584–598. [CrossRef]
4. Abraham, M.; Martins, F.; Mitchell, R.C. Algorithms for Skin Permeability Using Hydrogen Bond Descriptors: The Problem of Steroids. *J. Pharm. Pharmacol.* **1997**, *49*, 858–865. [CrossRef] [PubMed]
5. Todo, H. Transdermal Permeation of Drugs in Various Animal Species. *Pharmaceutics* **2017**, *9*, 33. [CrossRef] [PubMed]
6. Neupane, R.; Boddu, S.H.S.; Renukuntla, J.; Babu, R.J.; Tiwari, A.K. Alternatives to Biological Skin in Permeation Studies: Current Trends and Possibilities. *Pharmaceutics* **2020**, *12*, 152. [CrossRef]
7. El Tayar, N.; Tsai, R.-S.; Testa, B.; Carrupt, P.-A.; Hansch, C.; Leo, A. Percutaneous Penetration of Drugs: A Quantitative Structure–Permeability Relationship Study. *J. Pharm. Sci.* **1991**, *80*, 744–749. [CrossRef]
8. Anderson, B.D.; Raykar, P.V. Solute Structure-Permeability Relationships in Human Stratum Corneum. *J. Investig. Dermatol.* **1989**, *93*, 280–286. [CrossRef] [PubMed]
9. Barratt, M.D. Quantitative Structure-Activity Relationships for Skin Permeability. *Toxicol. Vitr.* **1995**, *9*, 27–37. [CrossRef]
10. Potts, R.O.; Guy, R.H. Predicting Skin Permeability. *Pharm. Res.* **1992**, *9*, 663–669. [CrossRef]
11. Chang, Y.-C.; Chen, C.-P.; Chen, C.-C. Predicting Skin Permeability of Chemical Substances Using a Quantitative Structure-Activity Relationship. *Procedia Eng.* **2012**, *45*, 875–879. [CrossRef]
12. Neely, B.J.; Madihally, S.V.; Robinson, R.L.; Gasem, K.A.M. Nonlinear Quantitative Structure-Property Relationship Modeling of Skin Permeation Coefficient. *J. Pharm. Sci.* **2009**, *98*, 4069–4084. [CrossRef] [PubMed]
13. Patel, H.; Ten Berge, W.; Cronin, M.T. Quantitative Structure–Activity Relationships (QSARs) for the Prediction of Skin Permeation of Exogenous Chemicals. *Chemosphere* **2002**, *48*, 603–613. [CrossRef]
14. Potts, R.O.; Guy, R.H. A Predictive Algorithm for Skin Permeability: The Effects of Molecular Size and Hydrogen Bond Activity. *Pharm. Res.* **1995**, *12*, 1628–1633. [CrossRef] [PubMed]

15. Alonso, C.; Carrer, V.; Espinosa, S.; Zanuy, M.; Córdoba, M.; Vidal, B.; Domínguez, M.; Godessart, N.; Coderch, L.; Pont, M. Prediction of the Skin Permeability of Topical Drugs Using in Silico and in Vitro Models. *Eur. J. Pharm. Sci.* **2019**, *136*, 104945. [CrossRef] [PubMed]
16. Fitzpatrick, D.; Corish, J.; Hayes, B. Modelling Skin Permeability in Risk Assessment—The Future. *Chemosphere* **2004**, *55*, 1309–1314. [CrossRef]
17. Geinoz, S.; Guy, R.H.; Testa, B.; Carrupt, P.-A. Quantitative Structure-Permeation Relationships (QSPeRs) to Predict Skin Permeation: A Critical Evaluation. *Pharm. Res.* **2004**, *21*, 83–92. [CrossRef]
18. Mitragotri, S.; Anissimov, Y.G.; Bunge, A.L.; Frasch, H.F.; Guy, R.H.; Hadgraft, J.; Kasting, G.B.; Lane, M.E.; Roberts, M.S. Mathematical Models of Skin Permeability: An Overview. *Int. J. Pharm.* **2011**, *418*, 115–129. [CrossRef]
19. Moss, G.P.; Dearden, J.C.; Patel, H.; Cronin, M.T.D. Quantitative Structure–Permeability Relationships (QSPRs) for Percutaneous Absorption. *Toxicol. Vitr.* **2002**, *16*, 299–317. [CrossRef]
20. Wilschut, A.; Ten Berge, W.F.; Robinson, P.J.; McKone, T.E. Estimating Skin Permeation. The Validation of Five Mathematical Skin Permeation Models. *Chemosphere* **1995**, *30*, 1275–1296. [CrossRef]
21. Jevric, L.R.; Podunavac Kuzmanovic, S.O.; Svarc Gajic, J.V.; Kovacevic, S.; Jovanovic, B.Z. RP-HPTLC Retention Datain Correlation with the In-Silico ADME Properties of a Series of s-Triazine Derivatives. *Iran. J. Pharm. Res.* **2014**, *13*, 1203–1211. [CrossRef]
22. Kovačević, S.; Jevrić, L.R.; Podunavac Kuzmanović, S.O.; Lončar, E.S. Prediction of In Silico ADME Properties of 1,2-O-Isopropylidene Aldohexose Derivatives. *Iran. J. Pharm. Res.* **2014**, *13*, 899–907. [CrossRef]
23. Barbato, F.; Cappello, B.; Miro, A.; La Rotonda, M.; Quaglia, F. Chromatographic Indexes on Immobilized Artificial Membranes for the Prediction of Transdermal Transport of Drugs. *Il Farmaco* **1998**, *53*, 655–661. [CrossRef]
24. Hidalgo-Rodríguez, M.; Soriano-Meseguer, S.; Fuguet, E.; Ràfols, C.; Rosés, M. Evaluation of the Suitability of Chromatographic Systems to Predict Human Skin Permeation of Neutral Compounds. *Eur. J. Pharm. Sci.* **2013**, *50*, 557–568. [CrossRef]
25. Lazaro, E.; Rafols, C.; Abraham, M.H.; Rosés, M. Chromatographic Estimation of Drug Disposition Properties by Means of Immobilized Artificial Membranes (IAM) and C18 Columns. *J. Med. Chem.* **2006**, *49*, 4861–4870. [CrossRef]
26. Nasal, A.; Sznitowska, M.; Buciński, A.; Kaliszan, R. Hydrophobicity Parameter from High-Performance Liquid Chromatography on an Immobilized Artificial Membrane Column and Its Relationship to Bioactivity. *J. Chromatogr. A* **1995**, *692*, 83–89. [CrossRef]
27. Turowski, M.; Kaliszan, R. Keratin Immobilized on Silica as a New Stationary Phase for Chromatographic Modelling of SkinPermeation. *J. Pharm. Biomed. Anal.* **1997**, *15*, 1325–1333. [CrossRef]
28. Waters, L.J.; Shahzad, Y.; Stephenson, J. Modelling Skin Permeability with Micellar Liquid Chromatography. *Eur. J. Pharm. Sci.* **2013**, *50*, 335–340. [CrossRef] [PubMed]
29. Martínez-Pla, J.J.; Martín-Biosca, Y.; Sagrado, S.; Villanueva-Camañas, R.M.; Medina-Hernández, M.J. Evaluation of the PH Effect of Formulations on the Skin Permeability of Drugs by Biopartitioning Micellar Chromatography. *J. Chromatogr. A* **2004**, *1047*, 255–262. [CrossRef]
30. Martínez-Pla, J.J.; Martín-Biosca, Y.; Sagrado, S.; Villanueva-Camañas, R.M.; Medina-Hernández, M.J. Biopartitioning Micellar Chromatography to Predict SkinPermeability. *Biomed. Chromatogr.* **2003**, *17*, 530–537. [CrossRef] [PubMed]
31. Ramadon, D.; McCrudden, M.T.C.; Courtenay, A.J.; Donnelly, R.F. Enhancement Strategies for Transdermal Drug DeliverySystems: Current Trends and Applications. *Drug Deliv. Transl. Res.* **2021**. [CrossRef]
32. Akhtar, N.; Singh, V.; Yusuf, M.; Khan, R.A. Non-Invasive Drug Delivery Technology: Development and Current Status of Transdermal Drug Delivery Devices, Techniques and Biomedical Applications. *Biomed. Eng. Biomed. Tech.* **2020**, *65*, 243–272. [CrossRef] [PubMed]
33. Sobańska, A.W.; Wanat, K.; Brzezińska, E. Prediction of the Blood-Brain Barrier Permeability Using RP-18 Thin Layer Chromatography. *Open Chem.* **2019**, *17*, 43–56. [CrossRef]
34. Pyzowski, J.; Brzezińska, E.; Sobańska, A.W. RP-18 Chromatographic-Based Study of the Blood—Brain Barrier Permeability of Selected Sunscreens and Preservatives. *JPC J. Planar Chromatogr. Mod. TLC* **2017**, *30*, 275–284. [CrossRef]
35. Sobańska, A.W.; Brzezińska, E. Application of RP-18 Thin-Layer Chromatography and Quantitative Structure–Activity Relationship Analysis for the Prediction of the Blood–Brain Barrier Permeation. *JPC J. Planar Chromatogr. Mod. TLC* **2016**, *29*, 287–298. [CrossRef]
36. Sobańska, A.W.; Robertson, J.; Brzezińska, E. Application of RP-18 TLC Retention Data to the Prediction of the Transdermal Absorption of Drugs. *Pharmaceuticals* **2021**, *14*, 147. [CrossRef] [PubMed]
37. Sobańska, A.W.; Hekner, A.; Brzezińska, E. RP-18 HPLC analysis of drugs' ability to cross the blood-brain barrier. *J. Chem.* **2019**, *2019*, e5795402. [CrossRef]
38. PreADMET, 209, Veritas A Hall, Yonsei University 85 Songdogwahak-ro, Yeonsu-gu, Incheon 21983, Republic of Korea. Available online: https://preadmet.bmdrc.kr/adme/ (accessed on 22 June 2021).
39. Klimová, Z.; Hojerová, J.; Pažoureková, S. Current Problems in the Use of Organic UV Filters to Protect Skin from Excessive Sun Exposure. *Acta Chim. Slovaca* **2013**, *6*, 82–88. [CrossRef]
40. Anderson, B.D.; Higuchi, W.I.; Raykar, P.V. Heterogeneity Effects on Permeability–Partition Coefficient Relationships in Human Stratum Corneum. *Pharm. Res.* **1988**, *5*, 566–573. [CrossRef]
41. Wang, L.; Chen, L.; Lian, G.; Han, L. Determination of Partition and Binding Properties of Solutes to Stratum Corneum. *Int. J. Pharm.* **2010**, *398*, 114–122. [CrossRef]

42. Johnson, M.E.; Blankschtein, D.; Langer, R. Evaluation of Solute Permeation through the Stratum Corneum: Lateral Bilayer Diffusion as the Primary Transport Mechanism. *J. Pharm. Sci.* **1997**, *86*, 1162–1172. [CrossRef] [PubMed]

43. Fu, X.C.; Wang, G.P.; Wang, Y.F.; Liang, W.Q.; Yu, Q.S.; Chow, M.S.S. Limitation of Potts and Guy's Model and a Predictive Algorithm for Skin Permeability Including the Effects of Hydrogen-Bondon Diffusivity. *Pharmazie* **2004**, *59*, 282–285. [PubMed]

44. Abraham, M.H.; Chadha, H.S.; Mitchell, R.C. The Factors That Influence Skin Penetration of Solutes. *J. Pharm. Pharmacol.* **1995**, *47*, 8–16. [CrossRef]

45. Ciura, K.; Nowakowska, J.; Pikul, P.; Struck-Lewicka, W.; Markuszewski, M.J. A Comparative Quantitative Structure-Retention Relationships Study for Lipophilicity Determination of Compounds with a Phenanthrene Skeletonon Cyano-, Reversed Phase-, and Normal Phase-Thin Layer Chromatography Stationary Phases. *J. AOAC Int.* **2015**, *98*, 345–353. [CrossRef]

46. Karadžić, M.Ž.; Jevrić, L.R.; Mandić, A.I.; Markov, S.L.; Podunavac-Kuzmanović, S.O.; Kovačević, S.Z.; Nikolić, A.R.; Oklješa, A.M.; Sakač, M.N.; Penov-Gaši, K.M. Chemometrics Approach Based on Chromatographic Behavior, in Silico Characterization and Molecular Docking Study of Steroid Analogs with Biomedical Importance. *Eur. J. Pharm. Sci.* **2017**, *105*, 71–81. [CrossRef]

47. Soczewiński, E.; Wachtmeister, C.A. The Relation between the Composition of Certain Ternary Two-Phase Solvent Systems and RM Values. *J. Chromatogr. A* **1962**, *7*, 311–320. [CrossRef]

48. Lien, E.J.; Gaot, H. QSAR Analysis of Skin Permeability of Various Drugs in Manas Compared to in Vivo and in Vitro Studies in Rodents. *Pharm. Res.* **1995**, *12*, 583–587. [CrossRef]

49. Clark, D.E. Rapid Calculation of Polar Molecular Surface Area and Its Application to the Prediction of Transport Phenomena. 1. Prediction of Intestinal Absorption. *J. Pharm. Sci.* **1999**, *88*, 807–814. [CrossRef]

50. Clark, D.E. Rapid Calculation of Polar Molecular Surface Area and Its Application to the Prediction of Transport Phenomena. 2. Prediction of Blood–Brain Barrier Penetration. *J. Pharm. Sci.* **1999**, *88*, 815–821. [CrossRef] [PubMed]

51. Bate-Smith, E.C.; Westall, R.G. Chromatographic Behaviour and Chemical Structure, I. Some Naturally Occuring PhenolicSubstances. *Biochim. Biophys. Acta* **1950**, *4*, 427–440. [CrossRef]

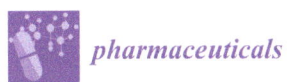 *pharmaceuticals*

Article

Capillary Liquid Chromatography for the Determination of Terpenes in Botanical Dietary Supplements

Henry Daniel Ponce-Rodríguez [1,2] , Jorge Verdú-Andrés [1] , Pilar Campíns-Falcó [1] and Rosa Herráez-Hernández [1,*]

[1] MINTOTA Research Group, Departament de Química Analítica, Facultat de Química, Universitat de València, Dr. Moliner 50, 46100 Burjassot, València, Spain; Henrypon@alumni.uv.es (H.D.P.-R.); Jorge.Verdu@uv.es (J.V.-A.); pilar.campins@uv.es (P.C.-F.)

[2] Departamento de Control Químico, Facultad de Química y Farmacia, Universidad Nacional Autónoma de Honduras, Ciudad Universitaria, Tegucigalpa 11101, Honduras

[*] Correspondence: rosa.herraez@uv.es; Tel.: +34-96-3544978

Abstract: Dietary supplements of botanical origin are increasingly consumed due to their content of plant constituents with potential benefits on health and wellness. Among those constituents, terpenes are gaining attention because of their diverse biological activities (anti-inflammatory, antibacterial, geroprotective, and others). While most of the existing analytical methods have focused on establishing the terpenic fingerprint of some plants, typically by gas chromatography, methods capable of quantifying representative terpenes in herbal preparations and dietary supplements with combined high sensitivity and precision, simplicity, and high throughput are still necessary. In this study, we have explored the utility of capillary liquid chromatography (CapLC) with diode array detection (DAD) for the determination of different terpenes, namely limonene, linalool, farnesene, α-pinene, and myrcene. An innovative method is proposed that can be applied to quantify the targets at concentration levels as low as 0.006 mg per gram of sample with satisfactory precision, and a total analysis time <30 min per sample. The reliability of the proposed method has been tested by analyzing different dietary supplements of botanical origin, namely three green coffee extract-based products, two fat burnings containing *Citrus aurantium* (bitter orange), and an herbal preparation containing lime and leaves of orange trees.

Keywords: natural products; plant materials; dietary supplements; terpenes; capillary liquid chromatography

Citation: Ponce-Rodríguez, H.D.; Verdú-Andrés, J.; Campíns-Falcó, P.; Herráez-Hernández, R. Capillary Liquid Chromatography for the Determination of Terpenes in Botanical Dietary Supplements. *Pharmaceuticals* **2021**, *14*, 580. https://doi.org/10.3390/ph14060580

Academic Editors: Jan Oszmianski and Sabina Lachowicz

Received: 2 June 2021
Accepted: 16 June 2021
Published: 17 June 2021

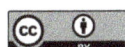
1. Introduction

Today, a wide variety of products are available intended to supplement the diet with the idea of promoting health and wellness. Dietary supplements are considered products at the interface between pharma and nutrition [1,2]. However, the regulations established for their preparation and distribution are not as strict as those set for pharmaceuticals [3]. Of particular concern are preparations that contain mixtures of plants, either in the whole form or as extracts, because they are perceived as safe for consumers due to their natural origin. Unlike homogeneous pharmaceuticals, supplements elaborated with similar ingredients may contain highly variable amounts of active compounds, depending on the plant sources and processes used during their production [4]. For these reasons, increasing attention is being paid to control the quality and efficacy of botanic dietary supplements through the analysis of their bioactive components [3,5]. In addition, adulteration and counterfeiting (such as the use of prohibited additives and incorrect botanical or geographical declaration) are frauds commonly detected in dietary supplements. Therefore, adequate analytical methods are required to detect such manipulations [6].

Plants are sources of several functional compounds, such as phenols, alkaloids, steroids, terpenes, and others. In particular, terpenes have been reported to exhibit diverse beneficial effects including anti-inflammatory, antimicrobial, anticarcinogenic or anti-aging [7–9]. Because of such properties, the levels of terpenes are gaining importance for assessing the biological activity of a variety of medicinal plants and dietary supplements [4,10]. Terpenoids are the main constituents of essential oils, and due to their volatility, they are responsible for the aroma. Some representative terpenes, such as linalool, have been proposed as biomarkers to detect adulterations and to control the safety of marketed products [11]. Due to its antimicrobial activity, limonene has been proposed as an ecological preservative in some food products [12].

Gas chromatography (GC) has been extensively used for the analysis of volatile terpenes in plants. The studies reported during the past years were mainly focused on establishing the terpenes profile of different vegetal species and fruit beverages [13–19]. Only a few works dealt with the determination of terpenes in products aimed at enhancing health. This is the case of the study reported by Mukazayire et al., who described a method for the characterization of essential oils in medicinal plants with notable antioxidant activity [20]; the investigation included some terpenic compounds. As most of those studies were aimed at establishing the volatile profile of the tested plants, GC with mass spectrometry (MS), or GC × GC-MS, often in combination with multivariate data treatment, were the analytical techniques used. Liquid chromatography (LC), on the other hand, is the predominant technique in the analysis of plants used as food and medicines, although its application to the analysis of terpenes is rare [10]. This can be explained by the fact that terpenes are volatile and thus, well suited for GC, and also because of the lack of chromophores in their structure, which can be a serious limitation considering that the levels of terpenes in this kind of samples are usually low (<1%) [4].

Recent progress in LC has resulted in miniaturized scale separations, such as capillary LC (CapLC) with enhanced resolution and sensitivity derived from the fact that the dispersion of the analytes during the separation is considerably reduced [21]. Miniaturized LC offers additional advantages such as lower consumption of mobile and stationary phases, and a reduction in the generation of wastes [22]. However, in the analysis of dietary supplements, CapLC has only been applied to a few compounds so far, mainly amino acids and peptides, fatty acids, and flavonoids [23]. Therefore, the potential of CapLC for the analysis of terpenes in dietary supplements remains unexplored. In a recent study, we demonstrated that CapLC is a valuable tool for estimating the content of terpenes of resins obtained from different trees. Because of the high sensitivity attained, the method could be applied to the analysis of limonene, amyrin, lupeol, and lupenone in microsamples of resins [24].

Taking advantage of its high sensitivity, in the present study we report for the first time the application of CapLC to the quantification of representative terpenes in dietary supplements. The target compounds selected were limonene, linalool, farnesene, α-pinene, and myrcene. The chemical structure and main biological effects of these compounds according to the literature are shown in Table 1. The analytes were previously extracted from the samples in methanol using an ultrasound-assisted extraction (UAE) protocol. The proposed approach has been applied to the analysis of different commercial products containing botanical species as main ingredients with a variety of claimed properties (stimulant, fat-burning, and relaxant).

Table 1. Chemical structure and main effects of the tested compounds.

Compound	Structure	Activity
Linalool		- Sedative [25] - Anti-inflammatory [8]
Myrcene		- Sedative [25] - Anti-inflammatory [8] - Geroprotective [9]
Limonene		- Anti-inflammatory [8] - Antimutagenic [8] - Cardioprotective [9] - Antibacterial [9,12,13] - Geroprotective [9]
α-Pinene		- Anti-inflammatory [8] - Antimutagenic [8] - Geroprotective [9] - Antibacterial [13]
Farnesene		- Anti-inflammatory [8] - Antimutagenic [26]

2. Results

2.1. Separation and Analytical Performance

Different chromatographic conditions were assayed to achieve a satisfactory resolution of the analytes from other plant constituents. As it can be deduced from Table 1, the target analytes do not have polar groups (e.g., -OH or -NH$_2$) in their chemical structure. As a result, they are quite hydrophobic substances; the log of their octanol-water partition coefficients ranges from 2.97 (linalool) to 7.10 (farnesene) [27]. Thus, they were expected to elute at high retention times under reversed-phase separation conditions. With this in mind, different experiments were carried out with standard solutions of the analytes and with methanolic extracts of the samples tested in order to select a gradient elution program adequate for the separation of the analytes from other plant constituents with polar groups (polyphenols, amines). Most matrix compounds were found in the first part of the chromatograms under the conditions selected (Section 4.2) whereas the analytes eluted in the 15–20 min time window, and they were satisfactorily resolved, as can be seen in Figure 1. In this figure are depicted the chromatograms obtained at 200 nm and 220 nm for a mixture of the tested terpenes (5 µg mL^{-1} each compound). Although myrcene exhibited higher absorptivity at 220 nm, the peak areas were higher for most compounds at 200 nm (detector saturation was observed for linalool at 200 nm). Therefore, 200 nm was selected as the working wavelength. The retention times are listed in Table 2.

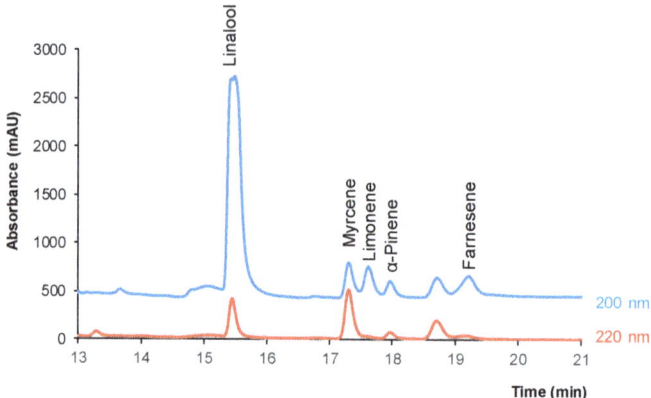

Figure 1. Chromatograms obtained under the selected conditions at 200 nm and 220 nm for a standard solution of the tested compounds (5 µg mL^{-1} each). For other experimental details, see text.

Table 2. Times of retention (t_r) and analytical parameters obtained with the proposed method.

Compound	t_r (min)	Concentration Interval (µg mL^{-1})	Linearity, n = 10 /R^2	LOD [1] (µg mL^{-1})	LOQ [2] (µg mL^{-1})	RSD [3], n = 3 (%)
Linalool	15.5	0.02–1.0	y = (20,200 ± 200) x + (67 ± 90) /0.999	0.005	0.02	11
Myrcene	17.3	0.05–2.5	y = (530 ± 20) x +(−20 ± 20) /0.992	0.01	0.04	2
Limonene	17.6	1.0–10.0	y = (920 ± 40) x +(−600 ± 300) /0.993	0.25	1.0	3
α-Pinene	18.0	1.0–10.0	y = (166 ± 6) x +(−60 ± 30) /0.993	0.25	1.0	11
Farnesene	19.3	1.0–5.0	y = (900 ± 40) x +(−200 ± 100) /0.991	0.25	1.0	11

[1] LOD—limit of detection; [2] LOQ—limit of quantification; [3] established at a concentration of 1 µg mL^{-1}.

Next, the analytical performance was evaluated by processing standard solutions of the analytes. The working concentration ranges were selected in order to obtain peak areas of about the same order for all the analytes at the working wavelength (200 nm). The results of this study are summarized in Table 2.

The linearity was evaluated for each compound by processing in duplicate five concentrations within the tested concentration range. Satisfactory linearity was observed in all instances. The limits of detection (LODs) and limits of quantification (LOQs) were established as the concentrations of analyte that resulted in signal-to-noise ratios of 3 and 10, respectively. These values were obtained by processing solutions with decreasing concentrations of the analytes; before analyzing each solution, water was processed to confirm the absence of contaminants and/or memory effects. The LODs ranged from 0.005 to 0.25 µg mL^{-1}, whereas the LOQs were in the 0.02–1.0 µg mL^{-1} interval. Finally, the precision was established through the successive injection of three replicates of standard solutions of the analytes. The relative standard deviations (RSDs) obtained were in the 2–11% range.

2.2. Sample Treatment

For sample treatment UAE was applied, using methanol as the extractive solvent. Portions of 25 mg of the homogenized samples were placed in glass vials. Then, 5 mL of methanol were added to the vials, and the resulting suspensions were first vortexed, and then placed in an ultrasonic bath for 5 min. The supernatant was separated from the solid residue and filtered. Finally, a portion of the extract was treated with 0.1% hydrochloric and injected into the chromatograph. No significant peaks were observed in the chromatograms obtained when the solid residues were further treated with a second 5-mL portion of methanol and subjected to the same extraction protocol.

The recoveries obtained under the proposed treatment were calculated by spiking a sample with known amounts of the analytes. The amount of each compound added to the sample was 0.25 μg g^{-1}. In this study sample GCE-3 was used because according to the label, it contained a greater number of ingredients. The recoveries were calculated by comparing the increments of the peak areas for the analytes in the spiked samples with those obtained for standard solutions containing an equivalent concentration of each compound. The values obtained are listed in Table 3. As observed, the recoveries ranged from 95% to 106%.

Table 3. Recovery and precision obtained in spiked green coffee. Values calculated for a spiked amount of the analytes of 0.25 mg g^{-1}.

Compound	Mean Recovery (%)	Precision, RDS (%)	
		Intra-Day (n = 3)	Inter-Day (n = 6)
Linalool	96 ± 5	5	4
Myrcene	106 ± 3	3	10
Limonene	95 ± 10	11	13
α-Pinene	98 ± 9	10	13
Farnesene	105 ± 7	7	6

In order to study the intra-day precision of the entire procedure, three portions of the samples were spiked with the analytes and processed consecutively; the inter-day precision was obtained from six replicates of the spiked samples processed on different days. The results are listed in Table 3. This table shows that the RSD values were of about the same order as those found for standard solutions of the analytes (Table 2).

2.3. Quantification of Terpenes in Dietary Supplements

The proposed method was applied to the analysis of different dietary supplements, namely three green coffee extracts-based products claimed to enhance physical performance, two fat burning products for losing weight, and herbal preparation (relaxant). Portions of 25 mg of the samples were treated with 5 mL of methanol as described above, and then the extracts were chromatographed. The presence of a compound in a sample was established from the concordance between the retention times and spectra of the suspected peak and those of a standard solution, and it was further confirmed by spiking the extract with such a compound. This is illustrated in Figure 2a for the peak identified as linalool in the chromatogram corresponding to the extract obtained for sample FB-1. This figure shows the chromatograms of the extract obtained for the sample and the same extract spiked with 1 μg mL^{-1} of linalool; this figure also shows the chromatogram obtained for a standard solution of linalool. The normalized spectra registered for linalool in the standard solution and the peak attributed to linalool in the sample are shown in Figure 2b. A good correlation between the two normalized spectra can be observed. The chromatogram obtained for sample FB-2 is depicted in Figure 2c.

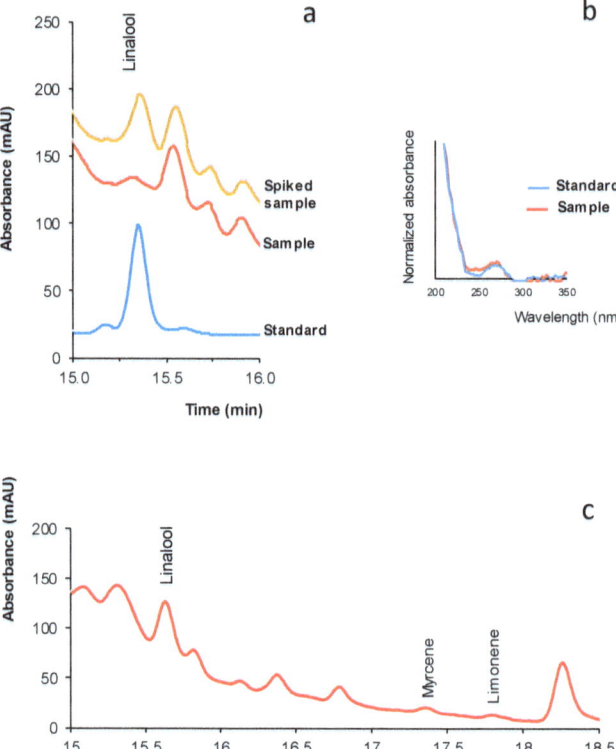

Figure 2. (**a**) Chromatograms obtained for a standard solution of linalool (5 μg mL^{-1}), for the extract of sample FB-1, and the same extract spiked with linalool (1 μg mL^{-1}). (**b**) normalized spectra of linalool and the peak attributed to linalool in the chromatogram of sample FB-1. (**c**) Chromatogram of the extract obtained for sample FB-2. For other experimental details, see text.

As an illustrative example of the signals of compounds present at very different concentrations, in Figure 3 are shown the peaks of the analytes found in sample HP for limonene, which corresponded to the highest concentration found for this compound throughout the study, and for farnesene and myrcene, both compounds present at the lowest concentrations in the sample.

For the quantitative study, the methanolic extracts obtained for each sample were chromatographed and the peak areas of the compounds found were calculated; if required, the extracts were previously diluted with water to adjust the peak areas of the analytes to their respective working linear intervals. The concentrations in the extracts were established from the calibration equations of Table 2, and then transformed into amounts of analyte in the samples taking into account the dilution factors (if applicable) and the recovery values of Table 3. The results obtained for all the samples tested are listed in Table 4.

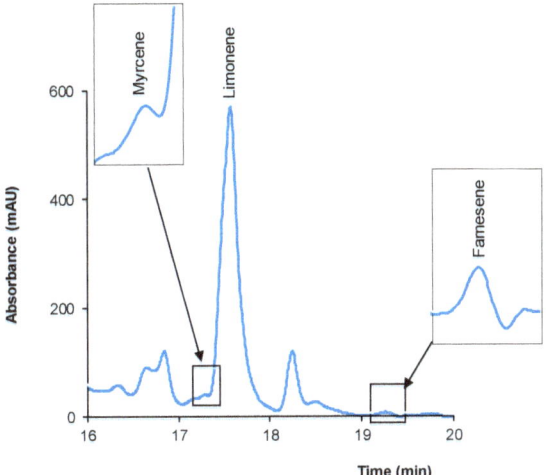

Figure 3. Peaks of limonene, myrcene, and farnesene in the chromatogram obtained for sample HP. For other experimental details, see text.

Table 4. Results obtained for the dietary supplements analyzed (n = 3).

Sample	Found Compounds	Found Amounts [1]	
		mg per unit (n = 3)	mg per g (n = 6)
GCE-1	Limonene	0.350 ± 0.004	0.318 ± 0.003
	Myrcene	0.059 ± 0.003	0.054 ± 0.003
GCE-2	-	-	-
GCE-3	Limonene	0.84 ± 0.01	1.68 ± 0.01
	Myrcene	1.3 ± 0.2	2.6 ± 0.3
FB-1	Limonene	0.129 ± 0.001	0.258 ± 0.002
	Linalool	0.0031 ± 0.0001	0.006 ± 0.001
	Myrcene	0.0200 ± 0.001	0.039 ± 0.003
FB-2	Limonene	0.130 ± 0.002	0.520 ± 0.005
	Linalool	0.003 ± 0.001	0.012 ± 0.001
	Myrcene	0.0030 ± 0.0005	0.012 ± 0.001
HP	Limonene	2.60 ± 0.05	1.90 ± 0.04
	Linalool	<LOQ	<LOQ
	Myrcene	0.150 ± 0.001	0.110 ± 0.001
	Farnesene	0.100 ± 0.003	0.070 ± 0.002

[1] Values expressed with digits known plus the first uncertain digit.

The results of Table 4 indicate that all samples tested contained limonene and myrcene, except sample GCE-2. Linalool was found in the fat burning and relaxant preparations, although in the later sample its concentration was below its LOQ. α-Pinene was not detected in any of the samples assayed.

As it can be deduced from the results of Table 4, most compounds were present in the samples at sub mg per gram of product levels. Relatively high amounts of limonene were found in some of the samples; a high content of myrcene was found in sample GCE-3. In contrast, none of the tested compounds was found in sample GCE-2. Considering the rest of the samples, the lowest content of terpenes corresponded to sample FB-1, which contained a total amount of 0.136 mg of the tested compounds per unit. The highest value was found in sample HP, with 2.85 mg of the terpenes tested per unit. Expressed in relative terms, the highest amount of terpenes was observed in sample GCE-3, with a total amount of 4.28 mg per g of sample (0.482%). A high value was also found in sample HP (2.1 mg per g of product), whereas for the rest of the samples, the total amount of terpenes was 0.3–0.5 mg per g of sample.

3. Discussion

Several studies have been carried out to establish the content of relevant terpenes in different vegetal species and beverages for a better characterization of their flavor characteristics and/or to assess their biological activity [12–14,18]. What all those studies have in common is that GC is the technique used for the analysis of the samples. However, since LC is the dominant technique in laboratories dealing with the phytochemical analysis of medicinal plants and dietary supplements, it would be useful to have analytical alternatives based on LC [10].

In the present study, we have explored the potential of CapLC as an alternative to GC for the analysis of terpenic compounds in dietary supplements of botanical origin. Figure 4 summarizes the main conclusions of this study, expressed in terms of the advantages and drawbacks of the proposed approach.

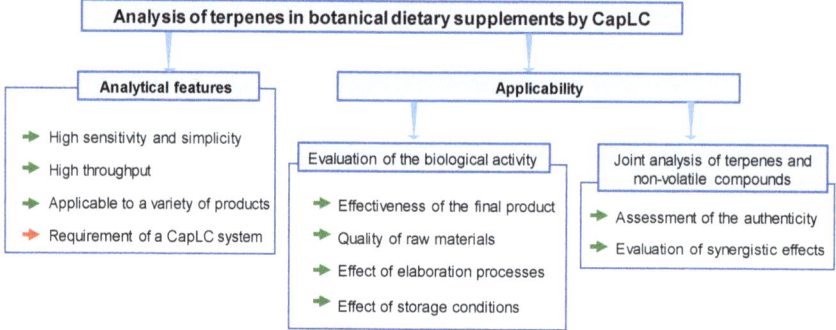

Figure 4. Analytical features and applicability of the method developed for the analysis of terpenes in botanical dietary supplements by CapLC; strengths in green; weaknesses in red.

First, from an analytical point of view, the proposed CapLC method allowed the quantification of the target compounds, even at sub mg per g levels, with suitable precision. The analytes were satisfactorily extracted from the samples by a simple UAE procedure. The high sensitivity and selectivity reached made unnecessary any preconcentration of purification steps; as a result, the whole analysis could be carried out in less than 30 min per sample. The selectivity was suitable so that the method could be applied to a variety of products that contained different botanical species as main ingredients. The requirement of a CapLC system is a limitation, although these kinds of systems are increasingly used in laboratories aimed at analyzing medicinal plants and dietary supplements. Moreover, unlike previous methods proposed for the analysis of terpenes in vegetal stuff, which in most instances involve MS detection, a simple UV detector is required.

As stated earlier, GC has been widely applied to the analysis of terpenes in plants and products elaborated from plants. However, in many cases, the real concentrations of the target compounds in the samples were not reported because the quantitative results were given as percentages of peak areas [15,17,19,20]. Kupska, et al. developed the GC x GC method with time-of-flight-MS detection to establish the terpenic profile of blue honeysuckle berries [13]. The volatile terpenes were previously isolated and concentrated by head-space solid-phase microextraction (HS-PSME). The concentrations measured in the sample extracts were lower than those measured in the present study. The concentrations of some terpenes, including linalool, in grapes, were measured by GC-MS in two studies. The target analytes were first extracted into a buffer, and then preconcentrated and purified by solid-phase extraction [14] or by HS-SPME [16]. Although the analytical performance of such methods was not reported, the concentrations of linalool measured were about the same order as those found in the present study (Table 4). Concentrations < 1 μg mL^{-1} of linalool were measured by He et al. in tea extracts by HS-SPME and GC-MS [18]. Compared with the proposed approach, the above results indicate that the concentrations of terpenes that can be measured by GC-MS are comparable or somewhat lower, although this can be partially attributed to the preconcentration achieved with the SPE or SPME treatments. The main advantages of the proposed CapLC method over GC-based assays are simplicity and speed.

As regards the utility, the proposed CapLC approach has been successfully used to establish the individual concentrations of representative terpenes in the methanolic extracts obtained from the samples assayed. Thus, the method can be applied to investigate the biological activity due to specific terpenes such as those included in the present study. It can be also used to compare the biological activities of different products through the calculation of the total amount of the selected terpenes. For example, from the results of Table 4, it can be deduced that the potential effects on health due to the presence of the selected terpenes in the products marketed as fat burnings are relatively low compared with the effects that can be expected for the other two types of products tested. Similar conclusions can be derived by comparing the contents of terpenes in products belonging to the same category. For example, the content of terpenes in sample GCE-3 was clearly superior to the amounts present in the other two products that contained green coffee extracts as the main ingredient; consequently, higher biological activity due to terpenes can be expected after the consumption of this product.

It must be remarked that none of the tested terpenes was found in sample GCE-2. The main ingredient of this product was decaffeinated green coffee extract, which suggests that the analytes were most probably lost during the industrial decaffeination process [28]. In contrast, sample HP contained four of the five terpenes included in the study, and a high amount of limonene; this is consistent with the fact that the manipulation of the ingredients involved in its production was clearly lower than that required to produce the other dietary supplements. Therefore, the proposed CapLC approach could be applied to evaluate the effect of the elaboration processes on the biological activity of the final products. It could be also used to estimate the sensory characteristics and the freshness of a product by determining the amounts of most volatile terpenes that remained in the sample after a period of storage.

Although in the present study the only compounds tested were terpenes, it has to be remarked that CapLC is a versatile technique that can be applied to the simultaneous determination of both volatile and non-volatile plant constituents. Thus, compounds with different physicochemical characteristics could be used as biomarkers to investigate the authenticity and safety of a given product in a single chromatographic run [11]. The technique could be also used to study possible synergistic effects on human health, which in many instances are not yet fully understood [6].

To summarize, CapLC is a versatile and useful tool that can be used to estimate the biological activity due to individual terpenes or a group of representative terpenes in dietary supplements elaborated from plant materials. The proposed method can be used as a reliable and versatile alternative to GC, and it can be easily implemented in laboratories dealing with the analysis of medicinal plants and dietary supplements, more familiarized with LC. The methodology used here offers advantages in terms of analytical performance and applicability, as can be deduced from Figure 4. The only limitation is the requirement of a CapLC system, although this may no longer be a problem considering that miniaturized techniques are increasingly used in laboratories devoted to the analysis of dietary supplements [23].

4. Materials and Methods

4.1. Chemicals and Solutions

All reagents used throughout the study were of analytical grade. Limonene, α-pinene, farnesene, myrcene, and linalool were obtained from Sigma-Aldrich (St. Louis, MO, USA). Hydrochloric acid (37%) was supplied by Scharlau (Barcelona, Spain). Methanol and acetonitrile (both HPLC grade) were purchased from VWR Chemicals (Randnor, PA, USA). Stock solutions of the analytes (1000 μg mL^{-1}) were prepared by dissolving the appropriate amounts of the commercial standards in methanol. Working solutions of the analytes and their mixtures were prepared by diluting the stock solutions with water.

Ultrapure water was obtained from an Adrona system (Adrona, Riga, Latvia). Water was filtered through 0.22 μm nylon membranes purchased from GVS (Sandford, ME, USA) before use. All solutions were stored at 4 °C until use.

4.2. Chromatographic Conditions

The chromatographic system consisted of a capillary pump (Agilent 1100 Series, Waldbronn, Germany) equipped with a Rheodyne model 7725 six-port injection valve and a photodiode array detector (Agilent 1200 Series). An Agilent HPLC ChemStation system was used for data acquisition and calculation. A 15-cm fused silica capillary with an internal volume of 12 μL was used as an injection loop. Working solutions were loaded into the loop by means of a 25 μL precision syringe.

A Zorbax SB C18 (150 mm × 0.5 mm id, 5 μm) column (Agilent) was used for the separation of the target compounds. The mobile phase was a mixture of water-acetonitrile in gradient elution mode. The percentage of acetonitrile was linearly increased from 15% at zero min to 20% at 5 min, to 50% at 9 min, and to 75% at 11 min. Finally, the percentage of acetonitrile was increased to 100% at 15 min and kept constant until the end of the run. The mobile phase flow rate was 10 μL min^{-1}. The analytical signal was recorded between 190 and 400 nm, and monitored at 200 nm unless otherwise stated.

The solvents were filtered through 0.22 μm nylon membranes (Teknokroma, Barcelona, Spain).

4.3. Analysis of Dietary Supplements

Different types of dietary supplements acquired in supermarkets located in the area of Valencia city (Spain) were analyzed: three green coffee extract-based products (GCE), two fat-burning formulations, and an orange herbal preparation. Sample GCE-1, marketed in the form of bags, contained unspecified amounts of *Carum carvi*, *Spiraea ulmaria*, *Paullinia cupana*, *Solidago virgaurea* L., *Foeniculum vulgare*, *Taraxacum dens leonis*, and *Coffea canephota*; the label declared the presence of limonene, although its concentration was not reported. The mean average mass of product per bag was 1.1 g. Sample GCE-2 contained 175 mg of decaffeinated green coffee extract (*Coffea arabica* L.) per capsule (0.40 g). Sample GCE-3 contained 200 mg of green coffee extract, 50 mg of green tea extract, 50 mg of *Citrus aurantium*, 10 mg of cayenne pepper, 12.5 mg of choline bitartrate, 12.5 mg of inositol, 0.7 mg of riboflavin, and 0.167 mg of chromium picolinate per capsule (mean average mass, 0.50 g). Sample FB-1 contained 125 mg of *Citrus aurantium*, 150 mg of *Raphanus sativus* L., and 125 mg of *Solidago Virgaurea* L. per capsule (0.50 g). Sample FB-2 contained 110 mg of *Citrus aurantium*, 55 mg of green tea, and 40 mg of cola nut extract per capsule (0.25 g). Finally, sample HP (1.40 g per bag) was a mixture of lime and leaves of orange trees intended marketed as a powder; linalool, α-pinene, and limonene were declared to be present, but their concentrations were not provided.

Accurately weighted portions of the samples (≈25 mg) were placed in 5 mL glass vials and treated with methanol. The mixture was vortexed for 1 min and then placed in an ultrasonic bath (300 W, 40 kHz, Sonitech, Guarnizo, Spain) for 5 min. Then the supernatants were removed and filtered with 0.22 μm nylon membranes. Finally, 90 μL of the extracts were placed in glass vials and mixed with 10 μL of a solution of 0.1% hydrochloric acid (*v/v*); if required, the extracts were previously diluted with water. Aliquots of the resulting mixtures (12 μL) were chromatographed.

All the experiments were carried out at room temperature.

5. Conclusions

In this work, we have applied for the first time CapLC to the determination of terpenes in dietary supplements elaborated with plant materials. The method offers high sensitivity and precision, making possible the quantification of the target compounds at concentrations ranging from 0.006 to 1.9 mg g^{-1}. Compared with GC-MS methods reported previously, the UAE-CapLC method is less sensitive but much simpler and quicker. The potential utility of the proposed method has been demonstrated by comparing the individual and total amounts of selected terpenes present in dietary supplements as a simple way to assess their biological activities. Given the promising results obtained, future applications of this technique in the analysis of dietary supplements and medicinal plants can be expected.

Author Contributions: Conceptualization, H.D.P.-R., J.V.-A., R.H.-H. and P.C.-F.; methodology, H.D.P.-R., J.V.-A., R.H.-H. and P.C.-F.; validation, H.D.P.-R., J.V.-A., R.H.-H. and P.C.-F.; investigation, H.D.P.-R., J.V.-A., R.H.-H. and P.C.-F.; data curation, H.D.P.-R., J.V.-A., R.H.-H. and P.C.-F.; writing—original draft preparation, H.D.P.-R., J.V.-A., R.H.-H. and P.C.-F.; supervision, H.D.P.-R., J.V.-A., R.H.-H. and P.C.-F.; project administration, P.C.-F.; funding acquisition, H.D.P.-R., J.V.-A., R.H.-H. and P.C.-F. All authors have read and agreed to the published version of the manuscript.

Funding: This research was funded by EU FEDER and MCIU-AEI (project CTQ2017-90082-P) of Spain, and the GENERALITAT VALENCIANA (PROMETEO 2020/078) for the financial support received. H.D.P.-R. expresses his gratitude to the UNIVERSIDAD NACIONAL AUTÓNOMA DE HONDURAS (Honduras) for the pre-doctoral grant received. The APC was funded by EU FEDER and MCIU-AEI (project CTQ2017-90082-P).

Institutional Review Board Statement: Not applicable.

Informed Consent Statement: Not applicable.

Data Availability Statement: The data presented in this study are available in this submission.

Conflicts of Interest: The authors declare no conflict of interest.

References

1. Kaur, S.; Das, M. Functional Foods: An Overview. *Food Sci. Biotechnol.* **2011**, *20*, 861–875. [CrossRef]
2. Eussen, S.R.B.M.; Verhagen, H.; Klungel, O.H.; Garssen, J.; van Loveren, H.; van Kranen, H.J.; Rompelberg, C.J.M. Functional Foods and Dietary Supplements: Products at the Interface Between Pharma and Nutrition. *Eur. J. Pharmacol.* **2011**, S2–S9. [CrossRef] [PubMed]
3. Sarma, N.; Giancaspro, G.; Venema, J. Dietary Supplements Quality Analysis Tools from the United States Pharmacopeia. *Drug Test. Anal.* **2016**, *8*, 418–423. [CrossRef]
4. Andrews, K.W.; Schweitzer, A.; Zhao, C.; Holden, J.M.; Roseland, J.M.; Brandt, M.; Dwyer, J.T.; Picciano, M.F.; Saldanha, L.G.; Fisher, K.D.; et al. The Caffeine Contents of Dietary Supplements Commonly Purchased in the US: Analysis of 53 Products with Caffeine-Containing Ingredients. *Anal. Bioanal. Chem.* **2007**, *389*, 231–239. [CrossRef]
5. Kowalski, R.; Baj, T.; Kowalska, G.; Pankiewicz, U. Estimation of Potential Availability of Essential Oil in Some Brands of Herbal Teas and Herbal Dietary Supplements. *PLoS ONE* **2015**, *10*, e0130714. [CrossRef] [PubMed]
6. Viana, C.; Zemolin, G.M.; Müller, L.S.; Dal Molin, T.R.; Seiffert, H.; de Carvalho, L.M. Liquid Chromatographic Determination of Caffeine and Adrenergic Stimulants in Food Supplements Sold in Brazilian e-Commerce for Weight Loss and Physical Fitness. *Food Addit. Contam. Part A* **2016**, *33*, 1–9. [CrossRef] [PubMed]
7. Cox-Georgian, D.; Ramadoss, N.; Dona, C.; Basu, C. Therapeutic and Medicinal Uses of Terpenes. In *Medicinal Plants. From Farm to Pharmacy*, 1st ed.; Joshee, N., Dhekney, S., Parajuli, P., Eds.; Springer: Cham, Switzerland, 2019; pp. 333–359. [CrossRef]
8. Kim, T.; Song, B.; Cho, K.S.; Lee, I.-S. Therapeutic Potential of Volatile Terpenes and Terpenoids from Forests for Inflammatory Diseases. *Int. J. Mol. Sci.* **2020**, *21*, 2187. [CrossRef]
9. Proshkina, E.; Plyusnin, S.; Babak, T.; Lashmanova, E.; Maganova, F.; Koval, L.; Platonova, E.; Shaposhnikov, M.; Moskalev, A. Terpenoids as Potential Geroprotectors. *Antioxidants* **2020**, *9*, 529. [CrossRef]
10. Zhao, J.; Ge, L.-Y.; Xiong, W.; Leong, F.; Huang, L.-Q.; Li, S.-P. Advanced Development in Phytochemicals Analysis of Medicine and Food Dual Purposes Plants Used in China (2011–2014). *J. Chromatogr. A* **2016**, *1428*, 39–54. [CrossRef] [PubMed]

11. Medina, S.; Pereira, J.A.; Silva, P.; Perestrelo, R.; Câmara, J.S. Food Fingerprints–A Avaluable Tool to Monitor Food Authenticity and Safety. *Food Chem.* **2019**, *278*, 144–162. [CrossRef]
12. Hąc-Wydro, K.; Flasiński, M.; Romańczuk, K. Essential Oils as Food Eco-preservatives: Model System Studies on the Effect of Temperature on Limonene Antibacterial Activity. *Food Chem.* **2017**, *235*, 127–135. [CrossRef]
13. Kupska, M.; Chmiel, T.; Jędrkiewicz, R.; Wardencki, W.; Namieśnik, J. Comprehensive Two-Dimensional Gas Chromatography for Determination of the Terpenes Profile of Blue Honeysuckle Berries. *Food Chem.* **2014**, *152*, 88–93. [CrossRef]
14. D'Onofrio, C.; Matarese, F.; Cuzzola, A. Study of the Terpene Profile at Harvest and During Berry Development of *Vitis vinifera* L. Aromatic Varieties Aleatico, Brachetto, Malvasia di Candia Aromatica and Moscato Bianco. *J. Sci. Food Agric.* **2017**, *97*, 2898–2907. [CrossRef]
15. Diaconeasa, Z.; Iuhas, C.I.; Ayvaz, H.; Rugină, D.; Stanilă, A.; Dulf, F.; Bunea, A.; Socaci, S.A.; Socaciu, C.; Pintea, A. Phytochemical Characterization of Commercial Processed Blueberry, Blackberry, Blackcurrant, Cranberry, and Raspberry and Their Antioxidant Activity. *Antioxidants* **2019**, *8*, 540. [CrossRef]
16. Pollon, M.; Torchio, F.; Giacosa, S.; Segade, S.R.; Rolle, L. Use of Density Sorting for the Selection of Aromatic Grape Berries with Different Volatile Profile. *Food Chem.* **2019**, *276*, 562–571. [CrossRef] [PubMed]
17. Duarte, L.M.; Amorim, T.L.; Grazul, M.L.; de Oliveira, M.A.L. Differentiation of aromatic, bittering and dual-purpose commercial hops from their terpenic profiles: An Approach Involving Batch Extraction, GC–MS and Multivariate Analysis. *Food Res. Int.* **2020**, *138*, 109768. [CrossRef]
18. He, F.; Qian, Y.L.; Qian, M.C. Flavor and Chiral Stability of Lemon-Flavored Hard Tea during Storage. *Food Chem.* **2018**, *239*, 622–630. [CrossRef]
19. Kim, M.K.; Jang, H.W.; Lee, K.-G. Sensory and Instrumental Volatile Flavor Analysis of Commercial Orange Juices Prepared by Different Processing Methods. *Food Chem.* **2018**, *267*, 217–222. [CrossRef] [PubMed]
20. Mukazayire, M.J.; Tomani, J.C.; Stévigny, C.; Chalchat, J.C.; Conforti, F.; Menichini, F.; Duez, P. Essential Oils of Four Rwandese Hepatoprotective Herbs: Gas Chromatography–Mass Spectrometry Analysis and Antioxidant Activities. *Food Chem.* **2011**, *129*, 753–760. [CrossRef]
21. Nazario, C.D.E.; Silva, M.R.; Franco, M.S.; Lanças, F.M. Evolution in Miniaturized Column Liquid Chromatography Instrumentation and Applications: An Overview. *J. Chromatogr. A* **2015**, *1421*, 18–37. [CrossRef]
22. Ponce-Rodríguez, H.D.; Verdú-Andrés, J.; Herráez-Hernández, R.; Campíns-Falcó, P. Innovations in Extractive Phases for In-Tube Solid-Phase Microextraction Coupled to Miniaturized Liquid Chromaography: A Critical Review. *Molecules* **2020**, *25*, 2460. [CrossRef] [PubMed]
23. Rocco, A.; Donati, E.; Touloupakis, E.; Aturki, Z. Miniaturized Separation Techniques as Analytical Methods to Ensure Quality and Safety of Dietary Supplements. *Trends Anal. Chem.* **2018**, *103*, 156–183. [CrossRef]
24. Ponce-Rodríguez, H.D.; Herráez-Hernández, R.; Verdú-Andrés, J.; Campíns-Falcó, P. Quantitative Analysis of Terpenic Compounds in Microsamples of Resins by Capillary Liquid Chromatography. *Molecules* **2019**, *24*, 4068. [CrossRef] [PubMed]
25. Mirghaed, A.T.; Ghelichpour, M.; Hoseini, S.M. Myrcene and Linalool as New Anesthetic and Sedative Agents in Common Carp, *Cyprinus carpio*-Comparison with Eugenol. *Aquaculture* **2016**, *464*, 165–170. [CrossRef]
26. Kiyama, R. Nutritional Implications of Ginger: Chemistry, Biological Activities and Signaling Pathways. *J. Nutr. Biochem.* **2020**, *86*, 108486. [CrossRef]
27. PubChem Database. Available online: https://pubchem.ncbi.nlm.nih.gov (accessed on 14 June 2021).
28. Kraujalytė, V.; Pelvan, E.; Alasalvar, C. Volatile Compounds and Sensory Characteristics of Various Instant Teas Produced from Black Tea. *Food Chem.* **2016**, *194*, 864–872. [CrossRef]

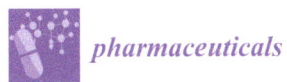 *pharmaceuticals*

Article

Quantification of 17 Endogenous and Exogenous Steroidal Hormones in Equine and Bovine Blood for Doping Control with UHPLC-MS/MS

Giovanni Caprioli [1], Michele Genangeli [1], Ahmed M. Mustafa [1,2], Riccardo Petrelli [1], Massimo Ricciutelli [1], Gianni Sagratini [1], Stefano Sartori [3], Fulvio Laus [4], Sauro Vittori [1] and Manuela Cortese [1,*]

1   School of Pharmacy, University of Camerino, 62032 Camerino, Italy; giovanni.caprioli@unicam.it (G.C.); michele.genangeli@unicam.it (M.G.); ahmed.mustafa@unicam.it (A.M.M.); riccardo.petrelli@unicam.it (R.P.); massimo.ricciutelli@unicam.it (M.R.); gianni.sagratini@unicam.it (G.S.); sauro.vittori@unicam.it (S.V.)
2   Department of Pharmacognosy, Faculty of Pharmacy, Zagazig University, Zagazig 44519, Egypt
3   Eureka Lab Division, 60033 Chiaravalle, Italy; sartori@eurekaone.com
4   School of Bioscience and Veterinary Medicine, University of Camerino, 62032 Camerino, Italy; fulvio.laus@unicam.it
*   Correspondence: manuela.cortese@unicam.it; Tel.: +39-07-3740-4506

Citation: Caprioli, G.; Genangeli, M.; Mustafa, A.M.; Petrelli, R.; Ricciutelli, M.; Sagratini, G.; Sartori, S.; Laus, F.; Vittori, S.; Cortese, M. Quantification of 17 Endogenous and Exogenous Steroidal Hormones in Equine and Bovine Blood for Doping Control with UHPLC-MS/MS. *Pharmaceuticals* **2021**, *14*, 393. https://doi.org/10.3390/ph14050393

Academic Editors: Jan Oszmianski and Sabina Lachowicz

Received: 25 March 2021
Accepted: 16 April 2021
Published: 21 April 2021

Publisher's Note: MDPI stays neutral with regard to jurisdictional claims in published maps and institutional affiliations.

Abstract: A simple and fast analytical method able to simultaneously identify and quantify 17 endogenous and exogenous steroidal hormones was developed in bovine and equine blood using UHPLC-MS/MS. A total amount of 500 μL of sample was deproteinized with 500 μL of a mixture of methanol and zinc sulfate and evaporated. The mixture was reconstituted with 50 μL of a solution of 25% methanol and injected in the UHPLC-MS/MS triple quadrupole. The correlation coefficients of the calibration curves of the analyzed compounds were in the range of 0.9932–0.9999, and the limits of detection and quantification were in the range of 0.023–1.833 and 0.069–5.5 ppb, respectively. The developed method showed a high sensitivity and qualitative aspects allowing the detection and quantification of all steroids in equine and bovine blood. Moreover, the detection limit of testosterone (50 ppt) is half of the threshold admitted in plasma (100 ppt). Once validated, the method was used to quantify 17 steroid hormones in both bovine and equine blood samples. The primary endogenous compounds detected were corticosterone (range 0.28–0.60 ppb) and cortisol (range 0.44–10.00 ppb), followed by androstenedione, testosterone and 11-deoxycortisol.

Keywords: HPLC-MS/MS; steroidal hormones; anti-doping; bovine blood; equine blood

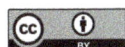
1. Introduction

This paper is a follow-up study of a method developed by Genangeli et al. for the simultaneous determination of steroids in horse serum [1]. Endogenous and exogenous steroids are abused in animal-related sports, and they have a major role in regulating a wide number of endogenous signals in the organism [2,3]. Anabolic steroids are synthetic compound derivatives from testosterone. The primary function of anabolic steroids can be summarized into reproductive and sexual differentiation, homeostasis, growth, development, and regulation of metabolism and nutrient supply [3–5]. Doping control in horse racing and animal-related events poses different challenges, in comparison with other sports where humans are involved, because both performance-enhancing and performance-impairing substances (or methods) can be used to manipulate and change the outcome of the competition while the controls are not standardized and rarely applied [6]. This may be more predominant in an animal competition where the bets reach high values leading to an abuse of illegal substances in order to ensure the winning [6]. Nowadays, competitions or events involving animals like cattle or horses are increasing in popularity. As previously reported from Genangeli et al. [1], only eleven compounds are present in the list of prohibited substances with international thresholds in both urine or plasma [7].

Apart from substances like theobromine, dimethyl sulfoxide or salicylic acid, testosterone is still the only steroid regulated in plasma, and its threshold in plasma horses is 100 ppt quantitated as free testosterone [7]. The performance improvement or health conditions camouflage in horses, or other animals, are common techniques used before an animal trading or during a race. These substances can cause severe harm to the animal. As reported from Kavitha et al., the following are the adverse effects of anabolic steroids by topic: cardiovascular, endocrine and metabolic, gastrointestinal, genitourinary, hematologic and oncologic, neuromuscular and skeletal, neuropsychiatric, dermatologic and renal [1,8]. Qualitative evaluation of steroidal hormones and their metabolites and quantitation of these molecules is crucial for the correct diagnosis and/or treatment of several diseases and conditions, such as disorders of puberty, amenorrhea, polycystic ovary syndrome, infertility, osteoporosis, adrenal insufficiency, hypogonadism, cognitive dysfunction, cardiovascular diseases and hormone-related malignancies [9]. At the moment, current analytical procedures regarding the matter are self-developed analysis, expensive, complicated or long and time-consuming to be replicated in clinical laboratories. Additionally, these methods are often based on immunohistochemical analysis, with reduced sensitivity and the high possibility of false positive responses or wrong quantitation [10–13]. Genye et al. developed a method to detect and analyze 13 steroids in human urine using a quadrupole-Orbitrap LC-MS/MS [14]. Tajudheen et al. studied the separation of two anabolic substances using a reversed phase chiral chromatography approach [15]. Brian et al. published an article regarding novel liquid chromatography-tandem mass spectrometry methods for measuring steroids [16]. Youwen et al. focused on the separation of 16 testosterone and nandrolone esters in equine plasma [17]. Colton et al. developed a method for fast screening of anabolic steroids in horse urine [18]. From literature, it appears that the majority of methods for endogenous and exogenous steroid analysis is mainly focused on human samples [19]. Additionally, these methods are developed using either high-performance liquid chromatography-tandem mass spectrometry (HPLC-MS/MS) or gas chromatography (GC-MS) where HPLC-MS/MS is the perfect technique due to its extreme specificity and high sensitivity [20–25]. The majority of the procedures existing in literature are oriented towards horses or horse racing; here, the importance of developing a general method able to precisely quantify and qualify several endogenous and exogenous steroids in blood from different animals, sensitive and reproducible, with a short analytical time that can provide reliable results. Thus, our work aimed to set up a new UHPLC-tandem mass-based method to detect and quantify seventeen hormones and metabolites in equine and bovine blood. Detectable and quantifiable compounds included in the proposed method are as follows: androsterone (AND), androstenedione (ANDD), dehydroepiandrosterone (DHEA), testosterone (TEST), cortisol (COR), corticosterone (CoCo), aldosterone (ALDO), 11-deoxycortisol (11-DOC), 11-deoxycorticosterone (11-DCC), dihydrotestosterone (DHT), nandrolone (NAN), boldenone (BOL), stanozolol (STA), dexamethasone sodium phosphate (Desa NaP), dexamethasone isonicotinate, (Desa-Iso), methylprednisolone (MePre) and pregnenolone (PRE). One deuterated hormone (testosterone-D3) was used as an internal standard in order to make the analytical method more robust. All the compounds included in this methodology are different from the molecules included in analytical procedures reported in the literature but currently adopted for doping purposes [22,26]. The proposed procedure is not time-consuming with clear and simple sample preparation. Additionally, the method resulted in being sensitive, accurate and robust after a full validation. Hence, it could bring faster and cheaper analysis easily applicable from any external laboratory. The proposed procedure was fully validated and applied to the analysis of blood samples from different kinds of animals (mares, stallions, geldings and cows).

2. Results and Discussion

2.1. Setup of the Chromatographic and Mass Analyzer Conditions

After testing different chromatographic conditions, the best results were obtained with a solution of water and 0.1% of formic (mobile phase A) and acetonitrile and 0.1% of formic acid (mobile phase B). The use of other solvents as mobile phase B led to a worse separation among peaks, and the presence of formic acid in the mobile phase enhanced the ionization of the analytes in the ESI source, resulting in a greater sensitivity of the overall method. Due to the different chemical structure of the analytes, several chromatographic-gradient conditions were tested. The complete baseline separation of all peaks in the shortest time was achieved by using the chromatographic condition listed in Table 1, and described in the section 'Liquid Chromatography-Tandem Mass Spectrometry'. A final column conditioning was also found to be essential for reproducibility of the retention time of the monitored compounds. A flow rate at 0.6 mL min^{-1} was the best option to achieve a good chromatographic separation in a short period of time. Different flow rates led to either a longer analytical time or an overlapping of peaks. As for the optimization of the chromatographic conditions, the mobile phases were chosen according to their influence in the ionization process occurring in the ESI source. The choice of acetonitrile and water with formic acid led to a significantly higher signal and ionization for all the compounds but also a good chromatography separation and resolution of peaks [27,28]. Additionally, papers in literature confirm that the addition of formic acid in a positive mode increases the response of target compounds [28,29]. In our case, we had an improvement of both ionization and chromatographic separation/resolution of peaks. The precursor and daughter ions obtained by injecting a standard solution of each compound are comparable with other methods found in the literature [16,18,22,26,30].

Table 1. Ultra-high-performance liquid chromatography-tandem mass spectrometry acquisition parameters (multiple reaction monitoring mode) used for the analysis of steroidal hormones and metabolites.

Compound	Abbreviation	Time Window (Minute)	Precursor Ion [a] (*m/z*)	Product Ion (*m/z*)	Fragmentor (V)	Collision Energy (V)	Dwell Time (Milli-Second)
Dexamethasone Sodium Phosphate	Desa-NA-P	2.0–3.7	473.11	435.2 355.2	97	8	200
Cortisol	CORT	2.0–3.7	363.01	121.1 327.2	136	24	200
Aldosterone	ALDO	2.0–3.7	361.41	343.2 315.2	116	16	200
Pregnenolone	PRE	2.0–3.7	361.41	343.2 105.0	87	4	200
Methylprednisolone	ME-PRE	3.7–5.5	375.01	357.2 323.2	92	4	180
11-Deoxycortisol	11-DOC	3.7–5.5	347.51	109.10 97.2	141	32	180
Corticosterone	COCO	3.7–5.5	347.01	329.2 329.2	111	12	180
Stanozolol	STA	3.7–5.5	329.51	81.10 95.10	170	50	180
Boldenone	BOL	3.7–5.5	287.41	121.00 135.00	107	24	180
Nandrolone	NAN	3.7–5.5	275.10	109.10 82.90	100	28	180
Dexamethasone isonicotinate	DESA-ISO	5.5–6.8	498.61	47.20 124.0	121	8	200
11-Deoxycorticosterone	11-DCC	5.5–6.8	331.01	97.10 109.1	117	20	200
Dihydrotestosterone	DHT	6.8–9.0	273.10	255.30 147.0	159	15	200
Testosterone	TESTO	5.5–6.8	289.01	97.10 109.1	131	20	100

Table 1. *Cont.*

Compound	Abbreviation	Time Window (Minute)	Precursor Ion [a] (*m/z*)	Product Ion (*m/z*)	Fragmentor (V)	Collision Energy (V)	Dwell Time (Milli-Second)
Androstenedione	ANDD	5.5–6.8	287.01	97.10 109.1	131	24	200
Dehydroepiandrosterone	DHEA	5.5–6.8	271.01	253.10 253.2	92	8	200
Androsterone	ANDRO	6.8–9.0	291.41	273.20 255.2	78	4	200
Testosterone–d3	d3-TESTO	5.5–6.8	292.00	97.00	135	25	120

[a] For every compound, the first product ion was used for quantitation and the second for qualification.

2.2. Method Validation

The proposed method was fully validated in terms of its analytical characteristics such as linearity, accuracy and precision, evaluation of the limit of detection (LOD) and limit of quantification (LOQ). Additionally, recovery and matrix were also investigated. The assessment of all these parameters is essential for the future application of the proposed method. All the concentrations were developed starting from the LOQ of every compound (Table 2).

Table 2. Values of the concentrations used for method validation for each analyte.

Compound	LOD	LOQ	C1	CM	C2	CU	U1
				ppb			
DESA-NA-P	0.333	1.00	10	50	100	500	1000
COR	0.183	0.55	11	55	110	550	1100
ALDO	0.183	0.55	11	55	110	550	1100
PRE	0.033	0.10	10	50	100	500	1000
ME-PRE	0.067	0.20	20	100	200	1000	2000
11-DOC	0.037	0.11	11	55	110	550	1100
COCO	0.167	0.50	10	50	100	500	1000
STA	0.033	0.10	10	50	100	500	1000
BOL	0.167	0.50	10	50	100	500	1000
NAN	0.333	1.00	10	50	100	500	1000
DESA-ISO	0.023	0.069	6.9	34.5	69	345	690
11-DCC	0.037	0.11	11	55	110	550	1100
TESTO	0.037	0.05	11	55	110	550	1100
ANDD	0.333	1.00	10	50	100	500	1000
DHEA	1.833	5.50	11	55	110	550	1100
ANDRO	0.733	2.20	22	110	220	1100	2200
DHT	1.833	5.50	11	55	110	550	1100

2.3. Evaluation of the Stability of Steroids in Glass and Plastic

Several endogenous and exogenous steroids were tested for stability in glass and plastic. A standard concentration of 200 ppb of the compounds listed in Table 3 was prepared, and an aliquot of the before mentioned mix was transferred into four plastic vials and four glass vials and stored at −4 °C. The first vial was immediately analyzed and the other four were analyzed over the following 3 days. As reported in Table 3, immediately after one day, the concentration of the steroids stored in the glass test tube dropped with a loss of >98%, suggesting an interaction of the analytes with the glass of the container.

Table 3. Loss of compounds in plastic vs. glass containers.

	DAY 1		DAY 2	
	Loss in Plastic (%)	Loss in Glass (%)	Loss in Plastic (%)	Loss in Glass (%)
COR	<1	99.63	<2%	>99.90
ALDO	<1	94.29	<2%	>99.90
11-DOC	<1	99.94	<2%	>99.90
COCO	<1	99.76	<2%	>99.90
11-DCC	<1	99.88	<2%	>99.90
PRE	<1	99.97	<2%	>99.90
ANDRO	<1	99.52	<2%	>99.90
TESTO	<1	99.85	<2%	>99.90
ANDD	<1	99.83	<2%	>99.90
DHT	<1	99.12	<2%	>99.90
DHEA	<1	99.65	<2%	>99.90

2.4. Precision and Linearity

Precision is known to be the closeness of agreement between independent test results obtained under stipulated conditions [1,31]. It is usually reported regarding standard deviation (SD) or relative standard deviation (RSD) [1,31]. The precision (intra-day and inter-day) was calculated from data obtained during a three-day validation (Table 4) of five daily repetitions using four concentrations from the LOQ to the U1 (LOQ, CM, CU and U1). The outcome is expressed according to the coefficient of variation (CV%). The CV resulted to be included in the range of 0.48–18.78% (Table 4). The inter-day precision ($n = 5$) expressed in relative standard deviation percent (RSD) was also satisfactory. The LOQ displayed RSD in the range of 10.86–18.37%, the CM resulted in an RSD of 2.62–18.78%, the CU showed an RSD of 3.52–18.40% and U1 had an RSD within 0.48–9.41% (Table 4). To calculate the linearity of the proposed method, two calibration curves were created using all the concentrations between LOQ and CU (low-range standard curve, 5 points, 5-day validation) and all the concentrations between the LOQ and U1 (high-range standard curve, 6 points, 5-day validation). The high-range curve was used to test the linearity in a more extense dynamic range. The linearity is expressed as the coefficient of linear regression (R^2), and it is higher than 0.99% (Table 4).

Table 4. Intra-day and inter-day precision expressed in CV% and linearity expressed in R^2.

Compound	Limit of Quantification		Medium Concentration		CU		U1		Linearity
	Intra-Day (CV%)	Inter-Day (CV%)	Intra-Day (CV%)	Inter-Day (CV%)	Intra-Day (CV%)	Inter-Day (CV%)	Intra-Day (CV%)	Inter-Day (CV%)	R^2
DESA-NA-P	10.86	14.16	6.74	7.58	2.62	4.12	1.02	1.48	0.99326
COR	16.47	18.49	9.50	10.35	6.49	8.24	3.56	4.49	0.99939
ALDO	14.45	17.52	6.95	8.40	6.79	7.63	6.07	6.85	0.99995
PRE	15.84	17.41	10.07	10.91	2.78	3.69	1.18	2.37	0.99922
ME-PRE	15.93	17.45	15.04	17.85	6.32	18.40	3.26	8.12	0.99912
11-DOC	17.10	17.87	6.63	7.72	6.93	7.53	5.48	6.73	0.99954
COCO	10.34	14.57	7.97	10.63	1.56	4.51	0.48	2.28	0.99991
STA	13.25	14.95	5.73	9.11	3.15	5.24	1.18	4.20	0.99941
BOL	15.83	17.89	11.85	16.66	3.71	18.05	2.03	6.97	0.99658
NAN	17.35	18.62	7.12	14.75	5.49	8.13	2.26	5.83	0.99861
DESA-ISO	17.43	18.37	9.77	18.99	7.88	9.65	4.49	6.41	0.99981
11-DCC	16.60	18.07	16.06	18.78	12.21	18.27	7.21	9.41	0.99953
TESTO	11.76	18.17	11.40	16.89	6.35	15.06	4.39	5.72	0.99841
ANDD	10.08	16.66	14.04	18.46	8.56	9.88	6.29	8.06	0.99987
DHEA	14.21	17.84	9.99	18.64	4.67	8.49	2.18	3.26	0.99970
ANDRO	16.81	17.77	5.34	8.23	4.30	4.80	2.93	3.21	0.99940
DHT	13.97	17.10	9.07	9.19	6.31	6.57	4.29	5.30	0.99997

The LODs and LOQs for all the compounds included in this analytical procedure displayed values in the range of 0.023–1.833 and 0.069–5.5 ppb, respectively. These values are similar and sometimes lower when compared with a limit of detection and quantification reported in the literature [22,26,32]. Additionally, the steroids and metabolites included in this procedure were chosen due to their frequency of usage and because they were partially included in procedure already present in the literature. Moreover, LOQ for testosterone is equal to 0.05 ppb, twice lower concerning 0.1 ppb (or 100 ppt), which is the threshold for plasma samples of young horses (geldings) [7].

2.5. Accuracy

Accuracy is known to be the closeness of agreement between a test result and the accepted reference value of the property being measured [1,33].

The intra and inter-day accuracy were calculated from the C1, C2 and U1 concentrations, from the data obtained during a three-day validation. The results are listed in Table S1 and expressed in terms of 'relative error percentage' (RE%). The RE% for all the analytes were within the range, 0.92–13.90% (Table S1). The inter-day ($n = 5$) accuracy was also satisfactory. Precisely, at the C1 concentration, the RE% values were in the range 6.08–13.64%; at the C2 concentration, the RE% values were 1.23–7.12%, and at the U1 concentration, the RE% values were 1.10–4.19%.

2.6. Recovery

Recovery was studied by spiking clean equine and bovine blood with a mixture standard of the 17 hormones. The recovery value was obtained using the following formula: $((A_{se} - As_{blank})/A_{std}) \times 100$, where A_{se} is the area about the serum enriched with a low concentration (C1 and CM) of all the compounds, A_{blank} is the area of analytes detected in the serum and A_{std} is the area of a mixture standard of all the compounds dissolved in methanol. The recoveries obtained by spiking the matrix at the CM concentration were in the range of 86.75–98.32%, with a CV lower than 5.04% (Table S2). Moreover, the recoveries at a concentration of C1 were in the range 85.60–99.39%, with a CV lower than 8.21% (Table S2).

2.7. Matrix Effect

Matrix is often responsible for a reduced or an increased signal/ionization (ion suppression/enhancement) in mass spectrometry [34]. These effects can strongly affect and compromise the quality and reproducibility of biological samples when injected and studied with LC-ESI-MS. To test the matrix effect, we performed a test known as "post-column infusion". This test, according to the literature, is one of the best techniques used to obtain qualitative information about matrix effects [35]. A methanol mixture of all the compounds at the medium concentration (CM) was injected in the ESI source using a micropump. Simultaneously, an injection of purified and deproteinized blood was performed. As shown in Figure 1, the signal is constant for almost all the chromatographic time, with the exception for a signal suppression at 9.5 min. All the compounds have a retention time shorter than 9.5 min; hence, the matrix does not cause ion suppression or enhancement effects in our method.

2.8. Specificity

In order to quantify the specificity of the proposed method, we controlled the retention time of parent/daughter ions for all the analytes over time. For each compound, we examined the chromatographic retention time regarding reproducibility, for a number of five times over a five-day period ($n = 25$). The RSD regarding the retention time was stable with an average percent value $\leq 0.97\%$. Specific parent/daughter ion transitions were identified for each steroid, and the MRM transitions with the most abundant product ion were selected for quantitation, and the other product ion was selected for qualification (Table 1). High specificity was achieved.

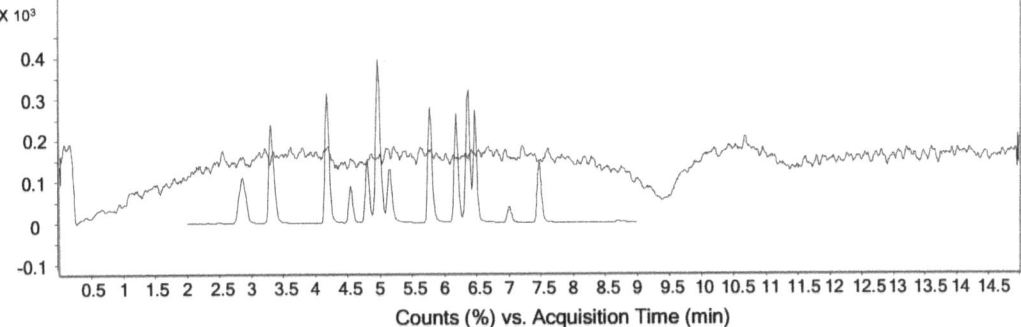

Figure 1. Post-column infusion of steroids serum-free and a mixture standard of all searched compounds in high-performance liquid chromatography-grade methanol.

2.9. Application and Testing of the Developed Method to Equine and Bovine Blood

The method described in this paper was successfully applied to thirty-three samples provided from four control agencies located in the south of Italy (Groups A, B, C, D). The high sensitivity and the quantitative aspects of the proposed method allowed the detection of most of the compound in the equine and bovine blood samples. The analysis was performed in blind, and due to privacy, we do not know if samples were bovine or equine. Due to the blind analysis and the thresholds changing between gender, species and age of the animals, we could not compare our results with international guidelines [36].

A total of thirty-three animals were analyzed in triplicate; percent RSDs in all cases were lower than 13.66%. Moreover, the mean values of the analytes found in the various samples are reported in Table 5. Only androsterone and DHEA were not detected in any samples. The main compounds found in the four groups of samples were cortisol (range 0.44–10.00 ppb), followed by corticosterone, androstenedione and dexamethasone isonicotinate. Overall, the level of exogenous steroids is below the thresholds from different guidelines and papers in the literature (pregnenolone, stanozolol and nandrolone < 1 ppb, boldenone < 15 ppb, testosterone < 20 ppb for geldings in plasma and <55 ppb for mares and fillies not in foal [6,37,38]). None of the samples showed levels of exogenous substances above 1 ppb, with the exception of ME-PRE in group C. Some animals showed traces of some of the exogenous steroids. In particular, DESA-NA-P is present only in the group A. PRE is present only in two samples belonging to group A. BOL was present only in three samples and not in group C. NAN was present in three samples belonging to group A and D. Our findings are the first step for a lager monitoring project on the presence of these exogenous compounds in mammals and their healthy effects.

Table 5. Content of endogenous and exogenous steroids in equine and bovine blood samples, expressed in ppb.

	Exogenous Steroids												Endogenous Steroids			
Animal	DESA-NA-P	PRE	ME-PRE	STA	BOL	NAN	DESA-ISO	11-DCC	TESTO	ANDD	DHEA	ANDRO	DHT	COR	ALDO	11-DOC	COCO
									ppb								
A 01	0.152	-	0.470	0.395	-	0.237	0.245	-	0.145	0.481	-	-	-	4.207	1.038	0.190	0.319
A 02	0.134	-	0.478	0.397	-	-	0.243	-	0.142	0.482	-	-	-	0.668	1.095	-	0.330
A 03	-	0.444	0.558	0.392	-	-	0.242	0.183	0.138	0.497	-	-	-	3.631	-	0.179	0.288
A 04	-	-	-	0.419	-	-	0.247	-	-	0.478	-	-	-	6.578	0.846	0.201	0.587
A 05	0.130	-	-	0.393	-	-	0.246	-	-	0.484	-	-	-	2.363	-	-	-
A 06	0.100	-	-	0.390	-	-	0.242	0.178	-	0.461	-	-	-	3.247	-	0.180	-

Table 5. *Cont.*

Animal	DESA-NA-P	PRE	ME-PRE	STA	BOL	NAN	DESA-ISO	11-DCC	TESTO	ANDD	DHEA	ANDRO	DHT	COR	ALDO	11-DOC	COCO
							Exogenous Steroids			Endogenous Steroids							
A 07	-	-	-	-	-	-	0.241	0.187	-	0.497	-	-	-	-	-	-	-
A 08	-	-	-	-	-	-	-	0.194	0.142	0.436	-	-	-	1.670	-	-	-
A 09	0.071	-	-	-	-	-	-	-	-	0.479	-	-	-	0.444	-	-	0.334
A 10	-	-	-	0.462	-	-	0.250	0.202	0.146	0.500	-	-	-	0.465	-	-	0.351
A 11	-	-	-	-	-	-	0.241	-	0.137	0.532	-	-	-	2.082	-	-	0.315
A 12	0.094	-	-	-	-	-	0.243	-	-	0.571	-	-	-	0.435	-	-	0.393
A 13	0.170	-	-	0.393	-	-	0.244	-	-	0.561	-	-	-	1.956	-	-	0.375
A 14	0.121	-	-	0.387	-	-	0.247	-	-	0.443	-	-	-	3.935	-	-	0.491
A 15	0.196	0,472	-	-	0.064	0.291	0.258	0.229	-	0.515	-	-	-	3.486	-	0.197	0.383
B 01	-	-	0.87	-	0.02	-	-	0.39	-	-	-	-	0.98	5.96	-	0.53	0.49
B 02	-	-	-	-	-	-	-	0.39	0.23	0.60	-	-	1.87	1.29	0.70	-	0.40
B 03	-	-	-	-	-	-	0.47	0.39	0.22	-	-	-	1.95	0.99	-	-	0.44
B 04	-	-	0.83	-	-	-	-	-	0.22	-	-	-	1.06	5.62	-	-	0.41
B 05	-	-	0.95	-	-	-	0.47	-	0.21	-	-	-	3.26	1.67	-	-	-
B 06	-	-	0.86	-	-	-	0.47	-	-	-	-	-	-	1.35	-	-	-
C 01	-	-	1.33	-	-	-	0.39	-	0.31	0.62	-	-	-	10.00	0.79	0.48	0.60
C 02	-	-	1.05	-	-	-	0.40	-	-	0.64	-	-	-	3.61	-	0.45	0.54
C 03	-	-	1.07	0.27	-	-	0.40	-	-	-	-	-	-	1.17	-	-	-
C 04	-	-	1.08	-	-	-	-	-	0.31	-	-	-	-	2.36	-	-	0.54
C 05	-	-	1.08	-	-	-	0.40	-	-	-	-	-	-	0.88	-	-	0.45
C 06	-	-	1.02	-	-	-	0.40	-	-	0.62	-	-	-	4.96	-	0.46	0.58
D 01	-	-	0.876	-	0.024	0.531	-	0.397	-	-	-	-	0.986	5.967	-	0.531	0.497
D 02	-	-	-	-	-	-	-	0.396	0.236	0.604	-	-	1.872	1.296	0.702	-	0.401
D 03	-	-	-	-	-	-	0.3	0.394	0.221	-	-	-	0.959	0.992	-	-	0.448
D 04	-	-	0.834	-	-	-	-	-	0.226	-	-	-	1.060	5.62	-	-	0.418
D 05	-	-	0.953	-	-	-	-	-	0.219	-	-	-	-	1.671	-	-	-
D 06	-	-	0.866	-	-	-	0.4	-	0.213	-	-	-	-	1.356	-	-	-

3. Materials and Methods

3.1. Disposable Chemicals and Materials

All the detected compounds used in this paper, including the internal standard, were ordered from Sigma-Aldrich (Milano, Italy) with a purity > 99%. An individual stock solution of each compound was prepared by the dissolution of 0.5 mg of every single molecule in 0.5 mL of HPLC-grade methanol (Carlo Erba, Milano, Italy). Other solutions were obtained from the dilution of the stock solutions in methanol. HPLC-grade acetonitrile was purchased from Carlo Erba (Milano, Italy). HPLC-grade formic acid (99%) was obtained from Merck (Darmstadt, Germany). Deionized water (>18 MΩ cm resistivity) was obtained by purification of water with a Milli-Q SP system (Millipore, Bedford, MA, USA). Sterile test tubes were purchased from Becton–Dickinson (Franklin Lakes, NJ, USA). The analytical procedures were carried out in polypropylene vials, test tubes and plastic centrifuge tubes in order to preserve the concentration and stability of the hormones. The glass has demonstrated that it could interfere with those molecules as reported in the section "*Evaluation of the stability of steroids in glass and plastic*" (Results and Discussion, Table 3).

3.2. Collection of Equine Blood

The equine and bovine blood used for the method optimization was collected from healthy horses and cows from the Unicam veterinary hospital in Matelica (MC) and stored in vials with EDTA or Lithium heparin. The blood was refined using activated charcoal to obtain a standard hormone-free-matrix and stored at −4 °C. The tested blood was obtained from several veterinary hospitals from the south of Italy, stored at −4 °C if analyzed within two days or stored at −20 °C if analyzed after two days.

3.3. Preparation of Steroids-Free Blood and Sample Preparation

The blood (50 mL) was kept under magnetic agitation overnight, with 1 g of charcoal to create steroids-free blood used in the development and validation steps, as reported by Genangeli et al. [1,39]. The solution was then let settle for 10 min, and the clear blood without visual residues of charcoal was transferred into a clean 50 mL plastic test tube. To obtain clean blood from the charcoal residues, this last step was repeated for additional time or until the no residues of charcoal were present on the bottom of the test tube. The hormone-free blood was stored at −20 °C.

A total of 500 μL of blood was denatured using 500 μL of a denaturing solution made of methanol (MeOH) and 5 g/L of zinc sulfate (ZnSO₄) and internal standard (testosterone d3, 1000 ppb) in Eppendorf tubes. The deproteinizing solution was prepared leaving the methanol and zinc sulfate under magnetic agitation overnight and then filtering the solution with a paper filter. The solution was then agitated with vortex for approximately 1 min to avoid the formation of blood clotting. The solution was centrifuged for 15 min at 13,000 rpm, and then the liquid was transferred into polypropylene test tubes. The obtained solution was evaporated under nitrogen gas flow, then rebuilt using 50 μL of 25% methanol and centrifuged again for 10 min at 13,000 rpm, and finally pipetted in high-recovery vials and injected in the UHPLC-ESI-MS/MS system.

3.4. UHPLC-ESI-MS/MS

The UHPLC system used was an Agilent 1290 infinity series coupled with an Agilent Technologies ESI-triple quadrupole 6420 (Santa Clara, CA, USA). The analytes were separated using a Zorbax RRHD C18 as an analytical column (50 × 2.10 mm, the internal diameter of 1.8 μm), also from Agilent Technologies (USA). The mobile phases adopted for the analysis are water (A) and acetonitrile (B) both containing 0.1% formic acid. The mobile phases were kept at a constant flow of 0.6 mL min^{-1} with a gradient elution of: 0 min 15% B, 2.5 min 25% B, 5 min 35% B, 7 min 50% B, 9 min 90% B and 11 min 15% B, and kept at 15% B until the end of the run (15 min). Five μL of samples were injected with an auto-sampler. The column was kept at 20 °C, and the drying gas in the ESI source 300 °C. The gas flow was 12 L min^{-1}, the pressure of the nebulizer was 40 psi, and the capillary voltage was 4000 V (negative and positive). Detection was performed in the 'multiple reaction monitoring' (MRM) mode dividing the runtime into four segments as reported in Table 1. The most abundant daughter ion was used for quantification purposes, and the rest of the daughter ions were used for qualification purposes. All the information regarding the compounds, abbreviation and settings of the mass analyzer are reported in Table 1.

3.5. Method Validation Settings

For the method evaluation and validation, seven concentrations of each analyte were used, starting from the limit of detection (LOD), limit of quantification (LOQ), then a series of low, medium and high concentrations (C1, CM, C2, CU). All the concentrations listed before, except for LOD, were used in the low-range standard curve (5 points); and for the high-range standard curve, one additional 'upper' concentrations (U1) was included (total of 6 points). All the concentrations divided by the compounds are summarized in Table 2.

Several concentrations were tested in order to find the LOQ. Precisely, ten concentrations were tested, and the LOQ values are in a range from 5.5 ppb for the DHEA and 0.069 ppb for the DESA ISO (data not shown).

3.6. Internal Standards

One deuterated internal standard was introduced as a control to increase the robustness of the method. The standard was added prior to the deproteinization step at the concentration of 1000 ppb.

4. Conclusions

A new UHPLC-MS/MS method was developed, permitting the detection of 17 endogenous and exogenous anabolic substances in equine and bovine blood samples. Most of the compounds in the current method are different from those reported in the literature, especially the ones of exogenous origin, and largely adopted to modify the condition of the considered animals. The high sensitivity of the method permitted the detection of several exogenous steroids in real samples, and can be considered the premise of a larger monitoring activity in order to obtain a robust statistical confirmation of our data, and evaluate the healthy effects of these species in the founded concentration levels. In addition, from the analytical point of view, the sample preparation is time-saving, fast and intuitive. With the proposed analytical method, it is possible to simultaneously monitor, quantify and qualify a large number of steroids presenting various steroid substructures in a short time (15 min chromatographic run) from blood samples. Moreover, the validation process demonstrated excellent performance regarding specificity, sensitivity (LOQ in the range of 0.069–5.5 ppb) and linearity. For the first time, a stability study of steroids was performed, revealing an interaction between our target analytes and the glassy wall of the storage container, then, the use of plastic materials is necessary for this purpose. The method was extended to detect most of the steroid esters in two animal species: horses and cattle. The results demonstrated the ruggedness of the method with respect to the biological variability of samples. The main steroids found in the four types of samples were cortisol, followed by corticosterone, androstenedione and dexamethasone isonicotinate. Androsterone and DHEA were not detected in any sample. In conclusion, the present method allows identification and quantification of steroids and performance increasing hormones, and it could be used when fraudulent use is suspected in racing animals, in an equine trade or to control the healthy state of these animals, including cattle.

Supplementary Materials: The following are available online at https://www.mdpi.com/article/10.3390/ph14050393/s1, Table S1: Intra-day and inter-day accuracy expressed in RE%, Table S2: Percent recovery and reproducibility at two fortification levels.

Author Contributions: Conceptualization, M.G., A.M.M. and M.R.; methodology, M.R., R.P. and M.C.; validation, M.G., A.M.M. and R.P.; investigation, M.G., G.C., F.L. and M.C.; resources, S.S. and S.V.; data curation, M.C. and A.M.M.; writing—original draft preparation, M.G., M.C. and A.M.M.; writing—review and editing, G.C. and M.C.; supervision, M.C. and G.S.; project administration, S.S. and S.V.; funding acquisition, S.V. and G.S. All authors have read and agreed to the published version of the manuscript.

Funding: This research received no external funding.

Institutional Review Board Statement: The study was approved from the Animal Welfare Body of the University of Camerino (project identification code: 1/2021, 2 April 2021).

Informed Consent Statement: Not applicable.

Data Availability Statement: Not applicable.

Conflicts of Interest: The authors declare no conflict of interest.

References

1. Genangeli, M.; Caprioli, G.; Cortese, M.; Laus, F.; Matteucci, M.; Petrelli, R.; Ricciutelli, M.; Sagratini, G.; Sartori, S.; Vittori, S. Development and application of a UHPLC-MS/MS method for the simultaneous determination of 17 steroidal hormones in equine serum. *J. Mass Spectrom.* **2017**, *52*, 22–29. [CrossRef]
2. Andrews, M.A.; Magee, C.D.; Combest, T.M.; Allard, R.J.; Douglas, K.M. Physical Effects of Anabolic-androgenic Steroids in Healthy Exercising Adults. *Curr. Sports Med. Rep.* **2018**, *17*, 232–241. [CrossRef] [PubMed]
3. Armstrong, J.M.; Avant, R.A.; Charchenko, C.M.; Westerman, M.E.; Ziegelmann, M.J.; Miest, T.S.; Trost, L.W. Impact of anabolic androgenic steroids on sexual function. *Transl. Androl. Urol.* **2018**, *7*, 483–489. [CrossRef] [PubMed]
4. Melo Junior, A.F.; Dalpiaz, P.L.M.; Sousa, G.J.; Oliveira, P.W.C.; Birocale, A.M.; Andrade, T.U.; Abreu, G.R.; Bissoli, N.S. Nandrolone alter left ventricular contractility and promotes remodelling involving calcium-handling proteins and renin-angiotensin system in male SHR. *Life Sci.* **2018**, *208*, 239–245. [CrossRef] [PubMed]

5. Büttler, R.M.; Martens, F.; Kushnir, M.M.; Ackermans, M.T.; Blankenstein, M.A.; Heijboer, A.C. Simultaneous measurement of testosterone, androstenedione and dehydroepiandrosterone (DHEA) in serum and plasma using Isotope-Dilution 2-Dimension Ultra High Performance Liquid-Chromatography Tandem Mass Spectrometry (ID-LC–MS/MS). *Clin. Chim. Acta* **2015**, *438*, 157–159. [CrossRef]
6. Wong, J.K.Y.; Wan, T.S.M. Doping control analyses in horseracing: A clinician's guide. *Vet. J.* **2014**, *200*, 8–16. [CrossRef]
7. IFHA. Available online: http://www.ifhaonline.org/default.asp?section=Racing&area=0#a6a (accessed on 25 March 2021).
8. Pellegrini, K.G.M.V. Anabolic Steroids. Available online: https://www.ncbi.nlm.nih.gov/books/NBK482418/#article-17499.s9 (accessed on 25 March 2021).
9. Caron, P.; Turcotte, V.; Guillemette, C. A chromatography/tandem mass spectrometry method for the simultaneous profiling of ten endogenous steroids, including progesterone, adrenal precursors, androgens and estrogens, using low serum volume. *Steroids* **2015**, *104*, 16–24. [CrossRef]
10. Görög, S. Recent Advances in the Analysis of Steroid Hormones and Related Drugs. *Anal. Sci.* **2004**, *20*, 767–782. [CrossRef]
11. Stanczyk, F.Z.; Jurow, J.; Hsing, A.W. Limitations of Direct Immunoassays for Measuring Circulating Estradiol Levels in Postmenopausal Women and Men in Epidemiologic Studies. *Cancer Epidemiol. Biomark. Prev.* **2010**, *19*, 903–906. [CrossRef] [PubMed]
12. Taieb, J. Testosterone Measured by 10 Immunoassays and by Isotope-Dilution Gas Chromatography-Mass Spectrometry in Sera from 116 Men, Women, and Children. *Clin. Chem.* **2003**, *49*, 1381–1395. [CrossRef] [PubMed]
13. Huang, X.; Yuan, D.; Huang, B. Determination of steroid sex hormones in urine matrix by stir bar sorptive extraction based on monolithic material and liquid chromatography with diode array detection. *Talanta* **2007**. [CrossRef] [PubMed]
14. He, G.; Wu, Y.; Lu, J. Doping control analysis of 13 steroids and structural-like analytes in human urine using Quadrupole-Orbitrap LC–MS/MS with parallel reaction monitoring (PRM) mode. *Steroids* **2018**, *131*, 1–6. [CrossRef] [PubMed]
15. Karatt, T.K.; Nalakath, J.; Perwad, Z.; Albert, P.H.; Abdul Khader, K.K.; Syed Ali Padusha, M.; Laya, S. Mass spectrometric method for distinguishing isomers of dexamethasone via fragment mass ratio: An HRMS approach. *J. Mass Spectrom.* **2018**, *53*, 1046–1058. [CrossRef]
16. Keevil, B.G. Novel liquid chromatography tandem mass spectrometry (LC-MS/MS) methods for measuring steroids. *Best Pract. Res. Clin. Endocrinol. Metab.* **2013**, *27*, 663–674. [CrossRef]
17. You, Y.; Uboh, C.E.; Soma, L.R.; Guan, F.; Li, X.; Liu, Y.; Rudy, J.A.; Chen, J.; Tsang, D. Simultaneous separation and determination of 16 testosterone and nandrolone esters in equine plasma using ultra high performance liquid chromatography–tandem mass spectrometry for doping control. *J. Chromatogr. A* **2011**, *1218*, 3982–3993. [CrossRef]
18. Wong, C.H.F.; Leung, D.K.K.; Tang, F.P.W.; Wong, J.K.Y.; Yu, N.H.; Wan, T.S.M. Rapid screening of anabolic steroids in horse urine with ultra-high-performance liquid chromatography/tandem mass spectrometry after chemical derivatisation. *J. Chromatogr. A* **2012**, *1232*, 257–265. [CrossRef] [PubMed]
19. Tuzimski, T.; Petruczynik, A. Review of Chromatographic Methods Coupled with Modern Detection Techniques Applied in the Therapeutic Drugs Monitoring (TDM). *Molecules* **2020**, *25*, 4026. [CrossRef] [PubMed]
20. Choi, T.L.S.; Kwok, K.Y.; Kwok, W.H.; Tsoi, Y.Y.K.; Wong, J.K.Y.; Wan, T.S.M. Detection of seventy-two anabolic and androgenic steroids and/or their esters in horse hair using ultra-high performance liquid chromatography-high resolution mass spectrometry in multiplexed targeted MS 2 mode and gas chromatography-tandem mass spectrometry. *J. Chromatogr. A* **2018**, *1566*, 51–63. [CrossRef] [PubMed]
21. Wong, J.K.Y.; Choi, T.L.S.; Kwok, K.Y.; Lei, E.N.Y.; Wan, T.S.M. Doping control analysis of 121 prohibited substances in equine hair by liquid chromatography–tandem mass spectrometry. *J. Pharm. Biomed. Anal.* **2018**, *158*, 189–203. [CrossRef] [PubMed]
22. Guan, F.; Uboh, C.E.; Soma, L.R.; Luo, Y.; Rudy, J.; Tobin, T. Detection, quantification and confirmation of anabolic steroids in equine plasma by liquid chromatography and tandem mass spectrometry. *J. Chromatogr. B* **2005**, *829*, 56–68. [CrossRef]
23. Hintikka, L. *Development of Mass Spectrometric Methods for Analysis of Anabolic Androgenic Steroids*; University of Helsinki: Helsinki, Finland, 2018.
24. Georgakopoulos, C.G.; Vonaparti, A.; Stamou, M.; Kiousi, P.; Lyris, E.; Angelis, Y.S.; Tsoupras, G.; Wuest, B.; Nielen, M.W.F.; Panderi, I.; et al. Preventive doping control analysis: Liquid and gas chromatography time-of-flight mass spectrometry for detection of designer steroids. *Rapid Commun. Mass Spectrom.* **2007**, *21*, 2439–2446. [CrossRef] [PubMed]
25. Gray, B.; Viljanto, M.; Menzies, E.; Vanhaecke, L. Detection of prohibited substances in equine hair by ultra-high performance liquid chromatography-triple quadrupole mass spectrometry-application to doping control samples. *Drug Test. Anal.* **2018**, *10*, 1050–1060. [CrossRef] [PubMed]
26. Kaabia, Z.; Dervilly-Pinel, G.; Hanganu, F.; Cesbron, N.; Bichon, E.; Popot, M.A.; Bonnaire, Y.; Le Bizec, B. Ultra high performance liquid chromatography/tandem mass spectrometry based identification of steroid esters in serum and plasma: An efficient strategy to detect natural steroids abuse in breeding and racing animals. *J. Chromatogr. A* **2013**, *1284*, 126–140. [CrossRef]
27. Annesley, T.M. Ion suppression in mass spectrometry. *Clin. Chem.* **2003**, *49*, 1041–1044. [CrossRef]
28. Harrison, A.G. *Chemical Ionization Mass Spectrometry*, 2nd ed.; CRC Press: Boca Raton, FL, USA, 1992; p. 208.
29. Shao, B.; Zhao, R.; Meng, J.; Xue, Y.; Wu, G.; Hu, J.; Tu, X. Simultaneous determination of residual hormonal chemicals in meat, kidney, liver tissues and milk by liquid chromatography–tandem mass spectrometry. *Anal. Chim. Acta* **2005**, *548*, 41–50. [CrossRef]

30. Yamashita, K.; Okuyama, M.; Nakagawa, R.; Honma, S.; Satoh, F.; Morimoto, R.; Ito, S.; Takahashi, M.; Numazawa, M. Development of sensitive derivatization method for aldosterone in liquid chromatography–electrospray ionization tandem mass spectrometry of corticosteroids. *J. Chromatogr. A* **2008**, *1200*, 114–121. [CrossRef]
31. Zuber, J.; Kroll, M.M.; Rathsack, P.; Otto, M. Gas Chromatography/Atmospheric Pressure Chemical Ionization-Fourier Transform Ion Cyclotron Resonance Mass Spectrometry of Pyrolysis Oil from German Brown Coal. *Int. J. Anal. Chem.* **2016**, *2016*, 5960916. [CrossRef]
32. You, Y.; Uboh, C.E.; Soma, L.R.; Guan, F.; Li, X.; Liu, Y.; Chen, J.; Tsang, D. Simultaneous Determination of Testosterone and Testosterone Enanthate in Equine Plasma by UHPLC-MS-MS. *Chromatographia* **2010**, *72*, 1097–1106. [CrossRef]
33. Prokai, L.; Stevens, S.M. Direct Analysis in Real Time (DART) of an Organothiophosphate at Ultrahigh Resolution by Fourier Transform Ion Cyclotron Resonance Mass Spectrometry and Tandem Mass Spectrometry. *Int. J. Mol. Sci.* **2016**, *17*, 116. [CrossRef] [PubMed]
34. Allis, O.; Dauphard, J.; Hamilton, B.; Ni Shuilleabhain, A.; Lehane, M.; James, K.J.; Furey, A. Liquid Chromatography−Tandem Mass Spectrometry Application, for the Determination of Extracellular Hepatotoxins in Irish Lake and Drinking Waters. *Anal. Chem.* **2007**, *79*, 3436–3447. [CrossRef]
35. Bonfiglio, R.; King, R.C.; Olah, T.V.; Merkle, K. The effects of sample preparation methods on the variability of the electrospray ionization response for model drug compounds. *Rapid Commun. Mass Spectrom.* **1999**, *13*, 1175–1185. [CrossRef]
36. Kaabia, Z.; Dervilly-Pinel, G.; Popot, M.A.; Bailly-Chouriberry, L.; Plou, P.; Bonnaire, Y.; Le Bizec, B. Monitoring the endogenous steroid profile disruption in urine and blood upon nandrolone administration: An efficient and innovative strategy to screen for nandrolone abuse in entire male horses. *Drug Test. Anal.* **2014**, *6*, 376–388. [CrossRef]
37. Available online: https://www.comsol.nl/multiphysics/the-joule-heating-effect (accessed on 25 March 2021).
38. Wang, Y.N.; Zhao, M.; Yu, Y.B.; Wang, M.; Zhao, C.J. Metabolic profile of Cortex Fraxini in rats using UHPLC combined with Fourier transform ion cyclotron resonance mass spectrometry. *RSC Adv.* **2016**, *6*, 39642–39651. [CrossRef]
39. Magnisali, P.; Dracopoulou, M.; Mataragas, M.; Dacou-Voutetakis, A.; Moutsatsou, P. Routine method for the simultaneous quantification of 17α-hydroxyprogesterone, testosterone, dehydroepiandrosterone, androstenedione, cortisol, and pregnenolone in human serum of neonates using gas chromatography–mass spectrometry. *J. Chromatogr. A* **2008**, *1206*, 166–177. [CrossRef] [PubMed]

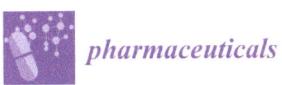

pharmaceuticals

Article

Development of a Rapid UHPLC-PDA Method for the Simultaneous Quantification of Flavonol Contents in Onions (*Allium cepa* L.)

Ana V. González-de-Peredo ⓘ, Mercedes Vázquez-Espinosa ⓘ, Ceferino Carrera ⓘ, Estrella Espada-Bellido ⓘ, Marta Ferreiro-González ⓘ, Gerardo F. Barbero *ⓘ and Miguel Palma ⓘ

Department of Analytical Chemistry, Faculty of Sciences, Agrifood Campus of International Excellence (ceiA3), University of Cadiz, IVAGRO, Puerto Real, 11510 Cadiz, Spain; ana.velascogope@uca.es (A.V.G.-d.-P.); mercedes.vazquez@uca.es (M.V.-E.); ceferino.carrera@uca.es (C.C.); estrella.espada@uca.es (E.E.-B.); marta.ferreiro@uca.es (M.F.-G.); miguel.palma@uca.es (M.P.)
* Correspondence: gerardo.fernandez@uca.es; Tel.: +34-956-01-6355

Citation: González-de-Peredo, A.V.; Vázquez-Espinosa, M.; Carrera, C.; Espada-Bellido, E.; Ferreiro-González, M.; F. Barbero, G.; Palma, M. Development of a Rapid UHPLC-PDA Method for the Simultaneous Quantification of Flavonol Contents in Onions (*Allium cepa* L.). *Pharmaceuticals* 2021, *14*, 310. https://doi.org/10.3390/ph14040310

Academic Editors: Sabina Lachowicz and Jan Oszmianski

Received: 6 March 2021
Accepted: 26 March 2021
Published: 1 April 2021

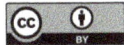
Abstract: Onion, one of the most consumed vegetables in the world, is also known to contain high levels of antioxidant compounds, with protective effects against different degenerative pathologies. Specifically, onion is rich in flavonols, mainly quercetin derivatives, which are compounds with high antioxidant and free radical scavenging power. For this reason, it is of the utmost importance to count on optimal analytical methods that allow for the determination and quantification of these compounds of interest. A rapid ultra-high performance liquid chromatography (UHPLC)-photo-diode array (PDA) method for the separation of the major flavonols in onions was developed using a Box–Behnken design in conjunction with multiresponse optimization on the basis of the desirability function. The conditions that provided a successful separation were 9.9% and 53.2% of phase B at the beginning and at the end of the gradient, respectively; 55 °C column working temperature; and 0.6 mL min^{-1} flow rate. The complete separation was achieved in less than 2.7 min with excellent chromatographic characteristics. The method was validated, and its high precision, low detection and quantification limits, good linearity, and robustness were confirmed. The correct applicability of the method improves the analysis of the raw material, increasing the quality of onions and its subproducts in terms of bioactive compounds and functional characteristics for consumers.

Keywords: *Allium cepa* L.; Box–Behnken; flavonoids; quercetin glycosides; liquid chromatography; multiresponse optimization; onion; phenolic compounds; UHPLC

1. Introduction

Onion (*Allium cepa* L.) is one of the most widely grown and consumed vegetables in the world [1]. This vegetable has shown a constant increasing production trend by more than 25% in the past few years [2]. Onion's pungent and unique taste makes it an ideal food condiment that is highly appreciated by consumers, favoring its trend increase. However, this increasing production tendency is also supported by the current awareness by consumers of its high content in non-nutrient bioactive compounds with preventive properties against some degenerative pathologies [3,4]. Specifically, onion presents antimicrobial, antioxidant, anticarcinogenic, antimutagenic, antiasthmatic, immunomodulatory, and cardiovascular properties [5,6]. The flavonols present in onions are some of the main contributors to these health-promoting properties. Every single type of onion (white, yellow, or red) is rich in flavonols, mainly quercetin derivatives, being recognized as one of the major dietary sources for quercetin [7]. Quercetin is a very interesting flavonol because of its antioxidant and free radical scavenging power, which gives onions their ability to protect against multiple diseases [8]. It should be highlighted that a recent research study has identified the natural compound quercetin as an inhibitor of severe acute respiratory syndrome coronavirus (SARS-CoV-2 3CLpro), one of the essential proteases for the replication of the coronavirus known as COVID-19 [9]. Specifically, quercetin has shown plenty of desirable characteristics and potential (inhibition constant Ki ~ 7 μM), allowing it to be considered an attractive candidate for further optimization and development in this field. With regards to onions, quercetin 3,4′-O-diglucoside and quercetin 4′-O-glucoside are the primary glucosides found in onion bulbs [10] since they account for about 95–99% of their total flavonol content [11]. The structures of these two particular flavonols and the rest of the flavonols present in onions can be referred to in Figure S1. A detailed analysis of these compounds is of great interest since it would allow for the evaluation of this vegetable's metabolomic profile. For this reason, it is of the utmost importance to count on optimal analytical methods that allow for the determination and quantification of these compounds of interest. Different techniques have been primarily employed for the determination of flavonols in onions. The analytical platform of choice for this study was ultra-high performance liquid chromatography (UHPLC) coupled to a photo-diode array (PDA). UHPLC represents a further advance in chromatographic techniques with additional advantages such as high-resolution separations using under 2 μm diameter solid-phase particles [12]. This implies high resolution and sensitivity in extremely short run times and, therefore, a lower cost on solvents [13]. Thus, UHPLC stands at a leading position for the analysis of phenolic compounds, and it has been widely used in numerous research studies on the phenolic contents that can be found in numerous natural matrices [14]. Regarding the detectors, as aforementioned, in this study, UHPLC system was coupled to a photo-diode array (PDA). PDA is one of the most commonly used detectors because of the wide range of molecules that can be analyzed, its relatively low price, and its availability in most food analysis laboratories. Specially this work wants to highlight the importance of using the PDA as an affordable detector for laboratories and food and quality industries. Most articles found in the literature use UHPLC coupled to mass spectrometry [15,16]. Mass spectrometry presents some substantial advantages, such as very high sensitivity and data collection on molecular mass and structural characteristics, but it is not always available to research groups or company laboratories in general because of its high costs. Furthermore, chromatographic methods that can be found in the literature require over 30 min to complete the successful separation of all the peaks [10,17,18]. In this work, the aim was to achieve the analysis of the main compounds of interest in minimum times, less than 5 min, separations that are difficult to achieve with mass spectrometry. This time reduction is an essential factor for any analysis procedure, and it is particularly interesting when intended to be used at an industrial scale, where time is critical.

According to some of the previous works published by our own research group [19,20], the use of UHPLC, without mass spectrometry and combined with a correct optimization of the chromatographic characteristics (solvent flow, gradient, etc.), allows for a successful analysis in a considerably shorter time. Analysis time and peak resolution are the two most important aspects to be taken into consideration for the optimization of a chromatographic method [14]. Both parameters depend mainly on gradient time and flow rate, and thus their influence on a successful separation is generally evaluated. In this work, it is intended to make use of the experiment designs combined with UHPLC for the study of flavonols in onion. Response surface methodology (RSM) is an excellent tool for studying and optimizing these variables. The use of RSM represents further advantages compared to conventional optimization methods in which only one variable is studied at the same time. Specifically, RSM allows for studying several variables and knowing both their individual and combined effect on the response variable, without the need to carry out a large number of experiments. This makes it a very useful tool without the need to involve high manufacturing costs [21]. Among the different RSM options, the Box–Behnken design (BBD) is often used for the statistics study, since a shorter number of runs is required when compared to other methodologies. This design saves time and avoids running experiments under extreme conditions, which might pose undesirable risks with regards to the reliability of the results. On the other hand, when the optimization procedure involves more than one response, each one of them cannot be optimized separately, since a number of solutions equal to the number of variables under study would be generated [20]. In such cases, a multiresponse optimization (MRO) with desirability functions is usually employed, which has been proven to be an effective statistical tool to solve multi-variable problems and to optimize either single or multiple responses [22]. Specifically, it has been proved to be useful for developing, improving, and optimizing processes, which was the objective of this study.

Therefore, the present work intended to develop and validate a rapid and reliable UHPLC-PDA methodology for the simultaneous separation of the flavonols present in onions by means of a BBD in conjunction with MRO and desirability functions. This method would allow laboratories, researchers, and companies to analyze the main flavonols found in onions without having to use mass spectrometry, doing so in a short time. A successful applicability of this methodology would improve analysis procedures and, therefore, would also favor the final quality of onions and their subproducts.

2. Results and Discussion

2.1. UHPLC Acquisition of the Responses

A BBD design was employed to determine the effect of three factors (the three independent variables) on the UHPLC-PDA separation. The factors studied were flow rate (X_1), solvent composition (% phase B) at the beginning of the gradient program (X_2), and solvent composition (% phase B) at the end of the gradient program (X_3). Specifically, the conditions studied for each variable were flow rate (mL min^{-1}): 0.4, 0.5, 0.6; %B at the beginning (%): 0, 5, 10; and %B at the end of the gradient program (%): 50, 75, 100. The onion extract was injected into the UHPLC system according to the BBD experiments (Table 1). The 15 experiments were carried out independent and randomly, while the values of the independent variables were the only variations between each other.

Table 1. Box–Behnken design matrix and experimental values obtained for resolutions and run time.

Run	Factors			Responses				
	X_1	X_2	X_3	Rs$_{3-4}$	Rs$_{4-5}$	Rs$_{5-6}$	Rs$_{6-7}$	Run Time (min)
1	0	0	0	1.50	3.62	3.34	1.74	2.761
2	1	0	1	1.22	3.68	2.72	1.31	2.326
3	0	0	0	1.77	4.53	4.10	2.02	2.775
4	0	−1	1	1.08	2.46	2.12	1.22	2.658
5	−1	0	−1	2.01	3.93	3.68	2.20	3.574
6	−1	0	1	1.00	2.83	2.79	1.27	2.659
7	0	1	1	1.18	3.53	3.08	1.47	2.210
8	0	0	0	1.36	3.62	2.89	1.41	2.759
9	0	1	−1	2.35	5.40	4.81	2.83	2.924
10	1	−1	0	1.25	3.60	3.49	1.75	2.892
11	0	−1	−1	1.80	3.88	4.01	2.35	3.699
12	−1	−1	0	1.13	3.38	3.05	1.61	3.242
13	−1	1	0	1.49	3.76	3.01	1.58	2.705
14	1	1	0	1.82	4.30	3.63	1.88	2.298
15	1	0	−1	2.02	4.33	4.91	2.92	3.199

With respect to the response variables (dependent variables), these were optimized according to the peak resolutions (Y_{Rs}), and the analyses run times (Y_{RT}). Resolution (R_S) is a numeric value that indicates how much a peak overlaps the adjacent peak from a perpendicular line crossing the trough. Most studies set a minimum resolution target of around 1.5 for a complete peak separation [23]. Resolution values of 1 imply a 4% overlap between the two adjacent peaks, while values of 1.5 result in an overlap of only 0.3%. Any value lower than 1 indicates a poor separation. In addition to the R_S, analysis run time (RT) was also considered as a variable response for the method optimization. This variable is related to the retention time of the final peak in the UHPLC chromatogram. Therefore, the final objective of the experimental design was to achieve maximum resolutions that did not imply exceedingly long analysis times. Among the seven major flavonols identified in the onion, quercetin 3,7,4'-O-triglucoside (peak 1) and quercetin 7,4'-O-diglucoside (peak 2) were discarded for the experimental design, since their peaks presented short retention times and therefore did not influence the analysis run time while achieving excellent separation in the 15 experiments that were carried out. Consequently, the resolutions of each one of the five major peaks identified (peak 3, peak 4, peak 5, peak 6, and peak 7) were considered for response variable optimization purposes. In particular, the four R_S values in this category were R_{S3-4}, R_{S4-5}, R_{S5-6}, and R_{S6-7}. The number corresponds to the elution order of the compounds in the column. The resolutions and the analysis run time resulting from each BBD experiment are shown in Table 1.

2.2. Optimization of the UHPLC Method

The MRO was used to determine the optimum chromatographic conditions for all the responses at the same time. Specifically, the effect of the three chromatographic working variables on the five responses were evaluated. Previous to this MRO, a RSM was employed to generate a separate model for each response. Then, the desirability function was constructed on the basis of the values obtained for each optimized response.

A total of five second-order mathematical models that represent the correlation between each independent variable and each response were generated. The resulting equations (Equations (1)–(5)) for the fitted models are as follows:

$$Y_{Rs3-4} = 1.56667 + 0.075X_1 + 0.2125X_2 - 0.4625X_3 - 0.120833X_1{}^2 + 0.05X_1X_2 \\ + 0.05X_1X_3 - 0.045833X_2{}^2 - 0.125X_2X_3 + 0.104167X_3{}^2 \tag{1}$$

$$Y_{Rs4-5} = 3.9 + 0.25X_1 + 0.45X_2 - 0.625X_3 - 0.1375X_1{}^2 + 0.075X_1X_2 + 0.125X_1X_3 \\ + 0.0125X_2{}^2 - 0.125X_2X_3 - 0.0875X_3{}^2 \tag{2}$$

$$Y_{Rs5-6} = 3.43333 + 0.275X_1 + 0.2375X_2 - 0.8375X_3 - 0.0666667X_1{}^2 + 0.025X_1X_2 \\ - 0.325X_1X_3 - 0.0916667X_2{}^2 + 0.05X_2X_3 + 0.158333\,X_3{}^2 \tag{3}$$

$$Y_{Rs6-7} = 1.7 + 0.15X_1 + 0.1125X_2 - 0.6125X_3 + 0.0X_1{}^2 + 0.025X_1X_2 - 0.175X_1X_3 \\ + 0.025X_2{}^2 - 0.05X_2X_3 + 0.225X_3{}^2 \tag{4}$$

$$Y_{RT} = 2.765 - 0.183125X_1 - 0.29425X_2 - 0.442875X_3 + 0.043X_1{}^2 - 0.01425X_1X_2 \\ + 0.0105X_1X_3 - 0.02375X_2{}^2 + 0.08175X_2X_3 + 0.1315X_3{}^2 \tag{5}$$

The different polynomial equations can be used to know what the value of the response variable will be if the value of the dependent variables is known. The greater the efficiency of these equations, the higher the correlation coefficient (R^2). The coefficients obtained ranged from 82.68% for R_{S4-5} to 99.94% for run time, which indicate a statistically significant agreement between the measured and the estimated responses.

An analysis of variance (ANOVA) was individually applied to evaluate the effect of the different factors on each response and the possible interactions between them. The factors and/or interactions that showed a p-value lower than 0.05 were considered to be significant factors with an influence on the response at the established level of significance (95%). With regards to the resolutions, all the responses showed p-values lower than 0.05 for percentage of phase B at the beginning of the gradient, which indicates that this factor had a significant effect on all the resolution responses. In particular, this factor had a negative effect, which means that the peak resolutions increased with a low %B at the beginning of the gradient. On the other hand, the percentage of phase B at the end of the gradient presented a positive relevant effect on both R_{S3-4} and R_{S4-5}, with a p-value < 0.05. With regard to the analysis run time, the three factors (flow rate, %B at the beginning, and %B at the end) had *p*-values lower than 0.05. The optimization target for this response variable was to minimize the analysis run time. In this sense, and on the basis of the ANOVA results, we concluded that in order to minimize the analysis time, a greater flow rate, a greater %B at the beginning of the gradient, and a greater %B at the end of the gradient, were necessary. Therefore, a high %B at the end of the gradient and a high flow rate favored the separation of the peaks and decreased the analysis time. On the other hand, the %B at the beginning had the opposite effect on the resolutions and run times. Such an opposite trend can be graphically observed in the three-dimensional (3D) surface plots that have been generated from the fitted model. The combined effects of %B at the end-%B at the beginning on the run time and R_{S1-2} are represented in Figure 1.

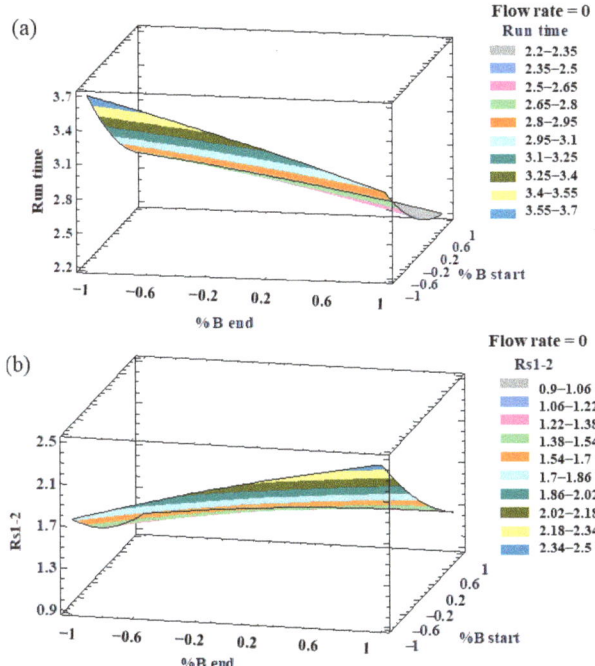

Figure 1. 3D surface plots of the Box–Behnken design to represent the influence of (**a**) %B at the end of the gradient–%B at the beginning of the gradient on the run time; (**b**) %B at the end of the gradient–%B at the beginning of the gradient on the resolution of peaks 1 and 2 (R_{S1-2}).

Subsequently, the MRO was used for the simultaneous optimization of the six responses. All the responses were considered to be equally important chromatographic characteristics for the separation and determination of the flavonols. The weight of each response in the computational analysis was determined by the impact coefficient that had been assigned to each response by the MRO. The run times obtained in the 15 BBD experiments varied between 2.210 and 3.699 min. This run time range was considered as acceptable for rapid separations, especially when compared to the analysis run times of the UHPLC methods for onion flavonols published in the literature. Although some methods require a time as relatively short as 15 min [24,25], most of them require at least 30 min to complete the correct separation of all the peaks [6,11], and some of them may even need as much as 60 min [17,18]. However, the impact for this variable was set to the highest relevance (5 impact), since one of the main objectives of this work was to develop a time-and-cost-saving multiple analysis UHPLC methodology. With regards to the resolutions, all the R_{S4-5} (ranging from 2.46 to 5.40) and R_{S5-6} (ranging from 2.12 to

4.91) obtained from the 15 BBD experiments were higher than 1.5, which is the minimum resolution required for a successful and complete separation. Therefore, the impact of these variables was set as lower importance (3 impact). Finally, R_{S3-4} (ranging from 1.00 to 2.35) and R_{S6-7} (ranging from 1.22 to 2.92) with resolutions under 1.5 in some of the BBD experiments were set at an intermediate relevance level (4 impact). Thus, the optimization defined by MRO was to maximize the resolution and minimize the run time.

From the MRO design, it was possible to extract information about the optimum values which show the maximum response for all the variables, that is, optimize the desirability function. Therefore, according to the MRO, the optimal values for the studied variables were as follows: 9.9% for %B at the beginning of the gradient, 53.2% for %B at the end of the gradient, and 0.6 mL min^{-1} for the flow rate. With regards to the flow rate, no higher flows were tested since they would imply really high pressure within the system. Thus, the maximum flow rate was restricted by the system pressure limit at 15,000 psi. The analysis time between the beginning of the gradient and the end of the gradient was 5 min. With these settings, the response variables generated a desirability index of 86.48%. For comparative purposes, Figure 2a,b shows the chromatograms obtained under a series of other conditions according to the BBD experiments.

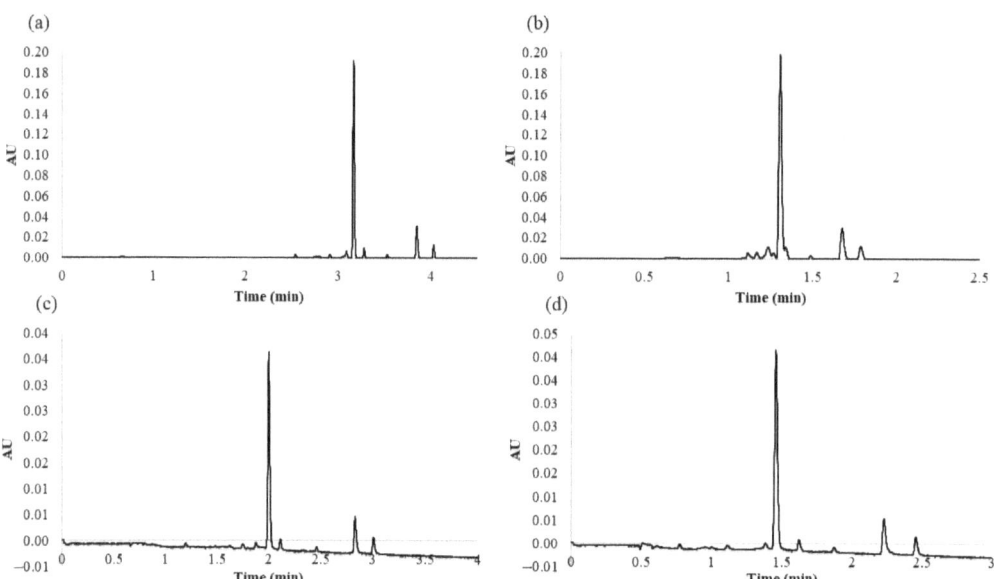

Figure 2. Different chromatograms obtained under different conditions: (**a**) chromatogram obtained from the 2° Box–Behnken design (BBD) experiment (analysis time longer than the established optimal conditions); (**b**) chromatogram obtained from the 11° BBD experiment (overlapping peaks); (**c**) chromatogram obtained at the lowest temperature, 35 °C (analysis times longer than the established optimal conditions); (**d**) chromatogram obtained at the highest temperature, 65 °C (poorer resolution than under the established optimal conditions).

Once the MRO had been performed, the desirability was plotted as a 3D contour plot that illustrates the result of the optimization of all the variables. The combined effects of %B at the beginning–%B at the end, %B at the start-flow rate, and %B at the end-flow rate are represented in Figure 3.

Once MRO had been applied, the effect that the column temperature had on the separation of the flavonols was also evaluated. For this purpose, and on the basis of the principles of column temperature changes, we gradually increased the temperature from 35 to 65 °C in 5 °C intervals in order to evaluate the effect of different column temperatures. Higher temperatures beyond the above-mentioned range were not tested, since according to Waters Corporation's recommendation, it may result in a shorter column lifetime. To compare the effect of the temperature on the separation of the five major compounds identified in the onion matrices, we evaluated peak resolution and analysis time. As the temperature was increased, the analysis time decreased. Higher temperatures had a positive effect, since they reduced the viscosity of the mobile phase, which in turn decreased column pressure and the compounds eluted at a greater speed (temperature (°C), t_R (min): 35, 3.01; 40, 2.92; 45, 2.83; 50, 2.71; 55, 2.65; 60, 2.54; 65, 2.46). These results confirmed that the method was more efficient at the highest temperatures within the studied range (55, 60, and 65 °C). Among these temperatures, 55 °C seemed to provide the best results in the separation of the seven major compounds identified in the red onion samples, since it resulted in narrow and very well resolved peaks in a very short run analysis time. At 60 and 65 °C, most of the peak chromatogram resolutions decreased (temperature (°C), resolution (R_{S4-5}): 55, 5.29; 60, 4; 65, 4.19); (temperature (°C), resolution (R_{S5-6}): 55, 5.36; 60, 4.28; 65, 4.83) due to the shortening of the total run analysis time. The chromatograms obtained at the lowest (35 °C) and highest (65 °C) temperatures within the range are shown in Figure 2c,d, respectively, to clearly observe the results previously described.

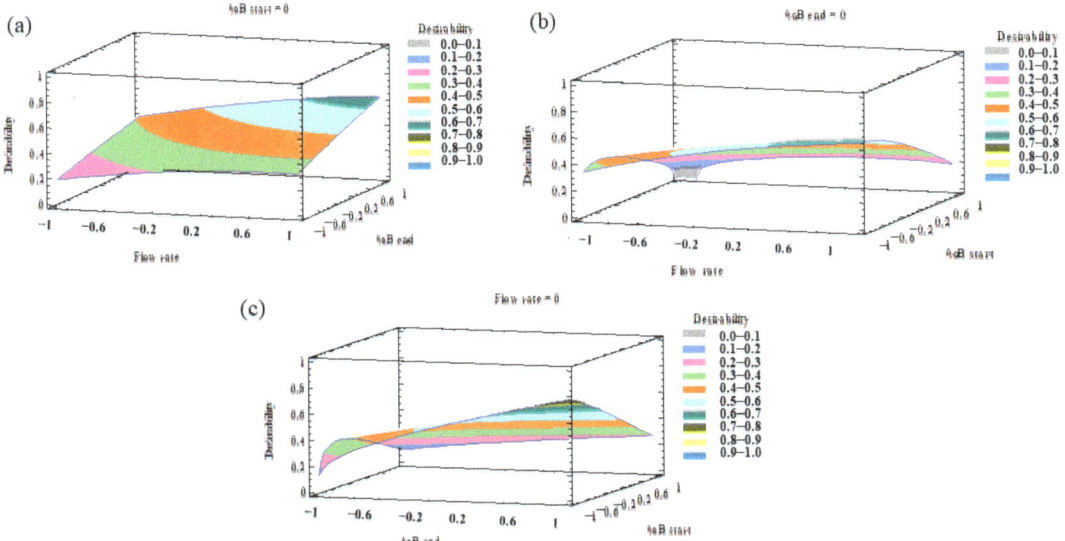

Figure 3. 3D surface plots of the multiresponse optimization (MRO) design representing the influence on the desirability function by (**a**) flow rate–%B at the end; (**b**) flow rate–%B at the beginning; (**c**) %B at the end–%B at the beginning.

2.3. Characteristics of the Developed Method

Finally, the optimum gradient of the UHPLC-PDA method developed in this study was as follows: 0.0 min, 9.9% B; 5.0 min, 53.2% B; 5.10 min, 100% B; 7.0 min, 100% B; 7.5 min, 9.9% B; 10 min, 9.9% B. The column temperature was maintained at 55 °C and the flow rate was 0.6 mL min^{-1}. The total analysis time (sample-to-sample) was 10.0 min, including the return to the initial conditions and the re-equilibration of the column, while the separation of the seven major compounds was completed in less than 2.7 min. A representative chromatogram employing PDA (λ = 360 nm) is presented in Figure 4.

It can be seen from the results that the compounds were correctly separated, with narrow peaks in a very short time. Thus, the selected conditions provided the best balance between reduced analysis time and successful separation of the seven peaks. Although there were articles in the bibliography that identified a greater number of compounds in onion, this work focused on the analysis of the seven onion flavonol majority. Only quercetin 3,4′-*O*-diglucoside and quercetin 4′-*O*-glucoside represented around 95–99% of the total flavonol content. This work aimed to provide an analytical utility for industries, wherein analyzing in less than 3 min the almost total percentage of flavonols is of greater interest than the analysis of minorities (<10%).

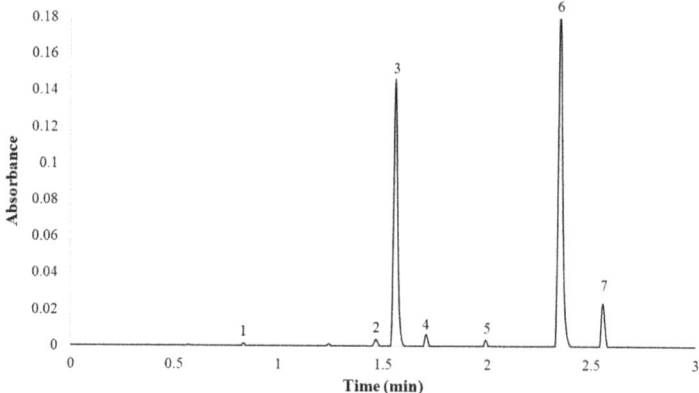

Figure 4. Red onion chromatogram at 360 nm. (1) Quercetin 3,7,4′-*O*-triglucoside; (2) quercetin 7,4′-*O*-diglucoside; (3) quercetin 3,4′-*O*-diglucoside; (4) isorhamnetin 3,4′-*O*-diglucoside; (5) quercetin 3-*O*-glucoside; (6) quercetin 4′-*O*-glucoside; (7) isorhamnetin 4′-*O*-glucoside.

The chromatographic properties evaluated were retention time (t_R), selectivity (α), retention factor (k), and resolution (Rs). The chromatographic properties obtained with the developed method are shown in Table 2.

Table 2. Chromatographic properties of the developed ultra-high performance liquid chromatography (UHPLC) method for flavonols in onions.

Peak	Compounds	t_R (min)	Width (W_b)	t'_R	Retention Factor (k)	Selectivity (α)	Resolution (R_s)
1	Quercetin 7,3,4′-*O*-triglucoside	0.945	2.85	0.448	1.36	-	-
2	Quercetin 7,4′-*O*-diglucoside	1.478	3.45	1.084	2.69	1.98	7.69
3	Quercetin 3,4′-*O*-diglucoside	1.688	4.10	1.174	3.22	1.19	2.15
4	Isorhamnetin 3,4′-*O*-diglucoside	1.835	2.40	1.315	3.59	1.11	1.93
5	Quercetin 3′-*O*-glucoside	2.119	2.55	1.599	4.30	1.20	4.56
6	Quercetin 4′-*O*-glucoside	2.478	5.65	1.951	5.19	1.21	3.68
7	Isorhamnetin 4′-*O*-glucoside	2.693	3.35	2.157	5.73	1.10	2.23

On the basis of the results obtained, we were able to conclude that the developed UHPLC method provides a successful separation of the chromatographic peaks with excellent resolutions, retention factors, and selectivities. Regarding the resolutions, all the values obtained were higher than 1.5, which implies an overlap of the peaks lower than 0.3%. With regards to the retention factor (k), $1 < k < 10$ is usually the target range [26]. The retention factor is a measure of the time that a compound remains in the stationary phase relative to the time that it remains in the mobile phase. Therefore, values greater than 10 do not imply a significant resolution increment but lead to excessively long retention times. Values significantly lower than 1 indicate that the analyte leaves the column when close to the dead time. In the case of this work, all the retention factor values were within the target range. Finally, in relation to selectivity, $\alpha > 1$ is usually the target range. A high α value indicates a clear separation between the peaks. In the case of this work, all the selectivity values were greater than 1.

2.4. Validation of the Developed Method

The developed method was validated in accordance with ICH Guideline Q2 (R1) [27]. Linearity, precision, limit of detection, and quantification as well as robustness were evaluated. The validation results are reported in Tables 3 and 4.

Table 3. Validation of the developed UHPLC method.

Peak	Compounds	Linear Equation	R^2	LOD (mg L^{-1})	LOQ (mg L^{-1})	CV [1] for Repeatability (%)		CV [1] for Intermediate Precision (%)	
						t_R	Rs	t_R	Rs
1	Quercetin 7,3,4'-O-triglucoside	y = 5069.90x + 8282.83	0.9997	0.0437	0.1454	2.33	-	2.80	-
2	Quercetin 7,4'-O-diglucoside	y = 6382.50x + 8282.83	0.9997	0.0347	0.1155	1.20	1.88	1.93	4.13
3	Quercetin 3,4'-O-diglucoside	y = 6382.52x + 8282.83	0.9997	0.0347	0.1155	1.17	3.89	1.91	4.59
4	Isorhamnetin 3,4'-O-diglucoside	y = 6247.89x + 8282.83	0.9997	0.0354	0.1181	0.95	2.52	1.76	2.72
5	Quercetin 3'-O-glucoside	y = 8610.35x + 8282.83	0.9997	0.0257	0.0857	0.96	4.88	1.70	4.90
6	Quercetin 4'-O-glucoside	y = 8610.35x + 8282.83	0.9997	0.0257	0.0857	0.88	1.53	3.17	3.65
7	Isorhamnetin 4'-O-glucoside	y = 8358.38x + 8282.83	0.9997	0.0265	0.0883	0.78	4.14	1.39	4.03

[1] CV: coefficient of variation.

Table 4. Robustness of the UHPLC method developed.

		Column Temperatures (°C)			Flow Rates (mL min^{-1})			Injection Volumes (μL)		
		52	55	58	0.57	0.60	0.63	2.8	3.0	3.2
Retention time (min)	Quercetin 7,3,4'-O-triglucoside	1.026 [a]	0.945 [b]	0.882 [c]	1.026 [a]	0.945 [b]	0.912 [c]	0.955 [a]	0.945 [a]	0.929 [a]
	Quercetin 7,4'-O-diglucoside	1.501 [a]	1.477 [a]	1.497 [a]	1.590 [a]	1.477 [b]	1.540 [b]	1.530 [a]	1.477 [a]	1.559 [a]
	Quercetin 3,4'-O-diglucoside	1.797 [a]	1.687 [b]	1.679 [b]	1.748 [a]	1.687 [b]	1.627 [c]	1.694 [a]	1.687 [a]	1.674 [a]
	Isorhamnetin 3,4'-O-diglucoside	1.936 [a]	1.835 [b]	1.804 [b]	1.887 [a]	1.835 [b]	1.775 [c]	1.839 [a]	1.835 [a]	1.823 [a]
	Quercetin 3'-O-glucoside	2.231 [a]	2.119 [b]	2.002 [c]	2.161 [a]	2.119 [b]	2.056 [c]	2.126 [a]	2.119 [a]	2.111 [a]
	Quercetin 4'-O-glucoside	2.591 [a]	2.478 [b]	2.357 [c]	2.512 [a]	2.478 [a]	2.417 [b]	2.484 [a]	2.478 [a,b]	2.471 [b]
	Isorhamnetin 4'-O-glucoside	2.797 [a]	2.693 [a]	2.574 [b]	2.721 [a]	2.692 [b]	2.633 [c]	2.697 [a]	2.693 [a,b]	2.683 [b]
Peak area	Quercetin 7,3,4'-O-triglucoside	1584 [a]	1749 [a]	1992 [a]	1815 [a]	1749 [a]	1846 [a]	1493 [a]	1749 [a]	2270 [b]
	Quercetin 7,4'-O-diglucoside	4073 [a]	4459 [a]	5070 [a]	5733 [a]	4459 [a]	5004 [a]	3246 [b]	4459 [a,b]	5251 [b]
	Quercetin 3,4'-O-diglucoside	104,048 [a]	112,705 [a]	123,675 [a]	123,884 [a]	112,705 [a]	122,463 [a]	88,187 [a]	112,705 [a]	140,119 [b]
	Isorhamnetin 3,4'-O-diglucoside	5073 [a]	5245 [a]	5931 [a]	5892 [a]	5245 [a]	5800 [a]	4233 [a]	5245 [a]	6905 [b]
	Quercetin 3'-O-glucoside	5045 [a]	4899 [a]	5396 [a]	5330 [a]	4899 [a]	5448 [a]	4015 [a]	4899 [a,b]	5811 [b]
	Quercetin 4'-O-glucoside	151,175 [a]	162,031 [a]	178,379 [a]	175,285 [a]	159,754 [a]	173,719 [a]	130,086 [a]	165,384 [a]	198,383 [b]
	Isorhamnetin 4'-O-glucoside	18,933 [a]	20,539 [a]	22,383 [a]	22,187 [a]	20,539 [a]	21,882 [a]	16,308 [a]	20,539 [a]	25,220 [b]

Table 4. *Cont.*

		Column Temperatures (°C)			Flow Rates (mL min⁻¹)			Injection Volumes (μL)		
Peak resolution	Quercetin 7,3,4′-O-triglucoside	-	-	-	-	-	-	-	-	-
	Quercetin 7,4′-O-diglucoside	6.22 [a]	7.69 [a]	6.94 [a]	6.95 [a]	7.69 [a]	7.68 [a]	7.62 [a]	7.69 [a]	8.15 [a]
	Quercetin 3,4′-O-diglucoside	2.89 [a]	2.15 [a,b]	1.6 [b]	1.62 [a]	2.15 [a]	0.810 [b]	1.80 [a]	2.15 [b]	1.20 [a]
	Isorhamnetin 3,4′-O-diglucoside	1.92 [a]	1.93 [a]	1.59 [a]	2.09 [a]	1.93 [a]	1.95 [a]	2.10 [a]	1.93 [a]	1.94 [a]
	Quercetin 3′-O-glucoside	4.54 [a]	4.56 [a]	2.9 [b]	4.60 [a]	4.72 [a]	4.56 [a]	4.48 [a]	4.56 [a]	4.44 [a]
	Quercetin 4′-O-glucoside	3.30 [a]	3.68 [a]	3.47 [a]	3.70 [a]	3.67 [a]	3.68 [a]	3.43 [a]	3.68 [a]	3.82 [a]
	Isorhamnetin 4′-O-glucoside	1.87 [a]	2.23 [b]	2.11 [a,b]	2.14 [a]	2.23 [a]	2.15 [a]	2.10 [a]	2.23 [a]	2.16 [a]

Same letter in the same row means that there were no significant differences as per the *t*-test ($p < 0.05$).

The linearity of the method was confirmed by the regression coefficient for quercetin 3-O-glucoside (r = 0.9997), which was obtained from the calibration curve of the commercially available standard constructed using six points (0.1–200 mg L⁻¹) in triplicate. The calibration curves for the rest of the compounds were estimated on the basis of the curve for quercetin 3-O-glucoside and each compound's molecular mass ratio and assuming that the seven flavonols have similar absorbance because of their similar chemical structures. This is a usual quantification procedure when the standard for any of the compounds of interest is not commercially available [14]. The R^2 showed values close to 1, which indicates that all the compounds identified in the onion matrices presented a good linearity within the target range (Table 3).

The repeatability and intermediate precision of the developed methodology were determined according to both retention time and chromatographic resolution. With respect to retention time, its repeatability and intermediate precision showed coefficients of variance (CV) lower than 3% for all the peaks. With regards to resolution, its repeatability and intermediate precision resulted in coefficients of variance (CV) lower than 5% for all the peaks (Table 3). It can be confirmed that in all the cases the CVs were within the acceptable limits (±10%) according to Association of Official Agricultural Chemists (AOAC) [28], and therefore support the accuracy of the developed UHPLC methodology.

The limit of detection (LOD) and limit of quantification (LOQ) for quercetin 3-O-glucoside were estimated as 3 and 10 times the signal-to-noise ratio, respectively. The LODs and LOQs of the rest of the compounds were calculated according to the corresponding values for quercetin 3-O-glucoside as well as each compound's molecular mass ratio. The LODs ranged from 0.0257 to 0.0437 mg L⁻¹ and the LOQs ranged from 0.0857 to 0.1454 mg L⁻¹ (Table 3).

Finally, the robustness of the method (Table 4) was evaluated by testing specific variations in flow rates, injection volumes, and column temperatures. Each parameter was tested at three different levels, and for each level, four repetitions were carried out. The effect of these variations on the retention times, the chromatographic resolution of the peaks, and the area of the chromatographic peaks were verified. The robustness results are reported in Table 4, where different letters (a, b, and c) in the same row indicate that significant differences were detected according to the *t*-test assuming equivalent variances (*p*-value < 0.05). No significant differences (*p*-values > 0.05) were found between the peak resolutions and areas resulting from the controlled variations, which allowed us to conclude that the controlled variations in temperature, flow rate, or injection volume did not give place to any relevant influences on peak resolution or area. The methodology was also proven to be robust ($p > 0.05$) with regards to retention time when the injection volume was varied. However, some of the compounds' retention times presented statistically relevant differences when the flow rate or the temperature were modified. This was to be expected, since retention time depends not only on the polarity of the specific molecule, but also on factors such as flow rate and temperature. For example, at a higher flow rate, the component molecules had less time to interact with the stationary phase as they were quickly pushed through the column. It is, therefore, necessary to keep an adequate control of the flow rate and the temperature by a proper balancing and conditioning of the equipment to provide an accurate resolution and a clear separation of the flavonols' peaks.

2.5. Application of the Developed Method to Different Onion Varieties

Once the UHPLC-PDA method for the analysis of flavonols in red onion had been optimized, an additional study was carried out to determine the flavonol content in different types of onions. This should demonstrate the applicability of the method to the analysis of different onions with different chemical compositions. Specifically, 13 onion varieties were studied: 6 white onions, 3 yellow onions, and 4 red onions. The results of the analyses are shown in Table 5 and the chromatograms obtained for a yellow, a red, and a white variety are also shown in Figure 5.

Table 5. Quantification of flavonols in white, yellow, and red onion varieties.

	Flavonol Composition (mg/10 g DW) [1]							
	Quercetin 7,3,4'-O-triglucoside	Quercetin 7,4'-O-diglucoside	Quercetin 3,4'-O-diglucoside	Isorhamnetin 3,4'-O-diglucoside	Quercetin 3'-O-glucoside	Quercetin 4'-O-glucoside	Isorhamnetin 4'-O-glucoside	Total
Spring white onion 1	0.09 ± 0.00	0.62 ± 0.00	14.31 ± 0.19	0.56 ± 0.00	0.56 ± 0.00	11.74 ± 0.14	1.11 ± 0.02	28.98
Sweet white onion 2	0.08 ± 0.01	0.12 ± 0.00	5.61 ± 0.06	0.23 ± 0.00	0.43 ± 0.02	2.50 ± 0.07	0.20 ± 0.00	9.17
Spring white onion 3	0.15 ± 0.00	0.51 ± 0.00	9.17 ± 0.06	0.48 ± 0.01	0.47 ± 0.00	7.36 ± 0.04	0.73 ± 0.01	18.88
Sweet white onion 4	0.11 ± 0.00	0.11 ± 0.03	5.58 ± 0.22	0.25 ± 0.00	3.77 ± 0.00	1.03 ± 0.10	0.40 ± 0.02	11.23
Sweet white onion 5	0.06 ± 0.03	0.12 ± 0.02	8.41 ± 0.15	0.12 ± 0.01	0.45 ± 0.00	9.42 ± 0.09	0.84 ± 0.00	19.42
Sweet white onion 6	0.07 ± 0.00	0.10 ± 0.01	7.28 ± 0.07	0.21 ± 0.00	0.12 ± 0.00	6.61 ± 0.05	0.98 ± 0.00	15.36
Yellow onion 1	0.21 ± 0.02	0.53 ± 0.03	12.32 ± 0.02	0.46 ± 0.02	0.52 ± 0.00	15.47 ± 0.00	0.65 ± 0.01	30.17
Yellow onion 2	0.29 ± 0.01	0.10 ± 0.02	7.13 ± 0.13	0.52 ± 0.03	0.40 ± 0.12	5.18 ± 0.01	0.91 ± 0.02	14.53
Yellow onion 3	0.18 ± 0.00	0.22 ± 0.01	8.13 ± 0.02	0.32 ± 0.00	5.00 ± 0.01	1.37 ± 0.05	0.13 ± 0.00	15.35
Red onion 1	0.36 ± 0.02	0.88 ± 0.06	25.58 ± 0.16	0.72 ± 0.01	0.57 ± 0.02	18.42 ± 0.15	1.47 ± 0.00	48.00
Red onion 2	0.34 ± 0.03	0.69 ± 0.04	16.36 ± 0.04	0.83 ± 0.01	0.57 ± 0.00	18.69 ± 0.03	2.44 ± 0.00	39.92
Red onion 3	0.28 ± 0.00	0.56 ± 0.00	17.60 ± 0.05	0.52 ± 0.03	0.92 ± 0.01	21.94 ± 1.03	1.03 ± 0.01	42.86
Red onion 4	0.29 ± 0.02	0.86 ± 0.02	24.97 ± 0.32	0.83 ± 0.02	0.56 ± 0.00	16.73 ± 0.91	1.99 ± 0.06	46.23

[1] Flavonoid composition expressed as mean of three replicates ± standard deviation (mg/10 g dry weight (DW) ± SD).

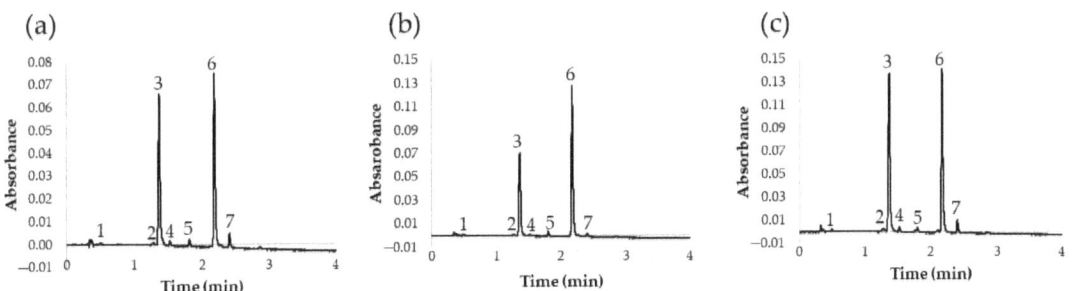

Figure 5. Chromatogram at 360 nm of different onion varieties: (**a**) white onion; (**b**) yellow onion; (**c**) red onion. (1) Quercetin 3,7,4'-O-triglucoside; (2) quercetin 7,4'-O-diglucoside; (3) quercetin 3,4'-O-diglucoside; (4) isorhamnetin 3,4'-O-diglucoside; (5) quercetin 3-O-glucoside; (6) quercetin 4'-O-glucoside; (7) isorhamnetin 4'-O-glucoside.

According to these results, we can conclude that the proposed UHPLC method was adequate for the analysis of different onion varieties, since it presented good chromatographic characteristics and short run times. This is of great interest, among other things, because it allows for the characterization of onion varieties according to their flavonol profile in a short time and with a high precision level. In fact, according to the resulting quantifications of flavonoids, it could be concluded that the major flavonols in red, yellow, and white varieties were quercetin 3,4'-O-diglucoside and quercetin 4'-O-glucoside, representing about 90% of their overall flavonol content. Furthermore, according to these results, the content of total flavonoids is considerably higher in red onions. Specifically, the red varieties presented nearly double flavonoid contents when compared to yellow or white onions. These results are in agreement with those already reported by other authors, who recommend the consumption of red varieties because of their greater flavonoid contents and health benefits [29]. On the other hand, flavonoid contents in white and yellow varieties were found to be very similar, and minor differences were mostly due to either specific variety (sweet, spring, etc.) or geographical origin.

3. Materials and Methods

3.1. Chemicals and Reagents

The solvent used for onion extraction was a mix of methanol and water. The methanol (Fischer Scientifics, Loughborough, United Kingdom) was HPLC-grade. The ultra-pure water was obtained from a Milli-Q water purification system (EMD Millipore Corporation, Bedford, MA, USA). For UHPLC analyses, acetonitrile (Panreac, Barcelona, Spain), water, and acetic and formic acid (Merck KGaA, Darmstadt, Germany) were used. The solvents were degassed and filtered through a 0.22 μm membrane (Nylon Membrane Filter, FILTER-LAB, Barcelona, Spain) before being used. The standard for the quantification of flavonols was quercetin 3-*O*-glucoside supplied by Sigma-Aldrich (Steinheim, Germany).

3.2. Plant Material

The plant material employed for the development of the method consisted of samples from red onion purchased from a local market in the province of Cadiz (Spain). The onions were subjected to a pretreatment in order to improve sample-solvent contact surface [30]. First, the onion bulbs were washed, cleaned, peeled, and cut using a knife. Then, the chopped bulbs were lyophilized in a freeze dryer LYOALFA (Azbil Telstar Technologies, Terrassa, Barcelona, Spain) and crushed in a knife mill GRINDOMIX (Retsch GM200, Haan, Germany). Furthermore, other different onion varieties, purchased from local markets in the province of Cadiz (Spain) and subjected to the same pretreatment, were also analyzed. Specifically, 6 white onion (spring and sweet), 3 yellow onion, and 4 red onion varieties were studied. Information about the characteristics of the different onions (origin, producer, caliber, etc.) are included in the Supplementary Materials (Table S1). Finally, all the samples were stored in a freezer at −20 °C.

3.3. Extraction Procedure

To extract the flavonols from the onions, we used ultrasound-assisted extraction. Specifically, a Sonopuls HD 2070.2 probe (BANDELIN electronic GmbH and Co KG, Heinrichstrabe, Berlin, Germany) was employed, coupled to a processor for amplitude (80% of the maximum amplitude) and cycle (0.5 s) adjustments. For temperature control (20 °C), a thermostatic bath (Frigiterm-10, Selecta, Barcelona, Spain) was employed. About 0.2 g of the lyophilized and homogenized onion was weighed into a Falcon tube, and 20 mL of 50:50 MeOH/H_2O mixture was added. The Falcon tube was placed in a double vessel through which the water from the thermostatic bath circulated. The extraction time was set at 10 min. After this time, the extracts were centrifuged at 7500 rpm (9.5 cm orbital radius, 5 min) and the supernatants were placed into a volumetric flask of 25 mL. The precipitates from the extraction were redissolved in 5 mL of the same extraction solvent and centrifuged again under the same conditions. The new supernatants were placed into volumetric flasks and topped up with the same solvent. The final extracts were stored at −20 °C for their correct conservation until further analysis. The ultrasound-assisted extraction (UAE) conditions that were set for the extractions were based on previous results obtained by our research group for phenolic compounds [31,32].

3.4. Identification of Flavonols by Liquid Chromatography Coupled to Mass Spectrometry

Because not all the standards were available for the group, we carried out a previous identification using liquid chromatography coupled to mass spectrometry. Specifically, the major flavonols present in *Allium cepa* L. were identified by ultra-high performance liquid chromatography (UHPLC) coupled to a photodiode array (PDA) detector (Waters Corporation, Milford, MA, USA) and a quadrupole-time-of-flight mass spectrometer (Q-ToF-MS) (Xevo G2 QTof, Waters Corp., Milford, MA, USA).

The column was a reverse-phase C18 analytical column with 1.7 μm particle size, 2.1×100 mm (ACQUITY UPLC CSH C18, Waters). The mobile phase A, 2% formic acid–water solution, and the mobile phase B, 2% formic acid–methanol solution, were used at a flow rate of 0.4 mL min^{-1}. The gradient employed was the following (time, % solvent B): 0.00 min, 15%; 3.30 min, 20%; 3.86 min, 30%; 5.05 min, 40%; 5.35 min, 55%; 5.64 min, 60%; 5.95 min, 95%; and 7.50 min, 95%. The total run time was 12 min: 8 min for the analysis and 4 additional minutes for re-equilibration. The mass spectra were acquired in negative ion mode under the following conditions: desolvation gas flow = 700 L h^{-1}, desolvation temperature = 500 °C, cone gas flow = 10 L h^{-1}, source temperature = 150 °C, capillary voltage = 700 V, cone voltage = 30 V, and collision energy = 20 eV. The ions were scanned from m/z 100 to m/z 1200.

Prior to their identification, all the UAE extracts were filtered through a 0.20 μm nylon syringe filter (Membrane Solutions, Dallas, TX, USA), and 3 μL was the volume injected. The compounds were individually identified on the basis of their retention time and molecular weight. The following 7 major flavonols were identified: compound 1, quercetin 3,7,4'-*O*-triglucoside (m/z = 787.1421); compound 2, quercetin 7,4'-*O*-diglucoside (m/z = 625.1396); compound 3, quercetin 3,4'-*O*-diglucoside (m/z = 625.1398); compound 4, isorhamnetin 3,4'-*O*-diglucoside (m/z = 639.1559); compound 5, quercetin 3-*O*-glucoside (m/z = 463.0886), compound 6, quercetin 4'-*O*-glucoside (m/z = 463.0873); compound 7, isorhamnetin 4-*O*'-glucoside (m/z = 477.1040). With respect to the PDA, the following maximum absorbance wavelengths were observed for each flavonol: quercetin 3,7,4'-*O*-triglucoside (346.7 nm), quercetin 7,4'-*O*-diglucoside (371.8 nm), quercetin 3,4'-*O*-diglucoside (343.2 nm), isorhamnetin 3,4'-*O*-diglucoside (346.7 nm), quercetin 3-*O*-glucoside (346.7 nm), quercetin 4'-*O*-glucoside (362.3 nm), and isorhamnetin 4'-*O*-glucoside (371.1 nm). The identified compounds coincide unequivocally with those reported by other authors in the bibliography [10,33–35]. The data corresponding to maximum absorbance wavelengths, mass spectra, theoretical and measured masses, and time of elution were included as Supplementary Material (Table S2). Once this preliminary identification has been carried out, the chromatographic method subsequently developed can be applied to other onion varieties, taking into account the retention times and absorbance spectra, without the need to apply masses. This is of interest because of the more time and effort involved in mass spectrometry and because it is not usually available for most food quality industries and research groups.

3.5. Separation and Quantification of Flavonols by UHPLC-PDA

The major flavonols found in the onions were separated and quantified by UHPLC by means of an ACQUITY UPLC H-Class system coupled to an ACQUITY UPLC Photodiode Array (PDA) detector. The PDA detector was set in the wavelength range of 210–400 nm for the 3D scan, with a data collection rate of 40 pts s^{-1}. However, all the flavonols were quantified by 2D scan, and the PDA was set at 360 nm, which is approximately the maximum absorbance wavelength of quercetin 3-*O*-glucoside, i.e., the commercially available flavonol standard. Since the rest of the standards were not available, the rest of the compounds were quantified according to the calibration curve of quercetin 3-*O*-glucoside, on the basis of the structural similarities between these molecules while taking into account their molecular weights.

The flavonols were separated by injecting a 3.0 μL sample into an Acquity UPLC BEH C18 column (50 mm × 2.1 mm i.d., 1.7 mm particle size, Waters Corporation, Milford, MA, USA). The temperature was set at 55 °C and the mobile phase was a binary solvent system.

Phase A was formed by 2% acetic acid in water and phase B by 2% acetic acid in acetonitrile. These conditions were selected in accordance with the expertise acquired by our research group from previous studies on this type of compounds [36–38]. The system was controlled by Empower3 Chromatography Data Software (Waters Corporation, Milford, MA, USA). The integration of flavonols was performed manually in the form "Valley-to-Valley".

3.6. Box–Behnken Design (BBD)

A BBD design was employed to determine the effect of 3 factors (the 3 independent variables) on the UHPLC-PDA separation. The factors studied were flow rate (X_1), solvent composition (% phase B) at the beginning of the gradient program (X_2), and solvent composition (% phase B) at the end of the gradient program (X_3). As these factors have different units and ranges, each factor was first normalized and forced into the range -1 to $+1$ [20]. Thus, a Box–Behnken design with 3 factors and 3 levels for each factor: low (-1), medium (0), and a high level (1), were set. Specifically, the studied ranges were as follows: flow rate (mL min^{-1}): 0.4, 0.5, 0.6; %B at the beginning (%): 0, 5, 10; and %B at the end (%): 50, 75, 100. The ranges for the study were selected on the basis of our team previous experience. The analysis time between the beginning and the end of the gradient was 5 min. The response variables (dependent variables) were optimized according to the peak resolutions (Y_{Rs}) and the analyses run time (Y_{RT}). The retention time of the last peak in the chromatogram was regarded as the analysis run time, while the peak resolutions were calculated according to Equation (6).

$$Rs = \frac{2\left(t_{R(B)} - t_{R(A)}\right)}{W_{b(A)} + W_{b(B)}}, \tag{6}$$

where $t_{R\,(A)}$ and $t_{R\,(B)}$ are the retention times of two adjacent peaks A and B, respectively, and $W_{b\,(A)}$ and $W_{b\,(B)}$ are the peak widths at the base of the same adjacent peaks. All of these parameters were calculated by means of Empower 3 Software (Waters Corporation, Milford, MA, USA).

On the basis of the number of factors and using the specific BBD equation, we obtained a design consisting of 15 experiments including 3 repetitions at their center point. The results obtained from the whole experimental design matrix were analyzed by response surface methodology. A mathematical model (Equation (7)) for each response can be built in which each response of the system was considered as a function of the corresponding factors and their corresponding interactions.

$$y = \beta_0 + \sum_{i=1}^{k} \beta_i X_i + \sum_{i=1}^{k} \beta_{ii} \cdot X_i^2 + \sum_{i} \sum_{i=1}^{k} \beta_{ij} X_{ij} + \varepsilon, \tag{7}$$

where y is the dependent variable; X_i and X_j are independent variables; β_0 is the regression coefficient for the intercept; β_i, β_{ii}, and β_{ij} are the regression coefficients for the linear, quadratic, and interactive terms, respectively; and ε is the error.

In order to find the optimum chromatographic conditions for the 3 responses (peak resolutions and analysis run time) at the same time, we performed an MRO together with their desirability functions. Firstly, the data were analyzed to generate a separate model for each response. Then, the predicted values obtained from each response surface were transformed into an individual desirability function, d_i. The scale of the desirability function ranges from 0 (for an unacceptable response value) to 1 (for a completely desirable one) [39]. D was calculated by combining the individual desirability values by applying the geometric mean (Equation (8)):

$$D = (d_1 \times d_2 \times \ldots d_m)^{\frac{1}{m}}, \tag{8}$$

where d_i indicates the desirability of the responses and m is the number of responses in the measure. The MRO methodology is a very useful tool for quality control and analytical laboratories since it can minimize analyses costs and time.

3.7. Validation Procedure and Chromatographic Properties

Once the UHPLC method had been developed for the determination of the major flavonols in onions, it was validated according to the recommendations of ICH Guideline Q2 (R1) [27] and then their chromatographic characteristics were measured.

For the validation of the method, we evaluated linearity, precision (repeatability and intermediate precision), robustness, and detection (LODs) and quantification limits (LOQs). The calculations were performed by means of Microsoft Office Excel 2013. A calibration curve for quercetin 3-*O*-glucoside, the commercially available standard, was plotted. The linearity of the calibration curve was evaluated by calculating its coefficient of determination (R^2). Since the rest of the standards were not available, these compounds were quantified according to the calibration curve of quercetin 3-*O*-glucoside, on the basis of the structural similarities between these molecules, while taking into account their molecular weights. The LODs and LOQs were obtained by dividing, respectively, 3 and 10 times the signal-to-noise ratios by the slope of the calibration curves that had been obtained. The repeatability and intermediate precision of the developed UHPLC method were evaluated according to the retention time and peak resolution of each compound. For this purpose, 9 replicates were completed on the same day. Regarding the intermediate precision, 21 replicates were completed on 3 different days. The precision was expressed as the coefficient of variance (CV) of each one of the above-mentioned parameters, where the acceptable CV limit was under 10%, in accordance with the AOAC manual for the Peer-Verified Methods program [28]. Finally, the robustness of the UHPLC method was also evaluated. For this purpose, specific variations in the range of the column temperature, the flow rate, and the injection volume were tested. For each parameter, 3 different variation levels were evaluated, and for each level, 4 repetitions were carried out. For the statistical analysis, two-tailed *t*-test assuming equal variances and a level of significance of 0.05 was employed.

With regards to the chromatographic properties, the retention time (t_R), the resolution (Rs), the retention factor (k) (Equation (9)), and the selectivity (α) (Equation (10)) were evaluated.

$$k = \frac{t'_R}{t_M}, \tag{9}$$

$$\alpha = \frac{t'_R(B)}{t'_R(A)} = \frac{K(B)}{K(A)}, \tag{10}$$

where $t_{R\,(A)}$ and $t_{R\,(B)}$ are the retention times of two adjacent peaks A and B, respectively; t_M is the column dead time; and t'_R is the adjusted retention time ($t'_R = t_R - t_M$). All of these parameters were calculated by means of Empower 3 Software (Waters Corporation, Milford, MA, USA).

4. Conclusions

A rapid and reproducible UHPLC-PDA methodology for the separation of the seven major flavonols that can be found in onions was developed. A BBD was used in conjunction with MRO to optimize the simultaneous separation of the seven flavonols of interest. The optimal conditions for a successful separation were 9.9% phase B at the beginning of the gradient, 53.2% phase B at the end of the gradient, 55 °C column working temperature, and 0.6 mL min^{-1} flow rate. The analysis time between the beginning of the gradient and the end of the gradient was 5 min. The complete separation was achieved in less than 2.7 min with excellent chromatographic characteristics (resolution, selectivity, and retention factor). The method has also been successfully validated, showing high repeatability and intermediate precision values (CV < 5%) for retention time and peak resolution, low limits of detection and quantification, as well as good linearity. Furthermore, the robustness of the methodology was satisfactorily tested against variations of injection volume, temperature column, and flow rate for most of the flavonols studied. The developed methodology saves time, solvent, and costs in comparison to other methods found in the bibliography. The method was also applied to the analysis of yellow, white, and red onions to successfully demonstrate its applicability to the analysis of different onion varieties. This method would allow laboratories, researchers, and companies to determine onion flavonol contents in a particularly short time, which in turn would contribute to improving the quality of onions and their sub-products when targeted to human consumption.

Supplementary Materials: The following are available online at https://www.mdpi.com/article/10.3390/ph14040310/s1: Figure S1: Structural types of analyzed flavonols. Table S1: Characteristics of the different onions studied. Table S2: Mass spectra information for the seven flavonols identified in onion bulbs by UHPLC–photo-diode array (PDA)–quadrupole-time-of-flight mass spectrometry (Q-ToF-MS) in negative ESI mode.

Author Contributions: Conceptualization, M.F.-G. and G.F.B.; methodology, A.V.G.-d.-P., M.V.-E. and C.C.; software, M.F.-G.; validation, A.V.G.-d.-P. and M.V.-E.; formal analysis, A.V.G.-d.-P., M.V.-E. and C.C.; investigation, A.V.G.-d.-P. and M.V.-E.; resources, M.P. and G.F.B.; data curation, E.E.-B., M.F.-G. and G.F.B.; writing—original draft preparation, A.V.G.-d.-P. and M.V.-E.; writing—review and editing, G.F.B. and E.E.-B.; visualization, G.F.B.; supervision, M.F.-G. and G.F.B.; project administration, G.F.B. and E.E.-B.; funding acquisition, G.F.B. and M.P. All authors have read and agreed to the published version of the manuscript.

Funding: This work has been supported by the project "EQC2018-005135-P" (Equipment for liquid chromatography by means of mass spectrometry and ion chromatography) of the State Subprogram of Research Infrastructures and Technical Scientific Equipment. This research was funded by University of Cadiz, by the INIA (National Institute for Agronomic Research) and FEDER (European Regional Development Fund), within the framework of the Operational Program under the Investment for Growth 2014–2020, Project RTA2014-00083-C03-03), and by the Ministry of Science and Innovation of Spain (FPU grant AP-2018-03811 to Ana Velasco González de Peredo).

Institutional Review Board Statement: Not applicable.

Informed Consent Statement: Not applicable.

Data Availability Statement: The data presented in this study is contained within the article or supplementary material.

Acknowledgments: The authors are grateful to the Instituto de Investigación Vitivinícola y Agroalimentaria (IVAGRO) for providing the necessary facilities to carry out the research. A special acknowledgement goes to Carmelo García Barroso (*in memoriam*) for his contribution to the scientific community in the area of phenolic compounds and oenology and his important inputs to this research.

Conflicts of Interest: The authors declare no conflict of interest.

References

1. Rodrigues, A.S.; Pérez-Gregorio, M.R.; García-Falcon, M.S.; Simal-Gándara, J.; Almeida, D.P.F. Effect of post-harvest practices on flavonoid content of red and white onion cultivars. *Food Control* **2010**, *21*, 878–884. [CrossRef]
2. FAO. *Global Forest Resources Assessment 2015*; Food and Agriculture Organization of the United Nations: Rome, Italy, 2016.
3. Block, E. The Organosulfur Chemistry of the Genus *Allium*—Implications for the Organic Chemistry of Sulfur. *Angew. Chem. Int. Ed. Engl.* **1992**, *31*, 1135–1178. [CrossRef]
4. Özcan, M.M.; Süleyma, D.; Nurhan, U. Effect of Species on Total Phenol, Antioxidant Activity and Phenolic Compounds of Different Wild Onion Bulbs. *J. Food Meas. Charact.* **2018**, *12*, 902–905. [CrossRef]
5. Ye, C.L.; Dai, D.H.; Hu, W.L. Antimicrobial and antioxidant activities of the essential oil from onion (*Allium cepa* L.). *Food Control* **2013**, *30*, 48–53. [CrossRef]
6. Park, M.J.; Ryu, D.H.; Cho, J.Y.; Ha, I.J.; Moon, J.S.; Kang, Y.H. Comparison of the Antioxidant Properties and Flavonols in Various Parts of Korean Red Oni, ons by Multivariate Data Analysis. *Hortic. Environ. Biotechnol.* **2018**, *59*, 919–927. [CrossRef]
7. Ferioli, F.; D'Antuono, L.F. Evaluation of Phenolics and Cysteine Sulfoxides in Local Onion and Shallot Germplasm from Italy and Ukraine. *Genet. Resour. Crop Evol.* **2016**, *63*, 601–614. [CrossRef]

8. Larson, A.J.; Symons, J.D.; Jalili, T. Quercetin: A Treatment for Hypertension?—A Review of Efficacy and Mechanisms. *Pharmaceuticals* **2010**, *3*, 237–250. [CrossRef] [PubMed]
9. Abian, O.; Ortega-Alarcon, D.; Jimenez-alesanco, A.; Ceballos-laita, L.; Vega, S.; Reyburn, H.T.; Velazquez-campoy, A. Structural Stability of SARS-CoV-2 3CLpro and Identification of Quercetin as an Inhibitor by Experimental Screening. *Int. J. Biol. Macromol.* **2020**, *164*, 1693–1703. [CrossRef]
10. Pérez-Gregorio, M.R.; Regueiro, J.; González-Barreiro, C.; Rial-Otero, R.; Simal-Gándara, J. Changes in Antioxidant Flavonoids during Freeze-Drying of Red Onions and Subsequent Storage. *Food Control* **2011**, *22*, 1108–1113. [CrossRef]
11. Ko, E.Y.; Nile, S.H.; Jung, Y.S.; Keum, Y.S. Antioxidant and Antiplatelet Potential of Different Methanol Fractions and Flavonols Extracted from Onion (*Allium cepa* L.). *3 Biotech* **2018**, *8*, 1–10. [CrossRef]
12. Jurinjak Tušek, A.; Benković, M.; Belščak Cvitanović, A.; Valinger, D.; Jurina, T.; Gajdoš Kljusurić, J. Kinetics and Thermodynamics of the Solid-Liquid Extraction Process of Total Polyphenols, Antioxidants and Extraction Yield from Asteraceae Plants. *Ind. Crop. Prod.* **2016**, *91*, 205–214. [CrossRef]
13. Tistaert, C.; Dejaegher, B.; Heyden, Y.V. Chromatographic Separation Techniques and Data Handling Methods for Herbal Fingerprints: A Review. *Anal. Chim. Acta* **2011**, *690*, 148–161. [CrossRef] [PubMed]
14. Stipcovich, T.; Barbero, G.F.; Ferreiro-González, M.; Palma, M.; Barroso, C.G. Fast Analysis of Capsaicinoids in Naga Jolokia Extracts (*Capsicum Chinense*) by High-Performance Liquid Chromatography Using Fused Core Columns. *Food Chem.* **2018**, *239*, 217–224. [CrossRef] [PubMed]
15. Moreno-Rojas, J.M.; Moreno-Ortega, A.; Ordóñez, J.L.; Moreno-Rojas, R.; Pérez-Aparicio, J.; Pereira-Caro, G. Development and Validation of UHPLC-HRMS Methodology for the Determination of Flavonoids, Amino Acids and Organosulfur Compounds in Black Onion, a Novel Derived Product from Fresh Shallot Onions (*Allium Cepa* Var. Aggregatum). *LWT-Food Sci. Technol.* **2018**, *97*, 376–383. [CrossRef]
16. Park, S.K.; Jin, D.E.; Park, C.H.; Seung, T.W.; Guo, T.J.; Song, J.W.; Kim, J.H.; Kim, D.O.; Heo, H.J. Ameliorating effects of ethyl acetate fraction from onion (*Allium cepa* L.) flesh and peel in mice following trimethyltin-induced learning and memory impairment. *Food Res. Int.* **2015**, *75*, 53–60. [CrossRef]
17. Lee, S.U.; Lee, J.H.; Choi, S.H.; Lee, J.S.; Ohnisi-Kameyama, M.; Kozukue, N.; Levin, C.E.; Friedman, M. Flavonoid content in fresh, home-processed, and light-exposed onions and in dehydrated commercial onion products. *J. Agric. Food Chem.* **2008**, *56*, 8541–8547. [CrossRef] [PubMed]
18. Majid, I.; Vikas, N. Instrumental Texture and FLavonoid Profile of Paste Developed from Sprouted Onion Varieties of Indian Origin. *Int. J. Food Prop.* **2017**, *20*, 2511–2526. [CrossRef]
19. González de Peredo, A.V.; Vázquez-Espinosa, M.; Piñeiro, Z.; Espada-Bellido, E.; Ferreiro-González, M.; Barbero, G.F.; Palma, M. Development of a Rapid and Accurate UHPLC-PDA-FL Method for the Quantification of Phenolic Compounds in Grapes. *Food Chem.* **2020**, *334*, 127569. [CrossRef]
20. Setyaningsih, W.; Saputro, I.E.; Carrera, C.A.; Palma, M.; Barroso, C.G. Multiresponse optimization of a UPLC method for the simultaneous determination of tryptophan and 15 tryptophan-derived compounds using a Box-Behnken design with a desirability function. *Food Chem.* **2017**, *225*, 1–9. [CrossRef] [PubMed]
21. Wani, T.A.; Ahmad, A.; Zargar, S.; Khalil, N.Y.; Darwish, I.A. Use of response surface methodology for development of new microwell-based spectrophotometric method for determination of atrovastatin calcium in tablets. *Chem. Cent. J.* **2012**, *6*, 134. [CrossRef]
22. Hu, Z.; Cai, M.; Liang, H.H. Desirability Function Approach for the Optimization of Microwave-Assisted Extraction of Saikosaponins from Radix Bupleuri. *Sep. Purif. Technol.* **2008**, *61*, 266–275. [CrossRef]
23. Zheng, J.; Polyakova, Y.; Row, K.H. Retention Factors and Resolutions of Amino Benzoic Acid Isomers with Some Lonic Liquids. *Biotechnol. Bioproc. E* **2006**, *11*, 477–483. [CrossRef]
24. Sharma, K.; Assefa, A.D.; Kim, S.; Ko, E.Y.; Lee, E.T.; Park, S.W. Evaluation of Total Phenolics, Flavonoids and Antioxidant Activity of 18 Korean Onion Cultivars: A Comparative Study. *J. Sci. Food Agric.* **2014**, *94*, 1521–1529. [CrossRef] [PubMed]
25. Turner, C.; Turner, P.; Jacobson, G.; Almgren, K.; Waldebäck, M.; Sjöberg, P.; Karlsson, E.N.; Markides, K.E. Subcritical Water Extraction and β-Glucosidase-Catalyzed Hydrolysis of Quercetin Glycosides in Onion Waste. *Green Chem.* **2006**, *8*, 949–959. [CrossRef]
26. Snyder, L.R.; Dolan, J.W. *High-Performance Gradient Elution*; Wiley-Interscience: Hoboken, NJ, USA, 2006.
27. ICH. *ICH Topic Q2 (R1) Validation of Analytical Procedures: Text and Methodology*; ICH: Geneva, Switzerland, 2005; Volume 1994.
28. AOAC. *AOAC Peer Verified Methods Program, Manual on Policies and Procedures*; AOAC International: Rockville, MD, USA, 2012.
29. Pérez-Gregorio, M.R.; García-Falcón, M.S.; Simal-Gándara, J.; Rodrigues, A.S.; Almeida, D.P.F. Identification and Quantification of Flavonoids in Traditional Cultivars of Red and White Onions at Harvest. *J. Food Compos. Anal.* **2010**, *23*, 592–598. [CrossRef]
30. Vallverdú-Queralt, A.; Medina-Remón, A.; Andres-Lacueva, C.; Lamuela-Raventos, R.M. Changes in Phenolic Profile and Antioxidant Activity during Production of Diced Tomatoes. *Food Chem.* **2011**, *126*, 1700–1707. [CrossRef] [PubMed]
31. Vázquez-Espinosa, M.; Espada-Bellido, E.; González de Peredo, A.V.; Ferreiro-González, M.; Carrera, C.; Palma, M.; Barroso, C.G.; Barbero, G.F. Optimization of Microwave-Assisted Extraction for the Recovery of Bioactive Compounds from the Chilean Superfruit (*Aristotelia Chilensis* (Mol.) Stuntz). *Agronomy* **2018**, *8*, 240. [CrossRef]

32. González de Peredo, A.V.; Vázquez-Espinosa, M.; Espada-Bellido, E.; Ferreiro-González, M.; Amores-Arrocha, A.; Palma, M.; Barbero, G.F.; Jiménez-Cantizano, A. Alternative Ultrasound-Assisted Method for the Extraction of the Bioactive Compounds Present in Myrtle (*Myrtus communis* L.). *Molecules* **2019**, *24*, 882. [CrossRef]
33. Bonaccorsi, P.; Caristi, C.; Gargiulli, C.; Leuzzi, U. Flavonol glucosides in *Allium* species: A comparative study by means of HPLC-DAD-ESI-MS-MS. *Food Chem.* **2008**, *107*, 1668–1673. [CrossRef]
34. Katsampa, P.; Valsamedou, E.; Grigorakis, S.; Makris, D.P. A green ultrasound-assisted extraction process for the recovery of antioxidant polyphenols and pigments from onion solid wastes using Box–Behnken experimental design and kinetics. *Ind. Crop. Prod.* **2015**, *77*, 535–543. [CrossRef]
35. Tedesco, I.; Carbone, V.; Spagnuolo, C.; Minasi, P.; Russo, G.L. Identification and Quantification of Flavonoids from Two Southern Italian Cultivars of *Allium cepa* L., Tropea (Red Onion) and Montoro (Copper Onion), and Their Capacity to Protect Human Erythrocytes from Oxidative Stress. *J. Agric. Food Chem.* **2015**, *63*, 5229–5238. [CrossRef] [PubMed]
36. de Souza Dias, F.; Lovillo, M.P.; Barroso, C.G.; David, J.M. Optimization and validation of a method for the direct determination of catechin and epicatechin in red wines by HPLC/fluorescence. *Microchem. J.* **2010**, *96*, 17–20. [CrossRef]
37. Piñeiro, Z.; Palma, M.; Barroso, C.G. Determination of Catechins by Means of Extraction with Pressurized Liquids. *J. Chromatogr. A* **2004**, *1026*, 19–23. [CrossRef] [PubMed]
38. Setyaningsih, W.; Saputro, I.E.; Carrera, C.A.; Palma, M.; García-Barroso, C. Fast Determination of Phenolic Compounds in Rice Grains by Ultraperformance Liquid Chromatography Coupled to Photodiode Array Detection: Method Development and Validation. *J. Agric. Food Chem.* **2019**, *67*, 3018–3027. [CrossRef]
39. Maran, J.; Manikandan, S.; Thirugnanasambandham, K.; Vigna Nivetha, C.; Dinesh, R. Box-Behnken Design Based Statistical Modeling for Ultrasound-Assisted Extraction of Corn Silk Polysaccharide. *Carbohydr. Polym.* **2013**, *92*, 604–611. [CrossRef]

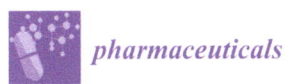

Article

Antioxidant and Antiproliferative Potentials of *Ficus glumosa* and Its Bioactive Polyphenol Metabolites

Moses Mutuse Mutungi [1,2,3], Felix Wambua Muema [1,2,3], Festus Kimutai [1,2,3], Yong-Bing Xu [1,2,3], Hui Zhang [1,2,3], Gui-Lin Chen [1,2,4] and Ming-Quan Guo [1,2,4,*]

1   CAS Key Laboratory of Plant Germplasm Enhancement and Specialty Agriculture, Wuhan Botanical Garden, Chinese Academy of Sciences, Wuhan 430074, China; mutungi.moses7@gmail.com (M.M.M.); fwambua83@mails.ucas.ac.cn (F.W.M.); festokim81@mails.ucas.ac.cn (F.K.); xuyongbing17@mails.ucas.ac.cn (Y.-B.X.); zhanghui183@mails.ucas.ac.cn (H.Z.); glchen@wbgcas.cn (G.-L.C.)
2   Sino-Africa Joint Research Center, Chinese Academy of Sciences, Wuhan 430074, China
3   University of Chinese Academy of Sciences, Beijing 100049, China
4   Innovation Academy for Drug Discovery and Development, Chinese Academy of Sciences, Shanghai 201203, China
*   Correspondence: guomq@wbgcas.cn; Tel.: +86-027-8770-0850

Citation: Mutungi, M.M.; Muema, F.W.; Kimutai, F.; Xu, Y.-B.; Zhang, H.; Chen, G.-L.; Guo, M.-Q. Antioxidant and Antiproliferative Potentials of *Ficus glumosa* and Its Bioactive Polyphenol Metabolites. *Pharmaceuticals* **2021**, 14, 266. https://doi.org/10.3390/ph14030266

Academic Editor: Jan Oszmianski

Received: 7 February 2021
Accepted: 5 March 2021
Published: 15 March 2021

Publisher's Note: MDPI stays neutral with regard to jurisdictional claims in published maps and institutional affiliations.

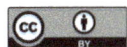

Abstract: *Ficus glumosa* Delile (Moraceae), a reputed plant that is used in herbal medicine, is of high medicinal and nutritional value in local communities primarily ascribed to its phytochemical profile. Currently, there are hardly any fine details on the chemical profiling and pharmacological evaluation of this species. In this study, the flavonoids and phenolics contents of the ethanol extracts and four extracted fractions (petroleum ether (PE), ethyl acetate (EA), *n*-butanol, and water) of the stem bark of *Ficus glumosa* were firstly quantified. Further, their antioxidant and antiproliferative potentials were also evaluated. The quantitative determination indicated that the EA and *n*-butanol fractions possessed the highest total flavonoids/phenolics levels of 274.05 ± 0.68 mg RE/g and 78.87 ± 0.97 mg GAE/g, respectively. Similarly, for the 2,2-diphenyl-1-picrylhydrazyl (DPPH), 2,2′-azino-bis-(3-ethylbenzothiazoline-6-sulfonic acid) (ABTS), and ferric-reducing antioxidant power (FRAP) assays, the EA fraction exhibited high potency in both DPPH and ABTS$^+$ scavenging activities with IC$_{50}$ values of 0.23 ± 0.03 mg/mL, 0.22 ± 0.03 mg/mL, and FRAP potential of 2.81 ± 0.01 mg Fe^{2+}/g, respectively. Furthermore, the EA fraction displayed high cytotoxicity against human lung (A549) and colon (HT-29) cancer cells. Additionally, the liquid chromatography coupled with electrospray ionization tandem mass spectrometry (LC-ESI-MS/MS) was employed in order to characterize the chemical constituents of the EA fraction of *Ficus glumosa* stem bark. Our findings revealed 16 compounds from the EA fraction that were possibly responsible for the strong antioxidant and anti-proliferative properties. This study provides edge-cutting background information on the exploitation of *Ficus glumosa* as a potential natural antioxidant and anti-cancer remedy.

Keywords: *Ficus glumosa*; polyphenols; HPLC-ESI-MS/MS; antiproliferative; antioxidant

1. Introduction

Ficus glumosa (Moraceae), which is also referred to as 'African rock fig', is a medium-sized tree, indigenous in semi-tropical and tropical African countries, and parts of West Asia [1]. It is a reputed species in African Traditional Medicine (ATM) for millennia and it serves a multipurpose use as food, healing diseases/ailments, and dye production. For instance, the leaves are boiled or eaten raw as vegetables in northern Nigeria [2], whilst the latex and figs as folk remedies, and the bark is used in the production of dye in the Southern, Eastern, and Western African countries [3]. Interestingly, the "swelling" trait of the latex makes it ideal as a potential disintegrant in tablet formulations [4]. Traditionally, figs and bark decoctions were used for the curing of rheumatoid arthritis, diarrhea, hemorrhoids, females sterility, and gingivitis [5,6], water retention, constipation, and liver complications [7]. The decoction from the leaves was orally administered for enhancement of weight loss, alleviate coughing, and helminths removal [8]. In Kenya, local communities use it for therapeutics and alimentation, for example, the figs are eaten as wild fruits and the latex is used to treat cancer complications and epilepsy [9].

Presently, some unraveled pharmacological activities of *Ficus glumosa* mainly include antidiabetic [10], antihypertension [11], hypolipidemia and antiatherogenic [12], antimalarial [13], antirheumatic [14], antioxidant [15], antibacterial [16], antifungal, and anticancer [17]. Further, studies on other *Ficus* species show substantial antiproliferative, anti-inflammatory, and antioxidant properties [18–20]. Previous studies linked the antioxidant, antibacterial, antitumor, and hypoglycemic properties of *Ficus glumosa* to its secondary metabolites profile, which is composed of alkaloids, flavonoids, saponins, triterpenoids, tannins, phenolic acids, steroids, and coumarins [21,22]. These polyphenols are naturally synthesized in plants as natural antioxidants and anticancer metabolites. They regulate cellular mechanisms that elicit antiproliferative activities. Further, they modulate the cumulative deleterious effects that are consequent of Reactive Oxygen and Nitrogen species (ROS/RNS) overproduction, growth factor receptors interaction, and pathways of cell signaling [23].

Antioxidants neutralize free radicals to suppress their oxidation potential by targeting signaling pathways, including phosphatidylinositide 3-kinases/protein kinase B (PI3K/Akt), among others [24]. Currently, there is an increased preference for natural antioxidants, as most synthetic antioxidants suffer a major setback of being carcinogenic [25]. The antioxidant and antiproliferative potentials of *Ficus glumosa* have been less explored, with a poor scientific elucidation of its medical utility. For instance, Ibrahim et al. [17] assayed the leaves of four species for antitumor properties (*F. glumosa*, *Holoptelea integrifolia*, *Ulmus parvifolia*, and *Rumex dantatus*), Madubunyi et al. [10] evaluated the antioxidant and antidiabetic potential of stem bark of *F. glumosa* in Nigeria, while Nana et al. [26] isolated chemical components from *F. glumosa* species and then assayed for their anticancer activities. Moreover, Olaokun et al. [27] screened for secondary metabolites, antioxidant properties, and inhibition of α-glucosidase and α-amylase enzymes of *Ficus glumosa*. The characterization of this species in Kenya is yet to be reported, despite having established that *Ficus glumosa* is rich in flavonoids, phenolic acids, fatty acids, and triterpenoids.

To this end, this study focused on evaluating the antioxidant and antiproliferative activities of ethanol extracts, ethyl acetate (EA), petroleum ether (PE), *n*-butanol, and water fractions of *Ficus glumosa*, and characterize its phytochemical profile. Meanwhile, the quantification of the total yield of flavonoids and phenolics of the ethanol extracts, PE, EA, *n*-butanol, and water fractions were performed. The high-performance liquid chromatography-electrospray ionization tandem mass spectrometry (HPLC-ESI-MS/MS) was further employed to identify the potential bioactive constituents in the EA fraction. Thus, this study will expand the scope of natural compounds screening and characterization, which serve as new entities in natural drug formulations.

2. Results and Discussion

2.1. Total Phenolics and Flavonoids Total Contents

Polyphenolics are ubiquitously synthesized in plants for growth and protection against invasion by predators and pathogens. They are similarly believed to have related effects on humans. For this reason, an evaluation of phenolics and flavonoids yield in this species was deemed to be necessary.

The total flavonoids and phenolics compositions (TFC & TPC) in *Ficus glumosa* ethanol extracts and fractions were determined while using two equations that were obtained from standard calibration curves: y = 1.535x − 0.0335, R^2 = 0.9982 for TFC, and y = 1.9908x − 0.0202, R^2 = 0.9993 for TPC. For TFC (Figure 1a), the EA fraction exhibited the highest content of 274.05 ± 0.68 mg RE/g, followed by *n*-butanol fraction with 185.34 ± 1.30 mg RE/g. Moreover, for TPC (Figure 1b), the *n*-butanol fraction showed the highest phenols accumulation of 78.87 ± 0.97 mg GAE/g, followed by the EA fraction with

70.99 ± 1.40 mg GAE/g. The observed trends of both TFC and TPC were in descending order of EA > *n*-butanol > ethanol extracts > PE > water, (8.44:5.71:3.96:1.14:1) and *n*-butanol > EA > ethanol extracts > water > PE, (5.56:5.01:3.67:1.10:1), respectively.

The present TPC yield in our study is lower when compared with that of methanol stem bark extract of *Ficus racemosa* that was obtained from Bangladesh, which was 242.97 mg GAE/g [28]. The TPC in *Ficus racemose* extracts from India was relatively lower, 39.03 ± 0.92 mg GAE/g extract [29]. Similarly, Abdel-Hameed [30] in a previous study on *Ficus decora*, and *Ficus afzelli* quantified TPC of 60.40 ± 3.06 and 70.96 ± 4.64 mg GAE/g in *n*-butanol fractions, 63.61± 3.70 and 97.30 ± 7.14 mg GAE/g in EA fractions, respectively. Further, the TFC levels of EA and *n*-butanol fractions of *Ficus glumosa* in the present study were higher than those of the same fractions of two *Ficus* species, *Ficus lyrata* and *Ficus sycomorous*, which were obtained from Egypt and Oman. They had TFC yields of 68.27 ± 4.17, 89.12 ± 6.88 mg RE/g, 153.52, and 123.54 mg QE/100g, respectively [30,31]. The extraction methodology and features of extracting solvents affect the solubility of different chemical components [32]. The TFC/TPC slight yields variation witnessed might be a consequence of the aforementioned factors, in addition to the difference in extraction procedures and geographical location.

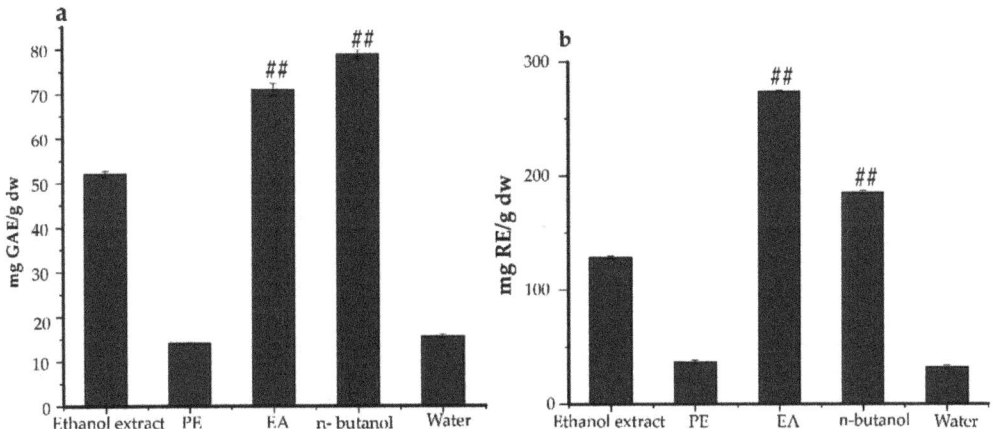

Figure 1. (**a**) (TPC) The total phenolics content and (**b**) (TFC) total flavonoids content of *Ficus glumosa*. The results are expressed in GAE (gallic acid equivalents) and RE (rutin equivalents) based on dry weight samples. ## $p < 0.01$ as compared to ethanol extracts. PE, Petroleum ether; EA, ethyl acetate.

2.2. Antioxidant Potential

Evaluating the antioxidant potential of compounds using only one assay is considered to be inconclusive due to the complex nature of polyphenols and divergent mechanisms of free radical scavenging [33]. Three antioxidant assays were used in this study, namely DPPH, ABTS, and FRAP were conducted to evaluate and compare the antioxidant power of the ethanol extracts, PE, EA, *n*-butanol, and water fractions of *Ficus glumosa*. A general observation was that the ethanol extracts, PE, EA, *n*-butanol, and water fractions expressed certain scavenging potentials against DPPH and ABTS assays (Figure 2a,b). The DPPH assay (Figure 3a) showed that the EA fraction exhibited the highest potential with an IC_{50} value of 0.23 ± 0.03 mg/mL. Similarly, in the ABTS assay (Figure 3b), the EA fraction presented significant scavenging activity with a lower IC_{50} value of 0.22 ± 0.03 mg/mL than the control, BHT, which had an IC_{50} value equal to 0.28 ± 0.02 mg/mL. Meanwhile, in the FRAP assay (Figure 3c), the EA fraction also displayed the strongest antioxidant potential with the IC_{50} value of 2.81 ± 0.01 mg Fe^{2+}/g, followed by *n*-butanol fraction and ethanol extracts. Generally, the EA fraction emerged as the most potent antioxidant in the three bioassays.

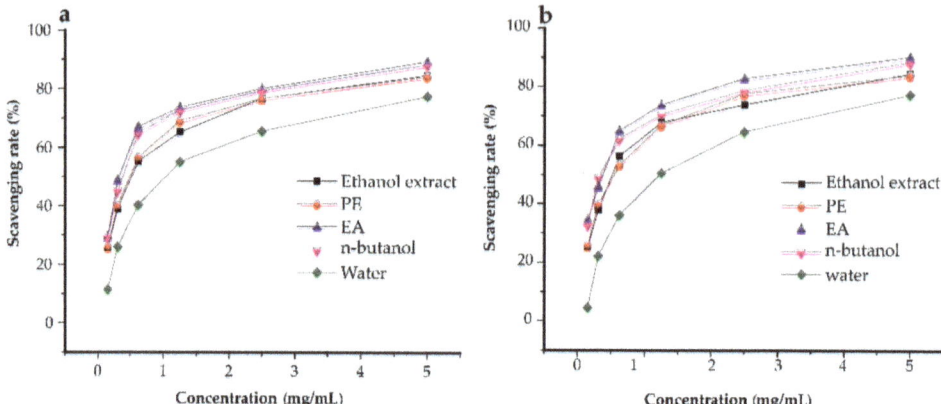

Figure 2. The percentage (%) scavenging rates of ethanol extracts, petroleum ether (PE), ethyl acetate (EA), *n*-butanol, and water fractions of *Ficus glumosa*. (**a**) The % radical scavenging rates of DPPH (2,2-diphenyl-1-picrylhydrazyl) assay, and (**b**) ABTS (2,2′-azino-bis (3-ethylbenzothiazoline-6-sulfonic acid) assay exhibited by ethanol extracts, PE, EA, *n*-butanol, and water fractions of *Ficus glumosa*.

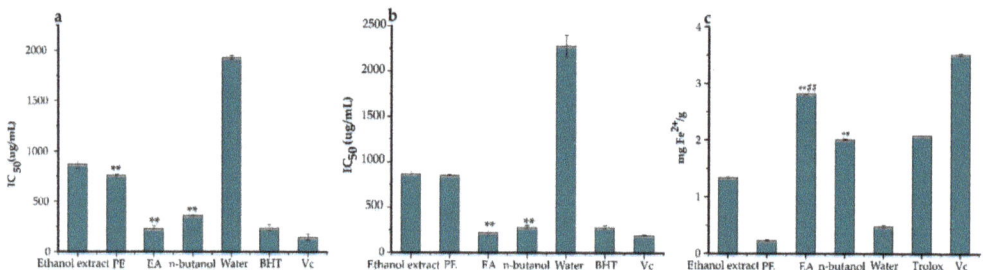

Figure 3. The antioxidant activities of ethanol extracts, petroleum ether (PE), ethyl acetate (EA), *n*-butanol, and water fractions of *Ficus glumosa* in IC_{50} and mg Fe^{2+}/g. (**a**) The IC_{50} values of DPPH (2,2-diphenyl-1-picrylhydrazyl) assay, (**b**) ABTS (2,2′-azino-bis (3-ethylbenzothiazoline-6-sulfonic acid) assay, and (**c**) FRAP (ferric-ion reducing power) assay exhibited by ethanol extracts, PE, EA, *n*-butanol, and water fractions of *Ficus glumosa*, and positive controls; BHT (butylated hydroxytoluene), Vc (vitamin c). ** $p < 0.05$ and ## $p < 0.05$ as compared to ethanol extracts and Trolox, respectively.

In previous studies on barks of four *Ficus* species, namely *F. glumosa* from Swaziland, *F. racemose* from Bangladesh, *F. racemose* from India, and *F. platyphylla* from Burkina Faso, displayed relatively lower DPPH IC_{50} values of 5.84 ± 1.53, 19, 5.99, and 1.93 ± 0.11 µg/mL, respectively [13,28,34,35]. Partly, our antioxidant results for DPPH and ABTS bear a close resemblance to those that were displayed by *Ficus* species from Yunnan, China [36]. They showed DPPH IC_{50} values, as follows; *Ficus virens var. verins* (1.03 mg/mL), *F. virens var. sublanceolata* (0.34 mg/mL), *F. callosa* (0.95 mg/mL), *F. oligodon* (2.54 mg/mL), *F. racemose* (1.11 mg/mL), *F. vasculosa* (0.97 mg/mL), and *F. auriculata* (0.29 mg/mL). Moreover, the same *Ficus* species exhibited ABTS IC_{50} values of 0.48, 0.23, 0.35, 0.86, 0.42, 0.69, and 0.25 mg/mL, respectively. Furthermore, our FRAP findings were consistent with previous studies that were reported by Madubunyi et al. [10] on *Ficus glumosa* bark extracts from Nigeria. The antioxidant activity correlates to the active metabolites in this sample fraction. The strong ability of polyphenols to donate H-atom to free radicals makes them suitable natural antioxidants [37]. In this regard, gallic acid, catechin, cinchonain I, cinchonain II, and procyanidin B2 are some well-known compounds with antioxidant potential that have been characterized in this study, hence being partly linked to the antioxidant results.

2.3. Antiproliferative Activity

Anticancer activity was related to antioxidant activity, because antioxidants can suppress the formation of cancers that arise from oxidative stress. The effective regulation of ROS via an antioxidant system could reduce cancer manifestation and also help in cancer treatment [38]. Upregulated ROS generation promotes oxidative stress, particularly on DNA molecules, by altering some gene sequences and/or activating proto-oncogenes, causing DNA damage and resulting in mutations [39]. Polyphenols elicit antiproliferative activities through the regulation of some transduction pathways, such as signal phosphatidylinositol 3-kinase (P13K), transducer and activating transcription (STAT-1), Nuclear factor-like 2 (erythroid-derived 2-) (Nrf2), Hypoxia-inducible factor (HIF)-1 Peroxisome proliferator-activated receptor (PRAR), and Mitogen-activated kinase-like protein (MAKP) [40]. Thus, it was important to assay the ethanol extracts, EA, *n*-butanol, PE, and water fractions of *Ficus glumosa* for antiproliferative activity on two cancer cells, namely lung carcinoma (A549) and colon carcinoma (HT-29) using SRB (sulforhodamine B) assay (Figure 4).

First of all, the cytotoxic effect of the ethanol extracts of *Ficus glumosa* was examined (for a concentration range from 3.7 to 300 μg/mL) on HT-29 and A549 cells over 72 h. It was revealed that the ethanol extracts exhibited dose-dependent inhibitory activities on HT-29 and A549 cells, with IC_{50} equal to 124.40 and 186.10 μg/mL, respectively. Aliquots of 100 μg/mL of ethanol extracts, PE, EA, *n*-butanol, and water fractions were evaluated for the antiproliferative activity. The PE and EA fractions displayed significant cytotoxicity, with an inhibition of 90.26% and 84.04% on HT-29 cells, and 88.38% and 82.10% on A549 cells, respectively, in comparison with the other fractions and ethanol extracts. The SRB assay of ethanol extracts on HFL-1 cells exhibited a high IC_{50} value of 232.66 μg/mL, which indicated low/no toxicity on a normal human lung. This indicated that the sample was biocompatible with the cell line. In regards to previous studies on stem barks of *Ficus* species (*F. fistulosa*, *F. hispida*, and *F. schwarzii*), they displayed relatively higher antiproliferative activities on A549 and HT-29 cells [41]. Similar findings were also reported in another study on *Ficus drupacea* stem bark extract against HT-29 cells, which unraveled an anticancer potential of IC_{50} 28. 9 ± 3.7 μg/mL [42]. Additionally, this study upholds the potential of this species to address a broad range of multifaceted diseases. Notably, the subject pharmacological potential of this species could be linked with the quality and quantity of structurally diverse secondary constituents' interaction with the test components.

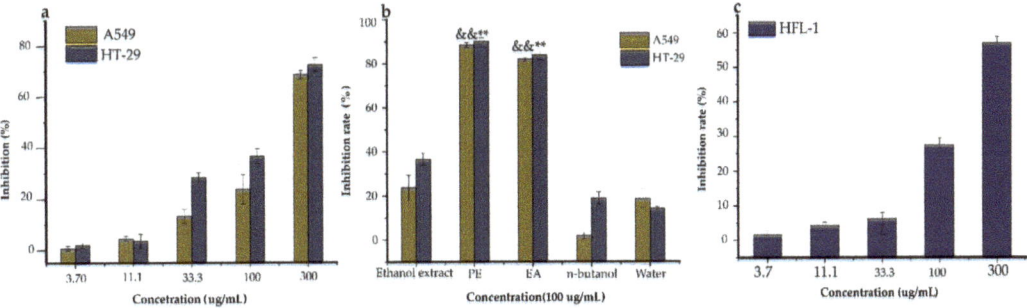

Figure 4. The antiproliferative activity of the ethanol extracts, PE (petroleum ether), EA (ethyl acetate), *n*-butanol, and water fractions of *Ficus glumosa*. (**a**) The (%) inhibition rates of HT-29 and A549 cells by different concentrations of ethanol extracts of *Ficus glumosa*. (**b**) The % inhibition rates of A549 and HT-29 cells treated with ethanol extracts, PE, EA, *n*-butanol, and water fractions of *Ficus glumosa*. (**c**) The toxicity of ethanol extracts of *Ficus glumosa* on normal lung (HFL-1) cells. && $p < 0.01$, ** $p < 0.01$ when compared to ethanol extracts.

2.4. HPLC Method Validation

The developed procedure was initially validated as ready for the quantification of the phenolic derivatives, phenolic acids, and flavonoids characterized in the EA fraction of *Ficus glumosa*. The calibration curves and correlation coefficients for the two standards were higher than $R^2 > 0.998$; an indication of good linearity within the examined ranges. Meanwhile, the LODs for both gallic acid and rutin were 1.84 and 1.93 μg/mL, whereas the LOQs were 5.58 and 5.85 μg/mL, respectively. This depicted a high sensitivity and reliability of the procedure for the effective quantification of analytes.

Further, our method was regarded to be repeatable, precise, and highly stable exhibited by the RSDs of intraday precision, repeatability, stability, and interday precision tests, which were all <2.5%. The recoveries ranged between 95–99% with RSDs of <2.43% indicating high accuracy and reproducibility. Table 1 provides the validation parameters results.

Table 1. Method validation for two compounds investigated.

Property	Analytes			
	Gallic Acid		Rutin	
Calibration equation	$y = 24.287x - 21.448$		$y = 16.298x + 3.3106$	
Linear ranges (μg/mL)	1–32		1.25–40	
Correlation coefficient (R^2)	0.9982		0.9988	
LOD	1.84		1.93	
LOQ	5.58		5.85	
Intraday precision (% RSD)	2.36		0.58	
Interday precision (% RSD)	1.69		0.47	
Repeatability (% RSD)	2.10		0.65	
Stability (% RSD)	2.49		0.56	
Recovery	Average recovery (%) 95.95	% RSD 2.43	Average recovery (%) 98.17	% RSD 0.55

y = peak area; × = concentration of analytes (μg/mL); R^2 = correlation coefficient; LOD/LOQ, limit of detection/quantification (S/N = 3.3/10); % RSD = percentage relative standard deviation.

2.5. HPLC-MS Analysis of EA Fraction of Ficus glumosa

In this study, for the first time, the qualitative analysis of the EA fraction of *Ficus glumosa* stem bark was achieved using HPLC-ESI-MS/MS (Figure 5). The HPLC method was first optimized to allow clear separation and maintain proper peak shapes in order to ensure a detailed investigation. An in-depth chromatographic investigation that was based upon retention time, the order of elution, and MS base peak led to the characterization of 16 compounds; three phenolic acids, a phenolic derivative, and 12 flavonoids, as in Table 2. The structures of the characterized compounds are shown in Figure 6.

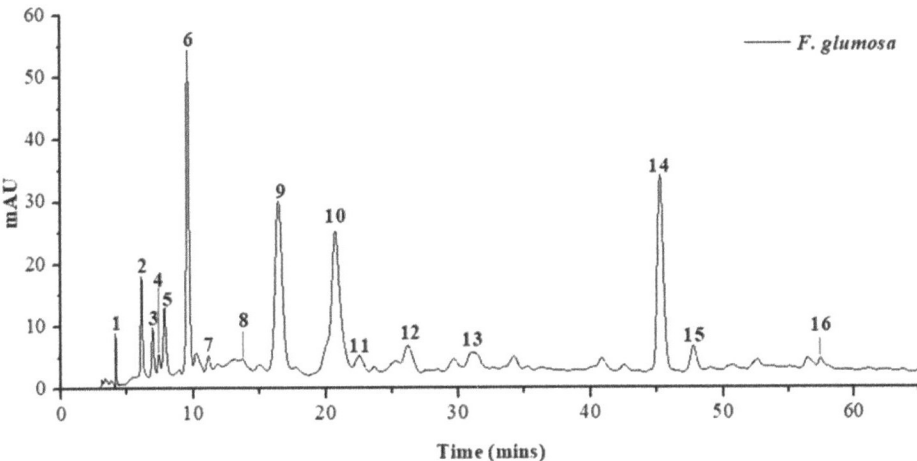

Figure 5. High-performance liquid chromatography-UV (HPLC-UV) chromatogram of EA fraction of *Ficus glumosa* at wavelength 280 nm.

Table 2. High-performance liquid chromatography-electrospray ionization tandem mass spectrometry (HPLC-ESI-MS/MS) data of compounds that were obtained from the EA fraction of *Ficus glumosa* stem bark.

Peak No.	Rt (min)	[M-H]–	MS/MS Fragments	Tentative Identification	Content (μg/g)	References
1	4.13	168.92	169, 125	Gallic acid	1.59	[43,44]
2	6.11	153.03	153, 109	Protocatechuic acid	3.83	[45]
3	6.96	353.08	191	Caffeoylquinic acid isomer	2.36	[46,47]
4	7.43	335.16	289, 245, 205, 203, 179, 151, 137, 125, 109	Epi-catechin	0.74	[48,49]
5	7.86	577.23	425, 407, 289, 245, 203, 161, 137, 125	Procyanidin B2 dimer	4.28	[50]
6	9.62	335.11	289, 245, 205, 203, 179, 165, 151, 137, 125, 109	Catechin	22.93	[48,49]
7	11.17	561.19	289, 273, 271, 245	(Epi)afzelechin-(4-8)-(epi)catechin	1.14	[51]
8	13.79	739.33	569, 459, 435, 417, 289, 177	Cinchonain II	0.32	[52,53]
9	16.50	739.38	739, 587, 569, 459, 435, 417, 339, 289, 245, 177	Cinchonain II isomer 1	30.86	[52,53]
10	20.75	451.16	341, 231, 217, 189, 177	Cinchonain I	22.82	[54]
11	22.50	739.29	569, 477, 459, 449, 435, 417, 339, 289, 177	Cichonain II isomer 2	2.24	[52,53]
12	26.18	451.15	341, 289, 231, 217, 189	Cinchonain I isomer 1	4.24	[54]
13	31.42	451.14	341, 231, 217, 189, 177	Cinchonain I isomer 2	0.29	[54]
14	45.29	451.13	341, 231, 217, 189, 177	Cinchonain I isomer 3	31.76	[54]
15	47.76	451.12	341, 217, 189, 177	Cinchonain I isomer 4	3.88	[54]
16	57.42	447.19	447, 403, 323, 295	Ellagic acid-rhamnoside	1.00	[55]

RT: retention time. Compounds were identified by comparing the mass spectra with literature data and available standards from databases (PubChem, ChemSpider, HDMB, and MassBank). The content of each compound is expressed as μg/g of dry weight.

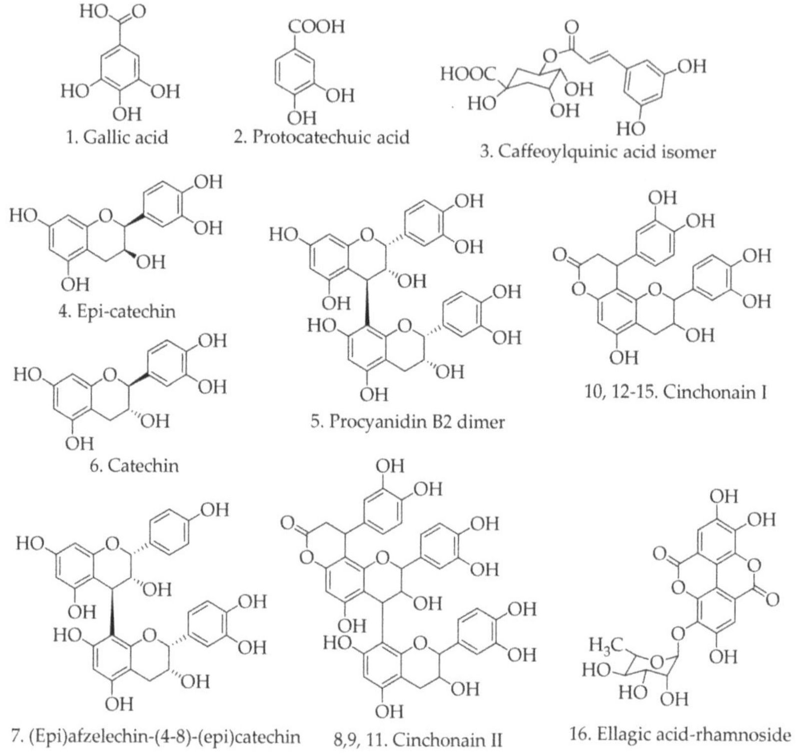

Figure 6. Structures of constituents tentatively identified in the EA fraction of *Ficus glumosa* stem bark.

Compound **1** produced the [M-H]⁻ at *m/z* 169, and the characteristic fragment ions at *m/z* 169 and 125, which signified a neutral loss of CO_2 molecule (44 Da). Thus, compound **1** was tentatively identified as gallic acid, as per recent reports [43,44]. Compound **2** displayed a precursor molecular ion [M-H]⁻ at *m/z* 153, and the loss of carboxyl group (44 Da) between the major fragment ions at *m/z* 153 and *m/z* 109 an indication of decarboxylation. The deprotonation of a molecule ion at *m/z* 153 led to the tentative identification of compound **2** as protocatechuic acid [45].

Compound **3** exhibited the [M-H]⁻ at *m/z* 353 and produced the fragment ion at *m/z* 191 [quinic acid-H]⁻ due to a loss of caffeoyl group ($C_9H_6O_3$). Compound **3** was tentatively identified as caffeoylquinic acid isomer, as earlier reported in xiao-er-qing-jie (XEQJ) granules and coffee [46,47].

Compounds **4** and **6** showed a similar protonated precursor ion at *m/z* 335 [M+HCOOH-H]⁻, which corresponds to formate adduct [M+HCOO]⁻ that formed from formic acid in the A-mobile phase. The MS^2 ion at *m/z* 289 generated fragments at *m/z* 245 [M-H-C_2H_4O]⁻, 205 [M-H-84]⁻, 203 [M-H-C_2H_4O-C_2H_2O]⁻, 179 [M-H-110]⁻, 165 [M-H-124]⁻, 151 [M-H-$C_7H_6O_3$]⁻, 137 [M-H-152]⁻, 125 [M-H-164]⁻, and 109 [M-H-180]⁻. The fragment ion at *m/z* 245 resulted from a loss of a C_2H_4O group. The cleavage of A ring produced the fragment ion at *m/z* 205. The elimination of a catechol group ($C_6H_6O_2$) yielded the ion at *m/z* 179. After heterocyclic ring fission (HRF), the B-ring was eliminated, generating fragment ion at *m/z* 165. The loss of rings A and C yielded ion at *m/z* 109. The ion at *m/z* 203 was produced from a molecular ion at *m/z* 245 after cleavage at the C-ring. Analyzing the elution order, retentions, and abundance of the fragments, the two compounds were concluded as isomers. When comparing the MS^2 spectra data and proposed fragmentation mechanism

(Figures 7 and 8) of these compounds with recent data reports, compound **4** and compound **6** were tentatively identified as epicatechin and catechin, respectively [48,49].

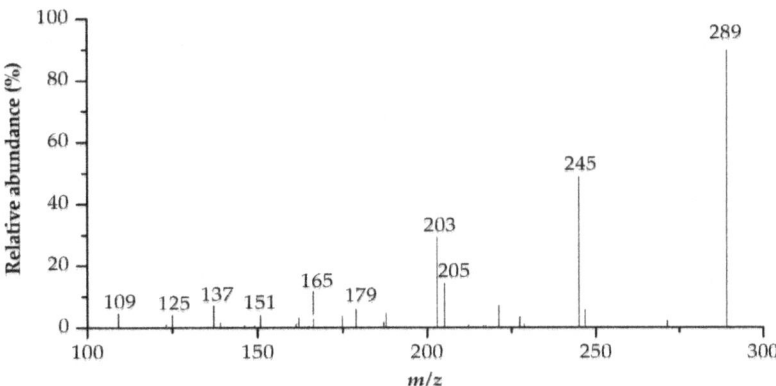

Figure 7. MS/MS spectra for catechin (peak **6**). The peak number corresponds to that in Table 2.

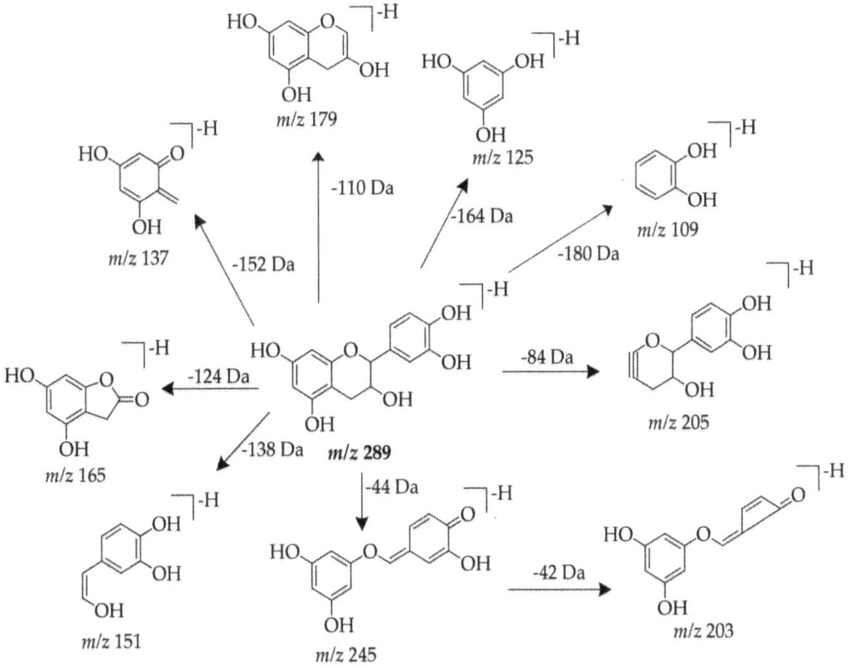

Figure 8. Proposed fragmentation pathway for catechin (peak **6**).

Compound **5** presented the [M-H]⁻ at m/z 577. Upon deprotonation, it yielded MS^2 at m/z 425, 407, 289, 245, 161, 137, and 125, respectively. The ion at m/z 425 resulted from the RDA (Retro-Diels-Alder) reaction losing 152 Da, then water (H_2O) was eliminated to form the molecular ion at m/z 407. The daughter ion at m/z 289 was consequent of the cleavage of quinone methide (QM) at the interflavan bond. The molecular ion at m/z 289 underwent further deprotonation to produce ions at m/z 245, 137, and 125, due to the neutral elimination of C_2H_4O molecule, RDA reaction, and a loss of 164 Da, respectively. The loss of 84 Da from ion at m/z 245 produced ion at m/z 161. When comparing the

MS/MS fragmentation of this compound with bibliographic data [50], compound **5** was tentatively identified as procyanidin B2 dimer.

Compound **7** showed the [M-H]$^-$ at *m/z* 561. After the RDA reaction that was characterized by a loss of 152 Da, it yielded ion at *m/z* 437. Further, MS^2 at *m/z* 289, 273, and 271 were generated as a result of quinone methide cleavage at interflavan bond. The molecular ion at *m/z* 289 suffered further deprotonation and released molecule ion at *m/z* 245 after losing a C_2H_4O group (44 Da). By analyzing this fragmentation mechanism, compound **7** was tentatively identified as (Epi)afzelechin-(4-8)-(epi)catechin, which was reported earlier in *Laurus nobilis* wood [51].

Compounds **8**, **9**, and **11** shared [M-H]$^-$ ions at *m/z* 739 with common MS/MS spectra at *m/z* 569, 459, 435, 417, 289, and 177, implying that they are isomers. The ion at *m/z* 569 [M-H-152-H_2O]$^-$ was produced as a consequence of RDA cleavage at the C ring characterized by 152 Da loss, and then followed by H_2O molecule loss. The fragment ion at *m/z* 459 [M-H-152-H_2O-$C_6H_6O_2$]$^-$ was generated due to the loss of dihydroxybenzene ($C_6H_6O_2$) from ion at *m/z* 569. Quinone methide fission generated ion at *m/z* 289, which also produced the daughter ion at *m/z* 177 after a loss of 112 Da. Repeated RDA cleavage at C-rings of lower and upper subunits led to the formation of the molecular ion at *m/z* 435. The ion at *m/z* 435 underwent a loss of H_2O molecule to form the fragment ion at *m/z* 417. Hence, compounds 8, 9, and 11 were concluded as cinchonain II isomers. To our expectation, similar compounds with identical fragmentation were reported in *Crataegus folium* and *Inula viscosa* species, respectively [52,53].

Compounds **10**, **12**, **13**, **14**, and **15** displayed the [M-H]$^-$ at *m/z* 451. They produced characteristic MS^2 fragments at *m/z* 341 [M-H-$C_6H_6O_2$]$^-$, *m/z* 231 [M-H-$2C_6H_6O_2$]$^-$, *m/z* 217 [M-H-$2C_6H_6O_2$-CH_2]$^-$, and *m/z* 189 [M-H-$2C_6H_6O_2$-C_2H_2O]$^-$, respectively, a confirmation that they were isomers. Besides, fragment ion at *m/z* 217 underwent further loss of 40 Da to generate predominant ion at *m/z* 177. Compounds **10**, **12**, **13**, **14**, and **15** were identified as cinchonain I isomers, which were earlier reported in *Acer palmatum* by Zhang et al. [54].

Compound **16** exhibited [M-H]$^-$ at *m/z* 447, and then released a series of MS^2 ions at *m/z* 403 [M-H-44]$^-$, 323 [M-H-124]$^-$, and 295 [M-H-124-CO]$^-$. By comparing this fragmentation mechanism with MS/MS data in previous literature, compound **16** was tentatively identified as ellagic acid-rhamnoside [55].

2.6. Quantification of Polyphenols in EA Fraction of Ficus glumosa

The biological assays and therapeutic effects of this species depend on the quantity of each secondary metabolite identified. Particularly, the efficacy of traditional drugs relies on the phytochemicals traits that elicit different biological activities.

The validated methods mentioned above were employed to investigate the quantities of the 16 bioactive constituents that were identified in the EA fraction of *Ficus glumosa*, as per the previous study. The secondary metabolites that were characterized in this fraction were polyphenols, known for their pharmacological properties. Each polyphenol was quantified based on two linear curves that were developed using external standards (gallic acid and rutin) and plotting the areas of established curves against concentrations. The phenolic derivatives and phenolic acids were given in terms of gallic acid, whereas the flavonoids were expressed as rutin. The quantities of the identified compounds in the EA fraction of *Ficus glumosa* stem bark were estimated and Table 2 provides their quantification results. As confirmed in the screening data, the flavonoids were mainly flavanols and they were the most chemical constituents in *Ficus glumosa* in this study. Cinchonain I isomer 3 (14) was the most abundant constituent, with 31.76 µg/g. Cinchonain II isomer 1 (9) was the second in abundance, with 30.86 µg/g, followed by catechin (6) (22.93 µg/g). Cinchonain I isomer 2 (13) was the least abundant, with 0.29 µg/g. Generally, cinchonain I isomers accounted for higher content, followed by cinchonain II isomers in this study. Phenolic acids occurred in trace amounts. In this class of compounds, protocatechuic acid displayed a higher content of 3.83 µg/g when compared to the other phenolic acids. Hence, it is suspected flavonoids accounted for the promising biological activities depicted by this fraction, owing to their abundance. It is worth noting that the quantification of each compound content was an estimation of occurrence in the analyzed sample.

The chemical and content variation in this species might affect further pharmacological explorations of *Ficus glumosa*. The geographical location and period of samples' collection might have influenced the content of bioactive constituents in this species. In addition to the aforementioned factors, perhaps there might be other factors affecting the chemical content that require extra investigations. Further, enhancing the efficacy, precision, and consistency in the preparation of herbal drugs, the validation of every step involved is recommended.

2.7. Biological Significance of Chemical Constituents in EA Fraction of Ficus glumosa

The pharmacological activities of this species could be linked with the quantity and quality of structurally diverse secondary constituents that interact and react with the test components. HPLC-ESI-MS/MS analysis of EA fraction revealed 16 polyphenolic compounds, mainly flavonoids and phenolic acids (Table 2). The aforementioned compounds are well known for their bioactivity significance.

Polyphenols are normally formed in plants for obvious roles; however, their increased synthesis is triggered as a counter mechanism to biotic/abiotic stresses [56]. Some of the identified compounds belong to phenolic acids, namely gallic acid (1), protocatechuic acid (2), and caffeoylquinic acid isomer (3). These are active metabolites that are widely reported with strong antioxidant and antitumor bioactivities [57,58]. The number of OH groups, the saturation degree, and other substitute groups dictate their potential in radical quenching/scavenging mechanism as well as their anticancer activity [59].

Flavonoids possess versatile health-promoting effects, as demonstrated in previous studies [60]. Majorly, flavanols constituted a higher percentage of components in the EA fraction. Bansal [61] highlighted that flavanols' biological properties tend to be influenced by the position and number of OH groups, the presence of catechol/pyrogallol groups on the B-ring, OH groups at positions C3, C5, and C7, and their degree of polymerization. In this regard, bioactivity decrease from trimers to monomers, whilst it increases from trimers to tetramers, whereas the ease of degradation varies with the type of interflavan bond in oligomers, with epicatechin being more easily oxidized than catechin [62]. In the present study, epicatechin (4), procyanidin B2 dimer (5), catechin (6), (epi)afzelechin-(4-8)-(epi)catechin (7), cinchonain II (8), and cinchonain I (10) were tentatively identified in this species and they were previously reported with some biological importance. They possess antioxidant, anti-inflammatory, and antiproliferative properties for the case of catechin (6) and epicatechin (4) [63], procyanidin B2 dimer (5) [64], and (epi)afzelechin-(4-8)-(epi)catechin (7) [65]. Further, cinchonain I (10) and II (8) compounds are reported to depict good antioxidant potential [66,67]. Ellagic acid-rhamnoside (16) was earlier assayed and found to exhibit high antioxidant and antibacterial properties [68,69].

Each of the identified compounds is believed to have interacted with the test components at different affinities that are reflected in the biological activities. Moreover, these identified phytochemicals showed lower potency than the standard controls that were used in the experimental tests. Hence, we recommend thorough screening and elucidation, followed by biological activity evaluation of each compound.

3. Materials and Methods

3.1. Chemicals and Reagents

China Medicine (Group) Shanghai Chemical Reagent Corp provided ethanol, ethyl acetate, petroleum ether, hexane, and *n*-butanol. (Shanghai, China). Acetonitrile and formic acid (HPLC grade solvents) were acquired from TEDIA Limited (Fairfield, OH, USA) and used with no further purification. The ultrapure water for LC-MS/HPLC analysis was generated using an EPED machine (Yeap Esselte Tech. Co., Nanjing, China). Sulforhodamine B (SRB), Dulbecco's Modified Eagle Medium (DMEM), streptomycin, and dimethyl sulfoxide (DMSO) were purchased from Gibco (New York, NY, USA). Millipore membranes (0.22 µm) were provided by Jinteng Instrument Corporation (China). Trolox, gallic acid (99%), rutin (98%), vitamin C, BHT, ABTS, DPPH, and TPTZ were bought from Sigma–Aldrich Corporation (St. Louis, MO, USA).

3.2. Plant Materials

The fresh stem barks of *Ficus glumosa* were harvested from a farm in Makueni County, Kenya in July 2019. The cultivated plant materials were identified and authenticated by a botanist from the East Africa Herbarium, National Museums of Kenya. A voucher specimen number EAHF001/2019 was deposited in the herbarium of East Africa.

These materials were washed, dried under a shed, pulverized, powdered, and then packed into polythene bags. They were stored at room temperature for further analysis.

3.3. Sample Extraction and Partitioning

The extraction process was performed as per a previous study [70] with some modifications. The 4.0 kg dried powdered *Ficus glumosa* stem bark was repeatedly extracted (30 min. for three times) using an ultrasound-assisted extraction method at 30 °C with 70% ethanol. The extracts were then combined and filtered. A rotatory evaporator was used to evaporate the filtered extracts at 45 °C under reduced pressure and then lyophilized for 48 h. The total dry ethanol extracts obtained was 435.5 g. From the dry ethanol extracts, 39.5 g was dissolved into 200 mL of H_2O. This solution was then subjected to subsequent liquid/liquid extraction using petroleum ether (PE), ethyl acetate (EA), *n*-butanol, and water in that order to obtain their corresponding PE, EA, *n*-butanol, and water fractions.

3.4. Preparation of Standard Solutions

Two reference compounds, rutin, and gallic acid, were prepared while using methanol, each at 1 mg/mL. The standard solutions were properly attenuated using methanol in a serial dilution to obtain working standards. The working solutions/standards ranged from 1.25 to 40 μg/mL for rutin and 1 to 32 μg/mL for gallic acid. Each of the external calibration curves was established using six working standards.

3.5. Method Validation for Quantitative Analysis

This analysis was conducted as per a recent study [71] with some modifications. The established procedure was used in determining the limit of detection and quantification (LOD/LOQ), precision, stability, and accuracy. Firstly, 10 μL of each of the working standards was analyzed using HPLC-UV (Agilent 1220 HPLC, Waldron, Germany) and chromatograms were obtained at 280 nm. Peak areas were plotted versus concentrations to obtain linear graphs. The LODs and LOQs were examined at a signal-to-noise ratio (S/N) of 3.3 and 10, respectively.

Intraday precision tests were conducted by analyzing one sample in six replicates within one day. The same sample was analyzed for three consecutively days in triplicate to evaluate for interday precision. For the repeatability test, five replicates of the sample extract were analyzed in a day. The stability test was conducted by examining one sample six times.

Two lots of three replicates of the sample extract were prepared to investigate for recovery. The first lot was analyzed. The second lot was spiked with a known concentration of the standards and then analyzed. Recovery (%) was calculated, as follows: [Detected amount—initial amount]/spiked amount × 100%. Eventually, precision, repeatability, stability, and recovery were given in RSD %.

3.6. Determination of Total Flavonoid Content (TFC)

This analysis was determined colorimetrically, as per [72] with few adjustments. Firstly, a freshly prepared sample was mixed well with 0.2 mL of 5% $NaNO_2$ in a 4 mL EP tube for 6 min. Afterward, 0.2 mL of 10% $AlCl_3 \cdot 6H_2O$ was added and the solution was allowed to settle. After 6 min., 1 mL of 4% NaOH solution was added. The contents were left for 15 min., after which the absorbance was observed at 510 nm with a UV-spectrophotometer (UV-11000, MAPADA Shanghai, China). This procedure was repeated using rutin in place of a sample extract. This test was performed in triplicate and the results were defined as mg of rutin equivalents per gram (mg RE/g) sample.

3.7. Determination of Total Phenolic Content (TPC)

The TPC was performed in accordance with the Folin–Ciocalteu guidelines [73], with some modifications. First, 50 μL of prepared sample extract together with 1.0 mL of 2% Na_2CO_3 solution were added in a 2.0 mL EP mixed, and then incubated for 6 min. After 50 μL Folin–Ciocalteu reagent addition, the solution was incubated in darkness for 40 min. Finally, the reaction absorbance was observed at 750 nm with a UV-spectrophotometer (UV-1100, MAPADA Shanghai, China). This method was repeated by replacing the sample extract with gallic acid. For each sample, this assay was conducted in triplicate, and the results were given as mg of gallic acid equivalents (mg GAE/g) per gram of sample.

3.8. In-Vitro Antioxidant Assays of Ficus Glumosa

3.8.1. DPPH Assay

The DPPH assay of the Ficus glumosa samples was evaluated as per the previous method [74] with little modifications. DPPH solution (0.1mM) was prepared using methanol. First, 10 μL of the prepared sample extract and positive controls were mixed each interchangeably with 190 μL of already prepared DPPH in a well-plate. The mixture was cultivated for 30 min. in the dark and the attained absorbance was observed at 517 nm using the multifunctional 96-well plate reader (Tecan, Infinite M20PRO, Switzerland). Methanol was used to correct the baseline as the blank. This assay was repeated three times. The percentage rate of the DPPH scavenging was calculated and then expressed, as follows: DPPH activity (%) = $[(C_O-C_1/C_O)] \times 100\%$, where Co is the control absorbance and C_1 is the sample extract/control absorbance.

3.8.2. ABTS Assay

This assay was performed as per [75] with minimal modifications. The ABTS solution (7 mM) was first prepared using ultrapure water. After that, $ABTS^+$ stock solution preparation was done by mixing equivalent volumes of ABTS (7 mM) with (2.45 mM) potassium persulfate (dissolved in water), and then the mixture was incubated for 16 h. Methanol was used to dilute the $ABTS^+$ stock until an absorbance of 0.70 ± 0.02 was achieved at 734 nm. The test samples were then appropriately attenuated to attain serial concentrations. Subsequently, 10 μL of the freshly prepared sample was mixed with 190 μL $ABTS^+$ solution and left covered for 30 min. The contents absorbance was observed and noted at 734 nm. Methanol was used to correct the baseline. This test was done three times. The ABTS calculation and results expression was in terms of IC_{50} similarly as in the DPPH assay that is described above.

3.8.3. FRAP Assay

The FRAP assay test of ethanol extracts, petroleum ether (PE), ethyl acetate (EA), n-butanol, and water fractions of Ficus glumosa was done as per [70] with minimal modifications. First, the stock solution, FRAP reagent (Fe^{3+}-TPTZ), was made up of 300 mM acetate buffer of pH 3.6 (sodium acetate, acetic acid plus water), $FeCl_3 \cdot 6H_2O$ solution, and 10 mM TPTZ (2,4,6-tri(2-pyridyl)-S-triazine) solution in 40 mM HCl in a ratio of 10:1:1 ($v/v/v$). It was heated first to attain 37 °C. In a 1.5 mL EP tube, 20 μL of the properly mixed sample was mixed with 60 μL H_2O and 520 μL fresh FRAP reagent. This solution was stored for 12 min. at 37 °C. Afterward, the absorbance of the mixture was read at 593 nm with a UV-spectrophotometer (UV-1100, MAPADA, China). Each test was repeated three times. The results were eventually given as milligrams Fe^{2+} per gram (mg Fe^{2+}/g) of the sample in mean values $\pm$ SEM. $FeSO_4 \cdot 7H_2O$ was used as the standard.

3.9. In-Vitro Anti-Proliferative Assay of Ficus glumosa

3.9.1. Cell Culture

Two human cancer cells for colon adenocarcinoma (HT-29) and lung adenocarcinoma (A549) were both purchased from China Centre for Type Culture Collection (Hubei, China). The DMEM (checked for contamination prior use) for the culture of cancer cells was composed of 100 μg/mL streptomycin-1% penicillin (100 U/mL), fetal bovine serum (10%), and L-glutamine (2 mM). The cells were cultured in an environment of 90% relative humidity (RH), 5% CO_2, and 37 °C for one week to achieve confluence. A hemocytometer was employed in order to check for the viable cells well suited for cytotoxicity assay with only those having over 80% confluence being the ones selected.

3.9.2. Anti-Proliferative Activity Analysis

The ethanol extracts, petroleum ether (PE), ethyl acetate (EA), n-butanol, and water fractions of *Ficus glumosa* were evaluated for antitumor activity against A549 and HT-29 cancer cells using the sulforhodamine (SRB) assay [76] with minimal modifications. Briefly, 100 μL monolayer cells (of specified density) that were contained in DMEM were inoculated in each 96-well-plate. The cells were incubated for 3 h in a well-humidified area at 90% RH, 37 °C, and then 5% CO_2 for another 24 h to regain confluence before the sample addition. At first, the extract samples were dissolved at high concentrations using DMSO, and later at a lower concentration using water and then allowed to dry at room temperature. DMEM was used to prepared different concentration samples in each well. The 96 well-plate was incubated for 72 h, and 5 μL of 10% cold (4 °C) trichloroacetic acid (TCA) was then added for 40 min. at 4 °C. The supernatant was washed and dried at 25 °C. Subsequently, the plates (dried) were stained in 1% CH_3CO_2H using 50 μL of 0.4% w/v SRB for 20 min. The 1% CH_3CO_2H was used to wash the plates and then allowed to dry. After drying, they were dissolved using 150 μL of 10 mM Tris base. The absorbance was taken at 510 nm wavelength. A medium with less than 0.1% DMSO was used as the control. This assay was conducted in triplicate and the results evaluated, as follows.

IC_{50} cell inhibition (%) = [OD mean of control − OD mean of extract/OD mean of control] × 100%, where OD is the absorbance value.

3.10. HPLC-ESI-MS/MS Analysis of EA Fraction of Ficus Glumosa

The analysis of *Ficus glumosa* was conducted using a Thermo Accela HPLC 600 connected with a mass spectrometer, TSQ-Quantum™ Access MAX (Thermo Fischer, San Jose, California, USA). The separation of the sample was achieved by Waters Symmetry RP-C18 column, 4.6 × 250 mm, 5 μm (Milford, USA) at 30 °C. The solvents (water/acetonitrile) were composed of formic (FA) acid (0.1%) in ultrapure water (A mobile phase) and 100% ACN (B mobile phase). The HPLC elution gradient was adjusted and set, as follows: 15–17% in 0–5 min., 17% in 5–15 min., 17–23% in 15–40 min., 23–25% in 40–45 min., and 25–33% in 45–65 min. Injected volume, 10 μL, 0.8 mL/min. as the flow rate, and online monitoring of UV-chromatogram was at 280 nm. The MS settings were adjusted, as below: negative full scan and dependent-data scan mode, capillary temperature, 350 °C, vaporizer temperature at 300 °C, sheath gas pressure (N_2) at 40 psi, auxiliary pressure (N_2) at 10 psi, and spray voltage at 3kV and mass range at 150–1500 m/z.

3.11. Statistical Analysis

All analyses were conducted, and their resulted values were given as mean ± standard deviations. The SPSS statistics 22 software (IBM Corporation, New York, USA) was used for data analysis. One way ANOVA with Duncan test was used for comparing multiple means and significance differences were considered at $p < 0.01$ and $p < 0.05$.

4. Conclusions

In this study, all of the bioassays conducted serve as evidence of the effects of *Ficus glumosa* on ABTS, DPPH, and FRAP, along with antiproliferative activities on A549 and

HT-29 cells. This is the first study to report on the phytochemical profile, antioxidant, and antiproliferative properties of the EA fraction of *Ficus glumosa* stem bark. The EA fraction depicted good potency in both antitumor and antioxidant activities, which reflected the polyphenols composition in this fraction. Notably, HPLC-ESI-MS/MS analysis led to the characterization of 16 compounds, which consisted of three phenolic acids, a phenolic derivative, and 12 flavonoids. Hence, this study comprehensively substantiates *Ficus glumosa* as a prospective remedy for cancer phytomedicine development. Meanwhile, detailed phytochemical fingerprinting work on this underexploited species not only provide a baseline for further investigations, but is also considered to be paramount in support of its pharmacological value, as justified in ethnopharmacological use.

Author Contributions: M.-Q.G. and G.-L.C. conceived of, designed, and supervised the study. M.M.M., F.W.M., F.K., Y.-B.X., and H.Z. performed the experiments, analyzed the data, and wrote the manuscript. All authors have read and agreed to the published version of the manuscript.

Funding: This work was partly supported by the Youth Innovation Promotion Association of Chinese Academy of Sciences (Grant No. 2020337 to G. Chen), and the Natural Science Foundation of Hubei Province (Grant No. 2019CFB254 to G. Chen). The funders played no roles in the study design, data collection and analysis, and decision to publish.

Data Availability Statement: Data sharing not applicable.

Conflicts of Interest: The authors declare no conflict of interest.

References

1. Beentje, H.J. Fig trees (*Ficus*, Moraceae) of Kenya. *J. East Afr. Nat. Hist. Soc. Ntl. Mus.* **1988**, *76*, 53–76.
2. Akpana, A.M.; Edward, M.J.; Henry, P.; Joseph, A. Mineral and vitamin composition of some lesser-known leafy vegetables consumed in northern senatorial district of Cross River State, Nigeria. *Am. J. Food. Nutr.* **2017**, *5*, 51–57.
3. Jansen, P.; Cardon, D. *Plant Resources of Tropical Africa 3. Dyes and Tannins*; PROTA Foundation: Wageningen, The Netherlands, 2005.
4. Ameh, P.O. Physicochemical properties and rheological behaviour of *Ficus glumosa* gum in aqueous solution. *Afr. J. Pure Appl. Chem.* **2013**, *7*, 35–43.
5. Telefo, P.B.; Lienou, L.L.; Yemele, M.D.; Lemfack, M.C.; Mouokeu, C.; Goka, C.S.; Tagne, S.R.; Moundipa, F.P. Ethnopharmacological survey of plants used for the treatment of female infertility in Baham, Cameroon. *J. Ethnopharmacol.* **2011**, *136*, 178–187. [CrossRef]
6. Masarirambi, M.T.; Zwane, P.E.; Surana, N.; Kunene, E.N.; Moyo, S.; Mabuza, L.L.; Makhanya, B.P. Indigenous dye plants of the Kingdom of Eswatini, traditional uses and new prospects. *Adv. Med. Plant Res.* **2019**, *7*, 8–14. [CrossRef]
7. Umar, Z.U.; Moh'd, A.; Tanko, Y. Effects of ethanol leaf extract of *Ficus glumosa* on fasting blood glucose and serum lipid profile in diabetic rats. *Niger. J. Physiol. Sci.* **2013**, *28*, 99–104.
8. Koné, W.M.; Atindehou, K.K. Ethnobotanical inventory of medicinal plants used in traditional veterinary medicine in northern Côte d'Ivoire (West Africa). *S. Afric. J. Bot.* **2008**, *74*, 76–84. [CrossRef]
9. Jeruto, P.; Mutai, C.; Ouma, G.; Lukhoba, C.; Nyamaka, R.L.; Manani, S.D. Ethnobotanical survey and propagation of some endangered medicinal plants from South Nandi district of Kenya. *J. Anim. Plant Sci.* **2010**, *8*, 1016–1043.
10. Madubunyi, I.I.; Onoja, S.O.; Asuzu, I.U. In vitro antioxidant and in vivo antidiabetic potential of the methanol extract of *Ficus glumosa* Del (Moraceae) stem bark in alloxan-induced diabetic mice. *Comp. Clin. Pathol.* **2010**, *21*, 389–394. [CrossRef]
11. Ntchapda, F.; Djedouboum, A.; Kom, B.; Nana, P.; Bonabe, C.; Maguirgue, K.; Talla, E.; Dimo, T. Diuretic activity of the aqueous extract leaves of *Ficus glumosa* Del. (Moraceae) in rats. *Sci. World J.* **2014**, *2014*. [CrossRef]
12. Ntchapda, F.; Djedouboum, A.; Talla, E.; Sokeng, D.S.; Nana, P.; Adjia, H.; Nguimbou, R.M.; Bonabe, C.; Gaimatakon, S.; Njintang, Y.N.; et al. Hypolipidemic and anti-atherogenic effect of aqueous extract leaves of *Ficus glumosa* (Moraceae) in rats. *Exp. Gerontol.* **2015**, *62*, 53–62. [CrossRef]
13. Sibandze, G.F. Pharmacological Properties of Swazi Medicinal Plants. Ph.D. Thesis, University of Witwatersrand, Johannesburg, South Africa, 2009.
14. Abubakar, M.S.; Musa, A.M.; Ahmed, A.; Hussaini, I.M. The perception and practice of traditional medicine in the treatment of cancers and inflammations by the Hausa and Fulani tribes of Northern Nigeria. *J. Ethnopharmacol.* **2007**, *111*, 625–629. [CrossRef]
15. Deepa, P.; Sowndhararajan, K.; Kim, S.; Park, S.J. A role of *Ficus* species in the management of diabetes mellitus: A review. *J. Ethnopharmacol.* **2018**, *215*, 210–232. [CrossRef]
16. Kwazo, H.A.; Faruq, U.Z.; Danggogo, S.M.; Malalmi, B.S.; Moronkola, D.O. Antimicrobial activity and phytochemical screening of crude water extract of the stem bark of *Ficus glumosa*. *Sci. Res Essays* **2015**, *10*, 177–183.
17. Ibrahim, M.T.; Shafei, A.A.; Mahrous, F. Phytochemical and biological studies of natural Egyptian recipe with anticancer effect. *IOSR J. Pharm. Biol. Sci.* **2017**, *12*, 29–39. [CrossRef]

18. Jasmine, R.; Manikandan, K.; Karthikeyan, K. Evaluating the antioxidant and anticancer property of *Ficus carica* fruits. *Afr. J. Biotechnol.* **2015**, *14*, 634–641. [CrossRef]
19. Purnamasari, R.; Winarni, D.; Permanasari, A.A.; Agustina, E.; Hayaza, S.; Darmanto, W. Anticancer activity of methanol extract of *Ficus carica* leaves and fruits against proliferation, apoptosis, and necrosis in Huh7it Cells. *Cancer Inform.* **2019**, *18*, 2576. [CrossRef]
20. Awolola, G.V. Phytochemical analyses and biological activities of four South African *Ficus* species (Moraceae). Ph.D. Thesis, University of Kwazulu-Natal, Durban, South Africa, 2015.
21. Barde, M.I.; Hassan, Y. Phytochemical screening and antioxidant potential of selected Nigerian vegetables. *Intern. Ann. Sci.* **2019**, *8*, 12–16.
22. Awolola, G.V.; Sofidiya, M.O.; Baijnath, H.; Noren, S.S.; Koorbanally, N.A. The phytochemistry and gastroprotective activities of the leaves of *Ficus glumosa*. *S. Afr. J. Bot.* **2019**, *126*, 190–195. [CrossRef]
23. Wahle, K.W.J.; Brown, I.; Rotondo, D.; Heys, S.D. Plant Phenolics in the Prevention and Treatment of cancer. In *Bio-Farms for Nutraceuticals*; Springer: Aberdeen, UK, 2010; pp. 36–51.
24. Khan, N.; Afaq, F.; Mukhtar, H. Cancer chemoprevention through dietary antioxidants: Progress and promise. *Antioxid. Redox Signal.* **2008**, *10*, 475–510. [CrossRef] [PubMed]
25. Lobo, V.; Patil, A.; Phatak, A.; Chandra, N. Free radicals, antioxidants and functional foods: Impact on human health. A review. *Pharmacogn. Rev.* **2010**, *4*, 118–126. [CrossRef]
26. Nana, F.; Sandjo, L.P.; Keumedjio, F.; Ambassa, P.; Malik, R.; Kuete, V.; Rincheval, V.; Choudhary, M.I.; Ngadjui, B.T. Ceramides and cytotoxic constituents from *Ficus glumosa* Del. (Moraceae). *J. Braz. Chem Soc.* **2012**, *23*, 482–487. [CrossRef]
27. Olaokun, O.O.; McGaw, L.J.; Eloff, J.N.; Naidoo, V. Evaluation of the inhibition of carbohydrate hydrolysing enzymes, antioxidant activity and polyphenolic content of extracts of ten African *Ficus* species (Moraceae) used traditionally to treat diabetes. *BMC Complement Altern. Med.* **2013**, *13*, 1–10. [CrossRef] [PubMed]
28. Sultana, J.; Kabir, A.S.; Hakim, M.A.; Abdullah, M.; Islam, N.; Reza, M.A. Evaluation of the antioxidant activity of *Ficus racemosa* plant extracts from north-western district of Bangladesh. *J. Life Earth Sci.* **2013**, *8*, 93–99. [CrossRef]
29. Yadav, S.; Gupta, V.K.; Gopalakrishnan, A.; Verma, M.R. Antioxidant activity analysis of *Ficus racemosa* leaf extract. *J. Entomol. Zool. Stud.* **2019**, *7*, 1443–1446.
30. Abdel-Hameed, E.-S.S. Total phenolic contents and free radical scavenging activity of certain Egyptian *Ficus* species leaf samples. *Food Chem.* **2009**, *114*, 1271–1277. [CrossRef]
31. Al-Matani, S.K.; Al-Wahaibi, R.N.S.; Hossain, M.A. Total flavonoids content and antimicrobial activity of crude extract from leaves of *Ficus sycomorus* native to Sultanate of Oman. *Karbala Intern. J. Mod. Sci.* **2015**, *1*, 166–171.
32. Siddhuraju, P.; Becker, K. Antioxidant properties of various solvent extracts of total phenolic constituents from three different agroclimatic origins of drumstick tree (*Moringa oleifera* Lam.) leaves. *J. Agric. Food Chem.* **2003**, *51*, 2144–2155. [CrossRef]
33. Singh, M.; Kaur, M.; Silakari, O. Flavones: An important scaffold for medicinal chemistry. *Eur. J. Med. Chem.* **2014**, *84*, 206–239. [CrossRef]
34. Veerapur, V.P.; Prabhakar, K.R.; Parihar, V.K.; Kandadi, M.R.; Ramakrishana, S.; Mishra, B.; Rao, B.S.S.; Srinivasan, K.K.; Priyadarsini, K.I.; Unnikrishnan, M.K. *Ficus racemosa* stem bark extract: A potent antioxidant and a probable natural radioprotector. *Evid. Based Complement. Alternat. Med.* **2009**, *6*, 317–324. [CrossRef]
35. Sawadogo, W.R.; Maciuk, A.; Banzouzi, J.T.; Champy, P.; Figadere, B.; Guissou, I.P.; Nacoulma, O.G. Mutagenic effect, antioxidant and anticancer activities of six medicinal plants from Burkina Faso. *Nat. Prod. Res.* **2012**, *26*, 575–579. [CrossRef]
36. Shi, Y.X.; Xu, Y.K.; Hu, H.B.; Na, Z.; Wang, W.-H. Preliminary assessment of antioxidant activity of young edible leaves of seven *Ficus* species in the ethnic diet in Xishuangbanna, Southwest China. *Food Chem.* **2011**, *128*, 889–894. [CrossRef]
37. Brewer, M.S. Natural antioxidants: Sources, compounds, mechanism of action, and potential applications. *Compr. Rev. Food Sci. Food Saf.* **2011**, *10*, 221–247. [CrossRef]
38. Reczek, C.R.; Chandel, N.S. The two faces of reactive oxygen species in cancer. *Annual. Rev. Cancer Biol.* **2017**, *1*, 79–98. [CrossRef]
39. Waris, G.; Ahsan, H. Reactive oxygen species: Role in the development of cancer and various chronic conditions. *J. Carcinog.* **2006**, *5*, 14. [CrossRef] [PubMed]
40. Bhullar, K.S.; Rupasinghe, H.P.V. Polyphenols: Multipotent therapeutic agents in neurodegenerative diseases. *Oxid. Med. Cell. Longev.* **2013**, *2013*. [CrossRef] [PubMed]
41. Abubakar, I.B.; Lim, K.H.; Loh, H.S. Alkaloid extracts of *Ficus* species and palm oil-derived tocotrienols synergistically inhibit proliferation of human cancer cells. *Nat. Prod. Res.* **2015**, *29*, 2137–2140. [CrossRef] [PubMed]
42. Yessoufou, K.; Elansary, H.O.; Mahmoud, E.A.; Skalicka-Woźniak, K. Antifungal, antibacterial and anticancer activities of *Ficus drupacea* L. stem bark extract and biologically active isolated compounds. *Ind. Crops Prod.* **2015**, *74*, 752–758. [CrossRef]
43. Mena, P.; Calani, L.; Dall'Asta, C.; Galaverna, G.; Garcia-Viguera, C.; Bruni, R.; Crozier, A.; Rio, D.D. Rapid and comprehensive evaluation of (poly)phenolic compounds in pomegranate (*Punica granatum* L.) juice by UHPLC-MSn. *Molecules* **2012**, *17*, 14821–14840. [CrossRef]
44. Wyrepkowski, C.C.; Gomes, D.L.M.C.; Sinhorin, A.P.; Vilegas, W.; De, R.A.G.; Resende, F.A.; Varanda, E.A.; Dos, L.C.S. Characterization and quantification of the compounds of the ethanolic extract from *Caesalpinia ferrea* stem bark and evaluation of their mutagenic activity. *Molecules* **2014**, *19*, 16039–16057. [CrossRef] [PubMed]

45. Chen, G.L.; Mutie, F.M.; Xu, Y.B.; Saleri, F.D.; Hu, G.W.; Guo, M.Q. Antioxidant, anti-inflammatory activities and polyphenolprofile of *Rhamnus prinoides*. *Pharmaceuticals.* **2020**, *13*, 55. [CrossRef]
46. Li, Y.; Liu, Y.; Liu, R.; Liu, S.; Zhang, X.; Wang, Z.; Zhang, J.; Lu, J. HPLC-LTQ-orbitrap MSn profiling method to comprehensively characterize multiple chemical constituents in xiao-er-qing-jie granules. *Anal. Methods.* **2015**, *7*, 7511–7526. [CrossRef]
47. Gómez-Juaristi, M.; Martínez-López, S.; Sarria, B.; Bravo, L.; Mateos, R. Bioavailability of hydroxycinnamates in an instant green/roasted coffee blend in humans. Identification of novel colonic metabolites. *Food Funct.* **2018**, *9*, 331–343. [CrossRef]
48. Ammar, S.; del Mar Contreras, M.; Belguith-Hadrich, O.; Bouaziz, M.; Segura-Carretero, A. New insights into the qualitative phenolic profile of *Ficus carica* L. fruits and leaves from Tunisia using ultra-high-performance liquid chromatography coupled to quadrupole-time-of-flight mass spectrometry and their antioxidant activity. *RSC Adv.* **2015**, *5*, 20035–20050. [CrossRef]
49. Kumar, S.; Singh, A.; Kushwaha, A.K.; Tiwari, R.; Chaudhary, L.B.; Srivastava, M.; Kumar, B. The UPLC–ESI–QqQLIT–MS/MS method for quantitative determination of phytochemicals in ethanolic extracts of different parts of eight *Ficus* species: Development and validation. *Int. J. Food Prop.* **2018**, *21*, 328–344. [CrossRef]
50. Rockenbach, I.I.; Jungfer, E.; Ritter, C.; Santiago-Schübel, B.; Thiele, B.; Fett, R.; Galensa, R. Characterization of flavan-3-ols in seeds of grape pomace by CE, HPLC-DAD-MSn and LC-ESI-FTICR-MS. *Food Res. Int.* **2012**, *48*, 848–855. [CrossRef]
51. Alejo-Armijo, A.; Tello-Abolafia, A.; Salido, S.; Altarejos, J. Phenolic compounds in laurel wood: A New source of proanthocyanidins. *J. Wood Chem. Technol.* **2019**, *39*, 436–453. [CrossRef]
52. Sendker, J.; Petereit, F.; Lautenschläger, M.; Hellenbrand, N.; Hensel, A. Phenylpropanoid-substituted procyanidins and tentatively identified procyanidin glycosides from Hawthorn (Crataegus spp). *Planta Med.* **2012**, *79*, 45–51. [CrossRef] [PubMed]
53. Brahmi-Chendouh, N.; Piccolella, S.; Crescente, G.; Pacifico, F.; Boulekbache, L.; Hamri-Zeghichi, S.; Akkal, S.; Madani, K.; Pacifico, S. A nutraceutical extract from *Inula viscosa* leaves: UHPLC-HR-MS/MS based polyphenol profile, and antioxidant and cytotoxic activities. *J. Food Drug Anal.* **2019**, *27*, 692–702. [CrossRef] [PubMed]
54. Zhang, L.; Tu, Z.C.; Xie, X.; Lu, Y.; Wang, Z.X.; Wang, H.; Sha, X.M. Antihyperglycemic, antioxidant activities of two *Acer palmatum* cultivars, and identification of phenolics profile by UPLC-QTOF-MS/MS: New natural sources of functional constituents. *Ind. Crops. Prod.* **2016**, *89*, 522–532. [CrossRef]
55. Biazotto, K.R.; De Souza, L.M.M.; Neves, B.V.; Braga, A.R.C.; Tangerina, M.M.P.; Vilegas, W.; Mercadante, A.Z.; De Rosso, V.V. Brazilian biodiversity fruits: Discovering bioactive compounds from underexplored sources. *J. Agric. Food Chem.* **2019**, *67*, 1860–1876. [CrossRef]
56. Sharma, A.; Shahzad, B.; Rehman, A.; Bhardwaj, R.; Landi, M.; Zheng, B. Response of phenylpropanoid pathway and the role of polyphenols in plants under abiotic Stress. *Molecules* **2019**, *24*, 2452. [CrossRef] [PubMed]
57. Gomes, C.A.; da Cruz, T.G.; Andrade, J.L.; Milhazes, N.; Borges, F.; Marques, M.P.M. Anticancer activity of phenolic acids of natural or synthetic origin: A structure-activity study. *J. Med. Chem.* **2003**, *46*, 5395–5401. [CrossRef] [PubMed]
58. Sarker, U.; Oba, S. Antioxidant constituents of three selected red and green color *Amaranthus* leafy vegetable. *Sci. Rep.* **2019**, *9*, 1–11. [CrossRef] [PubMed]
59. Goleniowski, M.; Bonfill, M.; Cusido, R.; Palazón, J. Phenolic Acids. In *Natural Products*; Springer: Berlin/Heidelberg, Germany, 2013; pp. 1951–1973. [CrossRef]
60. De Silva, A.B.K.H.; Rupasinghe, H.P.V. Polyphenols composition and anti-diabetic properties in vitro of haskap (*Lonicera caerulea* L.) berries in relation to cultivar and harvesting date. *J. Food Compos. Anal.* **2020**, *88*, 103402. [CrossRef]
61. Bansal, S.; Vyas, S.; Bhattacharya, S.; Sharma, M. Catechin prodrugs and analogs: A new array of chemical entities with improved pharmacological and pharmacokinetics properties. *Nat. Prod. Rep.* **2013**, *30*, 1438–1454. [CrossRef] [PubMed]
62. Aron, P.M.; Kennedy, J.A. Flavan-3-ols: Nature, occurrence and biological activity. A review. *Mol Nut Food Res.* **2008**, *52*, 79–104. [CrossRef] [PubMed]
63. Zanwar, A.A.; Badole, S.L.; Shende, P.S.; Hegde, M.V.; Bodhankar, S.L. Antioxidant role of catechin in health and disease. In *Polyphenols in Human Health and Disease*; Watson, R.R., Preedy, V.R., Eds.; Academic Press: San Diego, CA, USA, 2014; pp. 267–271.
64. Stevens, J.F.; Miranda, C.L.; Wolthers, K.R.; Schimerlik, M.; Deinzer, M.L.; Buhler, D.R. Identification and in vitro biological activities of hop proanthocyanidins: Inhibition of nNOS activity and scavenging of reactive nitrogen species. *J. Agric. Food Chem.* **2002**, *50*, 3435–3443. [CrossRef]
65. Pino, L.L.; Garcia, T.H.; Delgado-Roche, L.; Rodeiro, I.; Hernandez, I.; Vilegas, W.; Spengler, I. Polyphenolic profile by FIA/ESI/IT/MS(n) and antioxidant capacity of the ethanolic extract from the barks of *Maytenus cajalbanica* (Borhidi & O. Muniz) Borhidi & O. Muniz. *Nat. Prod. Res.* **2019**, *34*, 1481–1485.
66. Takara, K.; Kuniyoshi, A.; Wada, K.; Kinjyo, K.; Iwasaki, H. Antioxidative flavan-3-ol glycosides from stems of *Rhizophora stylosa*. *Biosci. Biotech. Biochem.* **2008**, *72*, 2191–2194. [CrossRef]
67. Xu, S.; Shang, M.Y.; Liu, G.X.; Xu, F.; Wang, X.; Shou, C.C.; Cai, S.Q. Chemical constituents from the rhizomes of Smilax glabra and their antimicrobial activity. *Molecules* **2013**, *18*, 5265–5287. [CrossRef]
68. Fontaine, B.M.; Nelson, K.; Lyles, J.T.; Jariwala, P.B.; Garcia-Rodriguez, J.M.; Quave, C.L.; Weinert, E.E. Identification of ellagic acid rhamnoside as a bioactive component of a complex botanical extract with anti-biofilm activity. *Front. Microbiol.* **2017**, *8*, 496. [CrossRef]
69. Oszmiański, J.; Wojdyło, A.; Nowicka, P.; Teleszko, M.; Cebulak, T.; Wolanin, M. Determination of phenolic compounds and antioxidant activity in leaves from wild Rubus, L. species. *Molecules* **2015**, *20*, 4951–4966. [CrossRef]

70. Zhu, M.Z.; Wu, W.; Jiao, L.L.; Yang, P.F.; Guo, M.Q. Analysis of Flavonoids in Lotus (*Nelumbo nucifera*) leaves and their antioxidant activity using microporous resin chromatography coupled with LC-MS and antioxidant biochemical assays. *Molecules* **2015**, *20*, 10553–10565. [CrossRef]
71. Zhu, M.; Wei, P.; Peng, Q.; Qin, S.; Zhou, Y.; Zhang, R.; Zhu, C.; Zhang, L. Simultaneous qualitative and quantitative evaluation of *Toddalia asiatica* root by using HPLC-DAD and UPLC-QTOF-MS/MS. *Phytochem. Anal.* **2018**, *30*, 164–181. [CrossRef] [PubMed]
72. Ru, Q.M.; Wang, L.J.; Li, W.M.; Wang, J.L.; Ding, Y.T. In vitro antioxidant properties of flavonoids and polysaccharides extract from tobacco (*Nicotiana tabacum* L.) leaves. *Molecules* **2012**, *17*, 11281–11291. [CrossRef]
73. Esmaeili, K.A.; Taha, R.M.; Mohajer, S.; Banisalam, B. Antioxidant activity and total phenolic and flavonoid content of various solvent extracts from in vivo and in vitro grown *Trifolium pratense* L. (Red Clover). *Biomed Res. Int.* **2015**, *2015*. [CrossRef]
74. Xu, Y.B.; Chen, G.L.; Guo, M.Q. Antioxidant and anti-inflammatory activities of the crude extracts of *Moringa oleifera* from Kenya and their correlations with flavonoids. *Antioxidants* **2019**, *8*, 296. [CrossRef] [PubMed]
75. Zou, Y.; Chang, S.K.C.; Gu, Y.; Qian, S.Y. Antioxidant activity and phenolic compositions of lentil (*Lens culinaris* var. Morton) extract and its fractions. *J. Agric. Food Chem.* **2011**, *59*, 2268–2276. [CrossRef] [PubMed]
76. Vichai, V.; Kirtikara, K. Sulforhodamine B colorimetric assay for cytotoxicity screening. *Nat. Protoc.* **2006**, *1*, 1112–1116. [CrossRef] [PubMed]

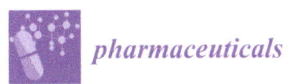 *pharmaceuticals*

Article

Comprehensive and Rapid Quality Evaluation Method for the Ayurvedic Medicine Divya-Swasari-Vati Using Two Analytical Techniques: UPLC/QToF MS and HPLC–DAD

Acharya Balkrishna [1,2], Sudeep Verma [1], Priyanka Sharma [1], Meenu Tomer [1], Jyotish Srivastava [1] and Anurag Varshney [1,2,*]

[1]   Drug Discovery and Development Division, Patanjali Research Institute,
      Haridwar 249 405, Uttarakhand, India; acharya.balkrishnapri@prft.in (A.B.); sudeep.verma@prft.in (S.V.);
      priyanka.sharma@prft.in (P.S.); meenu.tomer@prft.in (M.T.); jyotish.srivastava@prft.in (J.S.)
[2]   Department of Allied and Applied Sciences, University of Patanjali, Haridwar 249 405, Uttarakhand, India
*   Correspondence: anurag@prft.co.in; Tel.: +91-1334-244107 (ext. 7458)

Citation: Balkrishna, A.; Verma, S.; Sharma, P.; Tomer, M.; Srivastava, J.; Varshney, A. Comprehensive and Rapid Quality Evaluation Method for the Ayurvedic Medicine Divya-Swasari-Vati Using Two Analytical Techniques: UPLC/QToF MS and HPLC–DAD. *Pharmaceuticals* 2021, 14, 297. https://doi.org/10.3390/ph14040297

Academic Editors: Thomas Efferth, Jan Oszmianski and Sabina Lachowicz

Received: 12 February 2021
Accepted: 13 March 2021
Published: 27 March 2021

Publisher's Note: MDPI stays neutral with regard to jurisdictional claims in published maps and institutional affiliations.

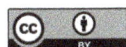

Abstract: Divya-Swasari-Vati (DSV) is a calcium-containing herbal medicine formulated for the symptomatic control of respiratory illnesses observed in the current COVID-19 pandemic. DSV is an Ayurvedic medicine used for the treatment of chronic cough and inflammation. The formulation has shown its pharmacological effects against SARS-CoV-2 induced inflammation in the humanized zebrafish model. The present inventive research aimed to establish comprehensive quality parameters of the DSV formulation using validated chromatographic analytical tools. Exhaustive identification of signature marker compounds present in the plant ingredients was carried out using ultra performance liquid chromatography-quadrupole time-of-flight mass spectrometry (UPLC/QToF MS). This was followed by simultaneous estimation of selected marker components using rapid and reliable high-performance liquid chromatography (HPLC) analysis. Eleven marker components, namely gallic acid, protocatechuic acid, methyl gallate, ellagic acid, coumarin, cinnamic acid, glycyrrhizin, eugenol, 6-gingerol, piperine and glabridin, were selected out of seventy-four identified makers for the quantitative analysis in DSV formulation. Validation of the HPLC method was evaluated by its linearity, precision, and accuracy tests as per the International Council of Harmonization (ICH) guidelines. Calibration curves for the eleven marker compounds showed good linear regression ($r^2 > 0.999$). The relative standard deviation (RSD) value of intraday and interday precision tests were within the prescribed limits. The accuracy test results ranged from 92.75% to 100.13%. Thus, the present inclusive approach is first of its kind employing multi-chromatographic platforms for identification and quantification of the marker components in DSV, which could be applied for routine standardization of DSV and other related formulations.

Keywords: Ayurveda; Divya-Swasari-Vati; herbal medicine; UPLC/QToF MS; HPLC; validation

1. Introduction

The world community is grappling with the devastating effects of the novel coronavirus disease (COVID-19) caused by Severe Acute Respiratory Syndrome Corona Virus 2 (SARS-CoV-2). The pandemic has caused a serious medical crisis, infecting more than 120 million people and leading to more than 2 million deaths [1]. The situation is considered to be more serious for patients suffering from respiratory syndromes. Infection with this respiratory virus is associated with robust inflammatory responses, which further worsen the condition [2]. The immune system plays an essential role in COVID-19 infection. Hence, enhancing the (natural body system) immunity may represent a major contribution as a prophylactic measure against multiple pathogenic conditions as well as maintaining optimum health [3].

Currently, the pandemic has entered a perilous phase where there are no specific drugs or other therapeutics against this viral outbreak [4]. The scientific community is working relentlessly to discover active pharmacological moieties that might provide new tools against this unabated transmission. Traditional, complementary and alternative medicines have emerged as the bright ray of hope in this regard [5]. Since immune dysfunction plays a vital role in disease progression, consumption of herbal medicines containing certain active compounds which have antimicrobial or antiviral, anti-inflammatory and immuno-stimulatory activities, might have potentials as effective prophylactic or even therapeutic against SARS-CoV-2 [6].

Divya-Swasari-Vati (DSV) is a calcio-herbal tablet formulation consisting of sixteen herbo-mineral ingredients (Table 1). The formulation is concocted using different parts of several medicinal plants which have a long history of usage for the treatment of respiratory infections and bronchitis. Herbal ingredients like roots of *Glycyrrhiza glabra* (licorice) have been used ethno-medicinally for the treatment of coughs, cold and COPD. Glycyrrhizin, a triterpenoid saponin from licorice has performed remarkably in inhibiting the replication of earlier SARS virus with very few side effects [7]. Eugenol, one of the abundant phenolics found in the buds of *Syzygium aromaticum* and bark of *Cinnamomum zeylanicum* (cinnamon), is very well known for its anti-inflammatory and free radical scavenging properties [8]. *Pistacia integerrima* (zebrawood) is known to exert anti-asthmatic action by mitigating TNFα activity [9]. *Cressa cretica* is known to have bronchodilatory and mast cell-stabilizing activity [10]. *Zingiber officinale* (ginger), has been used for ages as a home remedy for the treatment of common cold, asthma and bronchitis. A novel compound having structural similarities with 6-gingerol showed strong binding affinities SARS-CoV-2 viral receptors [11]. Piperine from the fruits of *Piper nigrum* (black pepper) and *Piper longum* (long pepper), has been shown to possess endothelial barrier protective and leukocyte migration suppressive effects [12]. Secondary metabolites from the roots of *Anacyclus pyrethrum* (Spanish chamomile) like saponins and tannins are known to exert immunomodulatory and immune-stimulating effects [13]. The ethno-medicinal uses of DSV ingredients have been recently validated in a mouse model of allergic asthma where the ingredients potentially suppressed the allergic asthma by modulating pro-inflammatory cytokines [14]. It is well established that the pathophysiology of SARS-CoV-2 infectivity involves different pro-inflammatory cytokines, which put the host immune system into overdrive. Thus, blocking the cytokine storm could represent a vital weapon for combating SARS-CoV-2 infectivity. Indeed, DSV successfully ameliorated SARS-CoV-2 spike protein-induced inflammation in a humanized zebrafish model by blocking the IL-6 and TNF α cytokine surge [15].

Plant extracts are exceedingly complex multicomponent mixtures. These wide arrays of phytochemical components may either function alone or in amalgamation with other components to yield the desired pharmacological effects [16]. Chromatographic fingerprinting and chemical profiling are very much essential for global acceptance of traditional herbal medicines (THMs); and have proved to be a favorable approach to ensure quality control of herbal preparations. Many agencies such as the World Health Organization (WHO), the Food and Drug Administration (FDA), and the European Medicines Agency (EMA) recommend the use of analytical modern analytical tools to monitor critical quality attributes of in-process materials in a timely manner. This approach is quintessential to verify the stability and consistency of THMs [17,18]. Poly-herbs of DSV consist of a myriad of secondary metabolites. Consequently, in order to standardize the formulation, and to help manufacturers to have consistent products, a suitable selection of analytical techniques becomes imperative.

Thus, for the comprehensive quality control of DSV, we describe herein the development of a simple, reliable, and sensitive high-performance liquid chromatography–diode array detection (HPLC–DAD) method for the simultaneous analysis of eleven marker components in the formulation. The intrinsic complexity of THMs with no obvious targets for quantification is one of the biggest challenges when it comes to ensuring their identity and quality. Ultra-performance liquid chromatography–mass spectrometry coupled with a quadrupole time of flight analyzer (UPLC/QToF MS) is one of the most powerful analytical tools which excels in the identification of ionisable moieties with high mass accuracy [19]. Seventy-four compounds were characterized in the DSV formulation using UPLC/QToF MS out of which eleven—gallic acid, protocatechuic acid, methyl gallate, ellagic acid, coumarin, cinnamic acid, glycyrrhizin, eugenol, 6-gingerol, piperine and glabridin—were chosen as the signature analytes of the formulation. A validated HPLC method was then successfully applied for the simultaneous quantification of target components in five different batches of DSV.

Table 1. Ingredients and Composition of Divya-Swasari-Vati (DSV) tablet formulation. Excipients: gum acacia (*Acacia arabica*) 4.62%, hydrated magnesium silicate 1.38% and colloidal silicon dioxide 1.38% are also present in the formulation.

S. No.	DSV Constituent's Scientific Name	Hindi Vernacular Name	% in Each DSV Tablet
1	*Pistacia integerrima*	Kakadasingi	11.66
2	*Glycyrrhiza glabra*	Mulethi	11.85
3	*Cressa cretica*	Rudanti	11.66
4	*Piper nigrum*	Marich	7.77
5	*Piper longum*	Choti pippal	7.77
6	*Zingiber officinale*	Sounth	7.77
7	*Cinnamomum zeylanicum*	Dalchini	5.92
8	*Syzygium aromaticum*	Lavang	5.92
9	*Anacylus pyrethrum*	Akarkara	5.92
10	Herbally processed ash from calcined shell of pearl oyster (*Pinctada fucata*)	Mukta- Shukti Bhasma	2.33
11	Herbally processed ash from rich gypsum	Godanti Bhasma	2.33
12	Herbally processed ash from calcined cowry shell of *Cypraea moneta*	Kapardak Bhasma	2.33
13	Herbally processed ash from calcined mica	Abharak Bhasma	2.33
14	Herbally processed ash from calcined form of alum	Sphatika Bhasma	2.33
15	Coral calcium powder processed with rose water	Praval Pishti	2.33
16	Herbally processed ash from calcined borax	Tankan Bhasma	2.33

2. Results

2.1. UPLC/QToF MS Analysis Characterized Chemical Markers in DSV

Peaks corresponding to chemical metabolites in DSV (Figure 1) were identified using the UPLC/QToF MS system and have been listed in Table 2. Fifty-nine compounds were identified in the positive mode of ionization (Figure 1A, Table 2) and forty-five compounds were identified in the negative mode of ionization (Figure 1B, Table 2). Thirty common compounds were found in both the ionization modes, i.e., positive and negative modes. Eleven markers (gallic acid, protocatechuic acid, methyl gallate, ellagic acid, coumarin, cinnamic acid, glycyrrhizin, eugenol, 6-gingerol, piperine and glabridin, Supplementary Figures S3 and S4) were selected out of seventy-four identified compounds as chemical markers to represent the herbal components in the DSV formulation. The identification of compounds relied on the mass fragmentation pattern data and accurate mass measurement of the selected chemical markers with the aid of a mass spectral library created in-house and reported literature values (Supplementary Figures S3 and S4). The triterpenoid glycyrrhizin and the isoflavonnoid glabridin were selected as the signature markers for *Glycyrrhiza glabra*. Eugenol, a phenylpropanoid derivative, and cinnamic acid were chosen for *Sygygium aromaticum* and *Cinnamomum zelanicum*, respectively. Methyl gallate, one of the active constituents present in the galls of *Pistacia integerrima*, was selected as its signature marker.

Coumarins are the biologically active constituents of the halophytic plant *Cressa cretica* hence coumarin was selected as the marker for that species. 6-Gingerol, a very well-known pungent phenol from *Zingiber officinale* was designated as the marker for this plant. The alkaloid piperine was chosen as the representative marker for *Piper nigrum* and *Piper longum*. Roots of *Anacylus pyrethrum* are rich in tannins, hence, the most popular tannins—gallic acid and ellagic acid—were selected for the same.

2.2. Establishment and Optimization of the HPLC–DAD Method:

Chromatographic separation seems to be a challenging task when it comes to structurally diversified phyto-components for these compounds possess very broad range of polarity. The aim was to separate the targeted components gallic acid, protocatechuic acid, methyl gallate, ellagic acid, coumarin, cinnamic acid, glycyrrhizin, eugenol, 6-gingerol, piperine and glabridin with a compatible solvent system. Compared with isocratic elution, gradient elution gave a shorter overall analysis and optimum resolution. After several trials, the best separation of all the marker components was found with a solvent system consisting 0.1% orthophosphoric acid in water adjusted to pH 2.5 with diethylamine (solvent A) and 0.1% orthophosphoric acid in acetonitrile: water (88:12) adjusted to pH 2.5 (solvent B) with gradient programming. Finally, optimized chromatographic conditions to ensure good separation were achieved by injecting 10 μL of standard and sample solution using a Shodex C18-4E (5 μm, 4.6 mm × 250 mm) maintained at 35 °C and subjected to binary gradient elution. The wavelengths at which all the signature analytes were detected were found to be 278 nm and 250 nm. The chromatograms, acquired with a flow rate of 1.0 mL/min showed effective separation of analytes (Figure 2).

2.3. Validation of the Developed and Optimized HPLC Method for Quantitative Analysis of Eleven Marker components in DSV

The HPLC method was validated by defining the linearity, limits of quantification and detection, accuracy, precision, robustness and ruggedness. Validation was performed on DSV (batch #B SWV117) of as per the requirements established by ICH guidelines [20].

2.3.1. Specificity, Linearity, Limits of Quantification and Detection

No interference was detected close to the retention times of the selected marker components indicating that the detected peaks were free from co-eluting interferents. The result indicates that the peak of the analyte was pure which confirmed the specificity of the method (Supplementary Figure S1). The linear regression analysis data for the calibration plot exhibited good linear relationship for all the compounds over the concentration range proposed. The correlation coefficient for the calibration curves of all the targeted signature analytes was found to be higher than 0.99 (Supplementary Figure S2). The results of regression equation, the correlation coefficient (r^2) along with the concentration range are listed in Table 3. The LOD of marker components was found to below the prescribed limit (NMT 33%) whereas, the LOQ values were also within the assigned permissible range (NMT 10%) (Table 3).

2.3.2. Accuracy and Precision

The recoveries of the eleven marker compounds at the three different concentrations were observed to be in the range from 92.75% to 100.13%. The results provided evidence that the established HPLC method is accurate for the simultaneous determination of eleven marker components in DSV (Table 3). Precision in interday and intraday runs are shown in Table 3. The values of the precision were within the permissible criteria of <2% for gallic acid, protocatechuic acid, methyl gallate, ellagic acid, coumarin, cinnamic acid, glycyrrhizin, eugenol, 6-gingerol, piperine and glabridin indicating that the method is sufficiently precise for them (Table 3).

(A)

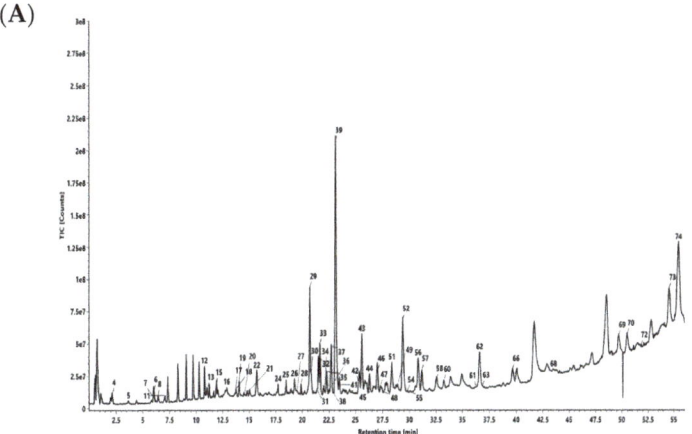

(B)

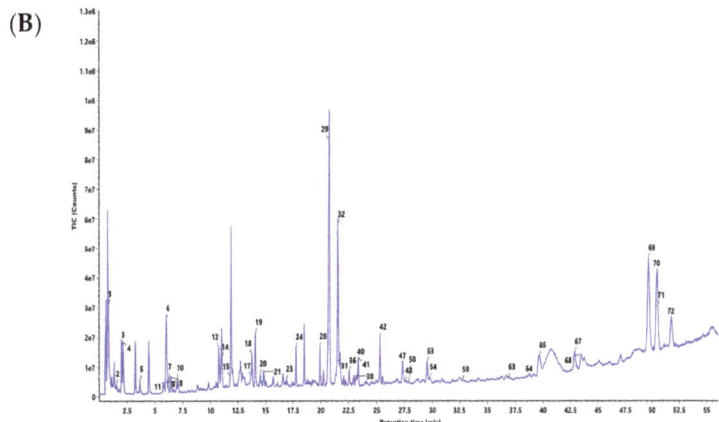

Figure 1. Total ion chromatogram of seventy-four compounds characterized in Divya-Swasari-Vati (DSV) in (**A**) positive mode and (**B**) negative mode using UPLC/QToF MS. The seventy-four compounds are, (1) quinic acid, (2) galloyl glucose, (3) gallic acid, (4) Theogallin, (5) protocaechuic acid, (6) methyl gallate, (7) 3, 4-di-O-galloylquinic acid, (8) chlorogenic acid, (9) 1,6-di-O-galloyl-glucose, (10) digallic acid, (11) cryptochlorogenic acid, (12) neoliquiritrin, (13) liquiritigenin, (14) ellagic acid, (15) quercetin-3-O-β-ᴅ-glucuronide, (16) coumarin, (17) kushenol O, (18) licurazide, (19) liquiritin apioside, (20) liquiritrin, (21) N-feruloyltyramine, (22) cinnamic acid, (23) 24-hydroxy licoricesaponin A3, (24) licoricesaponin A3 (25) glabrolide, (26) eugenol, (27) piperanine, (28) licoricesaponin G2, (29) glycyrrhizin, (30) piperyline, (31) 3-o-(β-ᴅ-glucoronopyranosyl (1-2)-β-ᴅ-galacto pyranosyl) glycyrrhetic acid, (32) licoricesaponin K2, (33) 6-gingerol, (34) 4,5-dihydropiperlonguminine, (35) piperlonguminine, (36) licoricesaponin J2, (37) feruperine, (38) licoricesaponin C2, (39) piperine, (40) shinpterocarpin, (41) licoricesaponin B2, (42) glabridin, (43) piperettine, (44) piperolein A, (45) dipiperamide E, (46) retrofractamide A, (47) glabrol, (48) 1- methoxyphaseollidin, (49) piperolactam-C9:1 (8E), (50) 1-methoxyphaseollin, (51) dehydropipernonaline, (52) pipernonaline, (53) 2-αhydroxyursolic acid, (54) licochalcone A, (55) dipiperamide-D, (56) piperolein B, (57) pipercide, (58) 10,11-dihydropipercide, (59) sophoranodichromane D, (60) piperundecalidine, (61) shinflavanone, (62) guineesine, (63) glycyrrhetic acid, (64) ursolic acid, (65) glycyrrhetol, (66) liquidambronal, (67) betulonic acid, (68) oleanonic acid, (69) deoxyglabrolide, (70) glypallidifloric acid, (71) 5-hydroxyeicosatetraenoic acid, (72) ginkgolic acid, (73) N-isobutyl-(2E,4E)-octadecadienamide, (74) pipnoohine.

Table 2. Identified metabolites in Divya-Swasari-Vati (DSV) on UPLC/QToF MS analysis.

Peak	Analyte	Formula	Neutral Mass (D)	Observed Mass (D)	RT (min)	Mode	Fragments
1	Quinic acid	$C_7H_{12}O_6$	192.0634	191.0555	0.80	−ve	$[C_7H_{12}O_6]^{-H}$, m/z 173.0445, m/z 149.0443, m/z 129.0184, m/z 113.0258, m/z 89.0267
2	Galloylglucose	$C_{13}H_{16}O_{10}$	332.0744	331.0665	1.50	−ve	$[C_{13}H_{16}O_{10}]^{-H}$, m/z 271.0442, m/z 211.0231, m/z 169.0130, m/z 151.0026
3	Gallic acid	$C_7H_6O_5$	170.0215	169.0136	1.95	−ve	$[C_7H_6O_5]^{-H}$, m/z 153.0177, m/z 137.0238, m/z 125.0238
4	Theogallin	$C_{14}H_{16}O_{10}$	344.0744	345.0821	2.13	+ve	$[C_{14}H_{16}O_{10}]^{+H}$, m/z 327.0714, m/z 247.0211, m/z 192.0607, m/z 153.0187, m/z 125.0239
				343.0667	2.00	−ve	$[C_{14}H_{16}O_{10}]^{-H}$, m/z 297.0600, m/z 271.0448, m/z 191.0550, m/z 166.9973, m/z 123.0092
5	Protocatechuic acid	$C_7H_6O_4$	154.0266	155.0340	3.65	+ve	$[C_7H_6O_4]^{+H}$, m/z 137.0237
				153.0185	3.61	−ve	$[C_7H_6O_4]^{-H}$
6	Methyl gallate	$C_8H_8O_5$	184.0372	185.0447	6.04	+ve	$[C_8H_8O_5]^{+H}$, m/z 169.0107, m/z 153.0186, m/z 139.0408
				183.0292	5.99	−ve	$[C_8H_8O_5]^{-H}$, m/z 168.0051, m/z 153.0181, m/z 124.0160, m/z 123.0079, m/z 106.0077
7	3,4-Di-O-galloylquinic acid	$C_{21}H_{20}O_{14}$	496.0853	497.0923	6.24	+ve	$[C_{21}H_{20}O_{14}]^{+H}$, m/z 327.0702, m/z 247.0232, m/z 153.0186, m/z 139.0408
				495.0775	6.18	−ve	$[C_{21}H_{20}O_{14}]^{-H}$, m/z 343.0652, m/z 245.0076, m/z 191.0547, m/z 166.9966
8	Chlorogenic acid	$C_{16}H_{18}O_9$	354.0951	355.1026	6.43	+ve	$[C_{16}H_{18}O_9]^{+H}$, m/z 319.0814, m/z 235.0602, m/z 205.0496, m/z 163.0395, m/z 130.0664
				353.0874	6.39	−ve	$[C_{16}H_{18}O_9]^{-H}$, m/z 275.0537, m/z 233.0444, m/z 205.0495, m/z 163.0388
9	1,6-Di-O-galloyl-glucose	$C_{20}H_{20}O_{14}$	484.0853	483.0775	6.64	−ve	$[C_{20}H_{20}O_{14}]^{-H}$, m/z 313.0547, m/z 271.0442, m/z 169.0129, m/z 169.0050
10	Digallic acid	$C_{14}H_{10}O_9$	322.0325	321.0246	6.94	−ve	$[C_{14}H_{10}O_9]^{-H}$, m/z 275.0173, m/z 257.0064, m/z 169.0130, m/z 168.0047, m/z 125.0237
11	Cryptochlorogenic acid	$C_{16}H_{18}O_9$	354.0951	355.1028	7.08	+ve	$[C_{16}H_{18}O_9]^{+H}$, m/z 319.0818, m/z 301.0712, m/z 235.0606, m/z 217.0499, m/z 149.0238
				353.0873	7.05	−ve	$[C_{16}H_{18}O_9]^{-H}$, m/z 335.0735, m/z 233.0442, m/z 217.0489, m/z 217.0489, m/z 191.0324, m/z 147.0429
12	Neoliquiritin	$C_{21}H_{22}O_9$	418.1264	419.1343	10.76	+ve	$[C_{21}H_{22}O_9]^{+H}$, m/z 389.1238, m/z 285.0760, m/z 257.0813, m/z 191.0330, m/z 137.0238, m/z 133.0863
				417.1192	10.73	−ve	$[C_{21}H_{22}O_9]^{-H}$, m/z 399.1010, m/z 297.0736, m/z 255.0651, m/z 254.0565, m/z 191.0328, m/z 135.0079
13	Liquiritigenin	$C_{15}H_{12}O_4$	256.0736	257.0814	11.03	+ve	$[C_{15}H_{12}O_4]^{+H}$, m/z 239.0707, m/z 215.0715, m/z 163.0399, m/z 137.0239, m/z 119.0498

Table 2. *Cont.*

Peak	Analyte	Formula	Neutral Mass (D)	Observed Mass (D)	RT (min)	Mode	Fragments
14	Ellagic acid	$C_{14}H_6O_8$	302.0063	300.9986	11.03	−ve	$[C_{14}H_6O_8]^{-H}$, m/z 283.9943, m/z 178.9969, m/z 151.0027, m/z 135.0080
15	Quercetin-3-O-β-D-glucuronide	$C_{21}H_{18}O_{13}$	478.0747	479.0826	11.81	+ve	$[C_{21}H_{18}O_{13}]^{+H}$, m/z 303.0506, m/z 245.0452, m/z 147.0448
				477.0677	11.77	−ve	$[C_{21}H_{18}O_{13}]^{-H}$, m/z 301.0336, m/z 299.0180, m/z 243.0281, m/z 151.0025
16	Coumarin	$C_9H_6O_2$	146.0368	147.0446	12.88	+ve	$[C_9H_6O_2]^{+H}$, m/z 131.0499
17	Kushenol O	$C_{27}H_{30}O_{13}$	562.1686	563.1763	13.67	+ve	$[C_{27}H_{30}O_{13}]^{+H}$, m/z 549.1600, m/z 387.1322, m/z 269.0813, m/z 237.0543, m/z 153.0719
				561.1619	13.65	−ve	$[C_{27}H_{30}O_{13}]^{-H}$, m/z 547.1428, m/z 401.0868, m/z 267.0648, m/z 252.0410, m/z 151.0391
18	Licurazide	$C_{26}H_{30}O_{13}$	550.1686	551.1762	13.77	+ve	$[C_{26}H_{30}O_{13}]^{+H}$, m/z 461.1421, m/z 419.1335, m/z 317.0667, m/z 257.0812, m/z 239.0705, m/z 137.0238
				549.1616	13.74	−ve	$[C_{26}H_{30}O_{13}]^{-H}$, m/z 417.1159, m/z 357.0962, m/z 255.0650, m/z 254.0566, m/z 135.0082
19	Liquiritin apioside	$C_{26}H_{30}O_{13}$	550.1686	551.1757	14.07	+ve	$[C_{26}H_{30}O_{13}]^{+H}$, m/z 453.1153, m/z 419.1333, m/z 389.1236, m/z 269.0813, m/z 257.0813, m/z 137.0238
				549.1614	14.04	−ve	$[C_{26}H_{30}O_{13}]^{-H}$, m/z 533.1630, m/z 399.1061, m/z 255.0651, m/z 165.0549, m/z 135.008
20	Liquiritin	$C_{21}H_{22}O_9$	418.1264	419.1344	14.51	+ve	$[C_{21}H_{22}O_9]^{+H}$, m/z 355.1184, m/z 257.0811, m/z 255.0655, m/z 147.0446
				417.1191	14.47	−ve	$[C_{21}H_{22}O_9]^{-H}$, m/z 343.1189, m/z 299.0544, m/z 255.0650, m/z 253.0490, m/z 163.0387, m/z 135.0079
21	N-feruloyltyramine	$C_{18}H_{19}NO_4$	313.1314	314.1395	14.83	+ve	$[C_{18}H_{19}NO_4]^{+H}$, m/z 177.0552, m/z 145.0289, m/z 121.0652
				312.1240	14.80	−ve	$[C_{18}H_{19}NO_4]^{-H}$, m/z 297.0988, m/z 178.0501, m/z 148.0520
22	Cinnamic acid	$C_9H_8O_2$	148.0524	149.0603	15.71	+ve	$[C_9H_8O_2]^{+H}$, m/z 131.0498
23	24-Hydroxy-licoricesaponin A3	$C_{48}H_{72}O_{22}$	1000.4515	999.4485	16.86	−ve	$[C_{48}H_{72}O_{22}]^{-H}$, m/z 939.4566, m/z 819.3776, m/z 485.3237, m/z 373.1632, m/z 179.0701
24	Licoricesaponin A3	$C_{48}H_{72}O_{21}$	984.4566	985.4633	17.71	+ve	$[C_{48}H_{72}O_{21}]^{+H}$, m/z 866.3528, m/z 809.4295, m/z 615.3875, m/z 453.3357, m/z 435.3246, m/z 153.0184
				983.4525	17.72	−ve	$[C_{48}H_{72}O_{21}]^{-H}$, m/z 645.3610, m/z 469.3300, m/z 351.0545, m/z 193.0348
25	Glabrolide	$C_{30}H_{44}O_4$	468.3240	469.3319	18.46	+ve	$[C_{30}H_{44}O_4]^{+H}$, m/z 439.3570, m/z 405.3154, m/z 315.1961, m/z 233.1539, m/z 175.1485, m/z 149.1327
26	Eugenol	$C_{10}H_{12}O_2$	164.0837	164.0838	19.26	+ve	$[C_{10}H_{12}O_2]^{-e}$, m/z 149.0603, m/z 131.0498, m/z 119.0497

Table 2. *Cont.*

Peak	Analyte	Formula	Neutral Mass (D)	Observed Mass (D)	RT (min)	Mode	Fragments
27	Piperanine	$C_{17}H_{21}NO_3$	287.1521	288.1608	19.40	+ve	$[C_{17}H_{21}NO_3]^{+H}$, m/z 256.1340, m/z 203.0709, m/z 171.0440, m/z 137.0604
28	Licoricesaponin G2	$C_{42}H_{62}O_{17}$	838.3987	839.4069	19.88	+ve	$[C_{42}H_{62}O_{17}]^{+H}$, m/z 582.2634, m/z 487.3414, m/z 469.3309, m/z 189.1641, m/z 175.1484
				837.3944	19.89	−ve	$[C_{42}H_{62}O_{17}]^{-H}$, m/z 793.3981, m/z 623.2339, m/z 431.2272, m/z 351.0551, m/z 193.0342
29	Glycyrrhizin	$C_{42}H_{62}O_{16}$	822.4038	823.4115	20.71	+ve	$[C_{42}H_{62}O_{16}]^{+H}$, m/z 700.4142, m/z 647.3781, m/z 453.3364, m/z 435.3262, m/z 272.1290, m/z 189.1645
				821.3994	20.69	−ve	$[C_{42}H_{62}O_{16}]^{-H}$, m/z 759.3939, m/z 645.3619, m/z 499.3038, m/z 351.0555, m/z 193.0348
30	Piperyline	$C_{16}H_{17}NO_3$	271.1208	272.1293	20.84	+ve	$[C_{16}H_{17}NO_3]^{+H}$, m/z 244.1349, m/z 242.1165, m/z 201.0551, m/z 171.0447, m/z 135.0449, m/z 122.0360
31	3-O-(β-D-Glucuronopyranosyl-(1-2)-β-D-galactopyranosyl) glycyrrhetic acid	$C_{42}H_{64}O_{15}$	808.4245	809.4319	21.41	+ve	$[C_{42}H_{64}O_{15}]^{+H}$, m/z 633.3987, m/z 439.3571, m/z 437.3407, m/z 241.0879, m/z 175.1114
				807.4197	21.42	−ve	$[C_{42}H_{64}O_{15}]^{-H}$, m/z 745.4132, m/z 485.3251, m/z 303.2322, m/z 187.0961
32	Licoricesaponine K2	$C_{42}H_{62}O_{16}$	822.4038	823.4114	21.51	+ve	$[C_{42}H_{62}O_{16}]^{+H}$, m/z 700.4185, m/z 647.3779, m/z 453.3364, m/z 435.3259, m/z 235.1698, m/z 189.1644
				821.3991	21.52	−ve	$[C_{42}H_{62}O_{16}]^{-H}$, m/z 807.4142, m/z 645.3607, m/z 485.3251, m/z 351.0550, m/z 193.0344
33	6-Gingerol	$C_{17}H_{26}O_4$	294.1831	317.1738	21.66	+ve	$[C_{17}H_{26}O_4]^{+Na}$, m/z 259.1702, m/z 177.0917, m/z 162.0680, m/z 137.0605
34	4,5-Dihydropiperlonguminine	$C_{16}H_{21}NO_3$	275.1521	276.1604	22.03	+ve	$[C_{16}H_{21}NO_3]^{+H}$, m/z 246.1507, m/z 203.0712, m/z 135.0446, m/z 131.0494
35	Piperlonguminine	$C_{16}H_{19}NO_3$	273.1365	274.1448	22.29	+ve	$[C_{16}H_{19}NO_3]^{+H}$, m/z 262.1438, m/z 201.0549, m/z 171.0446, m/z 135.0447, m/z 115.0992
36	Licoricesaponine J2	$C_{42}H_{64}O_{16}$	824.4194	825.4265	22.53	+ve	$[C_{42}H_{64}O_{16}]^{+H}$, m/z 613.3720, m/z 455.3516, m/z 409.3463, m/z 205.1061
				823.4147	22.53	−ve	$[C_{42}H_{64}O_{16}]^{-H}$, m/z 761.4095, m/z 597.2575, m/z 439.1797, m/z 351.0551, m/z 193.0346, m/z 175.0214
37	Feruperine	$C_{17}H_{21}NO_3$	287.1521	288.1602	22.72	+ve	$[C_{17}H_{21}NO_3]^{+H}$, m/z 270.1496, m/z 217.1090, m/z 203.0709, m/z 135.0447, m/z 124.0768
38	Licoricesaponin C2	$C_{42}H_{62}O_{15}$	806.4089	829.3991	22.94	+ve	$[C_{42}H_{62}O_{15}]^{+Na}$, m/z 560.3732, m/z 437.3411, m/z 396.2542, m/z 285.1852, m/z 173.0946
				805.4042	22.95	−ve	$[C_{42}H_{62}O_{15}]^{-H}$, m/z 743.3975, m/z 645.3662, m/z 501.3191, m/z 351.0552, m/z 167.0342

Table 2. Cont.

Peak	Analyte	Formula	Neutral Mass (D)	Observed Mass (D)	RT (min)	Mode	Fragments
40	Shinpterocarpin	$C_{20}H_{18}O_4$	322.1205	321.1135	23.28	−ve	$[C_{20}H_{18}O_4]^{-H}$, m/z 306.0883, m/z 265.0490, m/z 237.0542, m/z 175.0758, m/z 145.0290
39	Piperine	$C_{17}H_{19}NO_3$	285.1365	286.1449	23.13	+ve	$[C_{17}H_{19}NO_3]^{+H}$, m/z 258.1495, m/z 201.0552, m/z 171.0447, m/z 135.0449, m/z 112.0763
41	Licoricesaponin B2	$C_{42}H_{64}O_{15}$	808.4245	831.4131	23.34	+ve	$[C_{42}H_{64}O_{15}]^{+Na}$, m/z 731.3659, m/z 602.2705, m/z 485.3259, m/z 439.3567, m/z 279.1421, m/z 213.1123
				807.4201	23.35	−ve	$[C_{42}H_{64}O_{15}]^{-H}$, m/z 779.4222, m/z 695.3628, m/z 473.2729, m/z 351.0551, m/z 193.0343
42	Glabridin	$C_{20}H_{20}O_4$	324.1362	325.1445	25.28	+ve	$[C_{20}H_{20}O_4]^{+H}$, m/z 309.1130, m/z 270.0883, m/z 189.0916, m/z 173.0606, m/z 123.0447
				323.1292	25.26	−ve	$[C_{20}H_{20}O_4]^{-H}$, m/z 308.1037, m/z 268.0723, m/z 201.0915, m/z 135.0449
43	Piperettine	$C_{19}H_{21}NO_3$	311.1521	312.1605	25.59	+ve	$[C_{19}H_{21}NO_3]^{+H}$, m/z 294.1501, m/z 227.0709, m/z 197.0603, m/z 161.0602, m/z 138.0920
44	Piperolein A	$C_{19}H_{25}NO_3$	315.1834	316.1921	26.29	+ve	$[C_{19}H_{25}NO_3]^{+H}$, m/z 231.1025, m/z 194.1547, m/z 135.0448, m/z 131.0497
45	Dipiperamide E	$C_{34}H_{38}N_2O_6$	570.2730	571.2809	26.41	+ve	$[C_{34}H_{38}N_2O_6]^{+H}$, m/z 444.1771, m/z 286.1444, m/z 201.0520, m/z 173.0559
46	Retrofractamide A	$C_{20}H_{25}NO_3$	327.1834	328.1919	27.05	+ve	$[C_{20}H_{25}NO_3]^{+H}$, m/z 227.1072, m/z 187.0758, m/z 161.0602, m/z 131.0498
47	Glabrol	$C_{25}H_{28}O_4$	392.1988	393.2070	27.31	+ve	$[C_{25}H_{28}O_4]^{+H}$, m/z 337.1442, m/z 321.1129, m/z 281.0814, m/z 203.0708, m/z 149.0240, m/z 137.0604
				391.1922	27.29	−ve	$[C_{25}H_{28}O_4]^{-H}$, m/z 203.0707, m/z 187.1122, m/z 132.0577
48	1-Methoxyphaseollidin	$C_{21}H_{22}O_5$	354.1467	355.1551	27.58	+ve	$[C_{21}H_{22}O_5]^{+H}$, m/z 265.0494, m/z 189.0912, m/z 153.0557
				353.1397	27.55	−ve	$[C_{21}H_{22}O_5]^{-H}$, m/z 295.0591, m/z 201.0911, m/z 150.0315
49	Piperolactam-C9:1(8E)	$C_{20}H_{27}NO_3$	329.1991	330.2071	27.81	+ve	$[C_{20}H_{27}NO_3]^{+H}$, m/z 259.1323, m/z 208.1702, m/z 135.0446, m/z 133.0650
50	1-Methoxyphaseollin	$C_{21}H_{20}O_5$	352.1311	351.1239	27.86	−ve	$[C_{21}H_{20}O_5]^{-H}$, m/z 321.1108, m/z 267.0644, m/z 201.0913, m/z 146.0356
51	Dehydropipernonaline	$C_{21}H_{25}NO_3$	339.1834	340.1915	28.34	+ve	$[C_{21}H_{25}NO_3]^{+H}$, m/z 286.1445, m/z 227.1071, m/z 179.1310, m/z 161.0602, m/z 112.0761
52	Pipernonaline	$C_{21}H_{27}NO_3$	341.1991	342.2072	29.38	+ve	$[C_{21}H_{27}NO_3]^{+H}$, m/z 314.2119, m/z 229.1227, m/z 161.0601, m/z 135.0447, m/z 112.0761
53	2α-Hydroxyursolic acid	$C_{30}H_{48}O_4$	472.3553	471.3488	29.52	−ve	$[C_{30}H_{48}O_4]^{-H}$, m/z 423.3237, m/z 393.3123, m/z 279.2320
54	Licochalcone A	$C_{21}H_{22}O_4$	338.1518	339.1600	29.82	+ve	$[C_{21}H_{22}O_4]^{+H}$, m/z 276.0771, m/z 229.1227, m/z 189.0913, m/z 137.0602
				337.1449	29.79	−ve	$[C_{21}H_{22}O_4]^{-H}$, m/z 322.1187, m/z 267.0662, m/z 201.0910, m/z 175.0756, m/z 134.0369

Table 2. *Cont.*

Peak	Analyte	Formula	Neutral Mass (D)	Observed Mass (D)	RT (min)	Mode	Fragments
55	Dipiperamide D	$C_{36}H_{40}N_2O_6$	596.2886	597.2961	30.18	+ve	$[C_{36}H_{40}N_2O_6]^{+H}$, m/z 512.2070, m/z 334.1427, m/z 286.1444, m/z 186.0655
56	Piperolein B	$C_{21}H_{29}NO_3$	343.2147	344.2230	30.81	+ve	$[C_{21}H_{29}NO_3]^{+H}$, m/z 286.1447, m/z 222.1860, m/z 154.1234, m/z 135.0448
57	Pipercide	$C_{22}H_{29}NO_3$	355.2147	356.2231	31.16	+ve	$[C_{22}H_{29}NO_3]^{+H}$, m/z 283.1334, m/z 255.1387, m/z 234.1858, m/z 135.0448, m/z 133.1014
58	10,11-Dihydropipercide	$C_{22}H_{31}NO_3$	357.2304	358.2385	32.50	+ve	$[C_{22}H_{31}NO_3]^{+H}$, m/z 285.1489, m/z 191.1066, m/z 135.0445
59	Sophoranodichromane D	$C_{25}H_{28}O_5$	408.1937	407.1865	32.73	−ve	$[C_{25}H_{28}O_5]^{-H}$, m/z 350.1141, m/z 203.1064, m/z 148.0522
60	Piperundecalidine	$C_{23}H_{29}NO_3$	367.2147	368.2232	33.25	+ve	$[C_{23}H_{29}NO_3]^{+H}$, m/z 340.2281, m/z 255.1386, m/z 215.1071, m/z 135.0447, m/z 133.1011
61	Shinflavanone	$C_{25}H_{26}O_4$	390.1831	391.1912	36.31	+ve	$[C_{25}H_{26}O_4]^{+H}$, m/z 375.1594, m/z 257.0773, m/z 215.1072, m/z 189.0914, m/z 147.0810
62	Guineesine	$C_{24}H_{33}NO_3$	383.2460	384.2543	36.61	+ve	$[C_{24}H_{33}NO_3]^{+H}$, m/z 311.1648, m/z 283.1702, m/z 257.1535, m/z 175.0757, m/z 135.0447, m/z 131.0497
63	Glycyrrhetic acid	$C_{30}H_{46}O_4$	470.3396	471.3471	36.90	+ve	$[C_{30}H_{46}O_4]^{+H}$, m/z 407.3320, m/z 364.3158, m/z 229.1937, m/z 175.1489, m/z 173.1333
				469.3325	36.85	−ve	$[C_{30}H_{46}O_4]^{-H}$, m/z 451.3185, m/z 407.3289
64	Ursolic acid	$C_{30}H_{48}O_3$	456.3604	455.3538	38.72	−ve	$[C_{30}H_{48}O_3]^{-H}$, m/z 389.3044, m/z 331.2605, m/z 125.0969
65	Glycyrrhetol	$C_{30}H_{48}O_3$	456.3604	455.3538	39.61	−ve	$[C_{30}H_{48}O_3]^{-H}$, m/z 407.3301
66	Liquidambronal	$C_{30}H_{46}O_2$	438.3498	439.3578	39.68	+ve	$[C_{30}H_{46}O_2]^{+H}$, m/z 408.3381, m/z 297.2555, m/z 255.2120, m/z 203.1800, m/z 191.1800, m/z 135.1173
67	Betulonic acid	$C_{30}H_{46}O_3$	454.3447	453.3387	42.87	−ve	$[C_{30}H_{46}O_3]^{-H}$, m/z 301.2136, m/z 247.2058
68	Oleanonic acid	$C_{30}H_{46}O_3$	454.3447	455.3511	43.51	+ve	$[C_{30}H_{46}O_3]^{+H}$, m/z 409.3453, m/z 343.2649, m/z 261.2222, m/z 203.1799, m/z 177.1643
				453.3384	43.44	−ve	$[C_{30}H_{46}O_3]^{-H}$, m/z 422.2805
69	Deoxyglabrolide	$C_{30}H_{46}O_3$	454.3447	455.3522	49.70	+ve	$[C_{30}H_{46}O_3]^{+H}$, m/z 437.3415, m/z 353.2489, m/z 321.2565, m/z 215.1799, m/z 189.1644, m/z 161.1330
				453.3387	49.60	−ve	$[C_{30}H_{46}O_3]^{-H}$, m/z 393.3134, m/z 317.2845, m/z 245.1536, m/z 177.0910, m/z 153.1281
70	Glypallidifloric acid	$C_{30}H_{46}O_3$	454.3447	455.3521	50.49	+ve	$[C_{30}H_{46}O_3]^{+H}$, m/z 437.3417, m/z 353.2487, m/z 297.2582, m/z 203.1800, m/z 161.1330, m/z 135.1175
				453.3388	50.40	−ve	$[C_{30}H_{46}O_3]^{-H}$, m/z 393.3133, m/z 167.1100

Table 2. *Cont.*

Peak	Analyte	Formula	Neutral Mass (D)	Observed Mass (D)	RT (min)	Mode	Fragments
71	5-Hydroxyeicosatetraenoic acid	$C_{20}H_{32}O_3$	320.2351	319.2287	50.50	−ve	$[C_{20}H_{32}O_3]^{-H}$, m/z 275.2378, m/z 273.2217, m/z 205.1217, m/z 153.1275
72	Ginkgolic acid	$C_{22}H_{34}O_3$	346.2508	347.2590	51.83	+ve	$[C_{22}H_{34}O_3]^{+H}$, m/z 329.2486, m/z 233.1530, m/z 189.0919, m/z 161.0603, m/z 133.0294
				345.2442	51.73	−ve	$[C_{22}H_{34}O_3]^{-H}$, m/z 301.2531, m/z 299.2372, m/z 203.1433, m/z 175.1123, m/z 133.0651
73	N-Isobutyl-1-(2E,4E)-octadecadienamide	$C_{22}H_{41}NO$	335.3188	336.3278	54.54	+ve	$[C_{22}H_{41}NO]^{+H}$, m/z 322.3121, m/z 280.2647, m/z 182.1551, m/z 154.1237, m/z 135.1176
74	Pipnoohine	$C_{24}H_{43}NO$	361.3345	362.3438	55.42	+ve	$[C_{24}H_{43}NO]^{+H}$, m/z 348.3279, m/z 306.2809, m/z 264.2334, m/z 191.1805, m/z 154.1238, m/z 135.1178

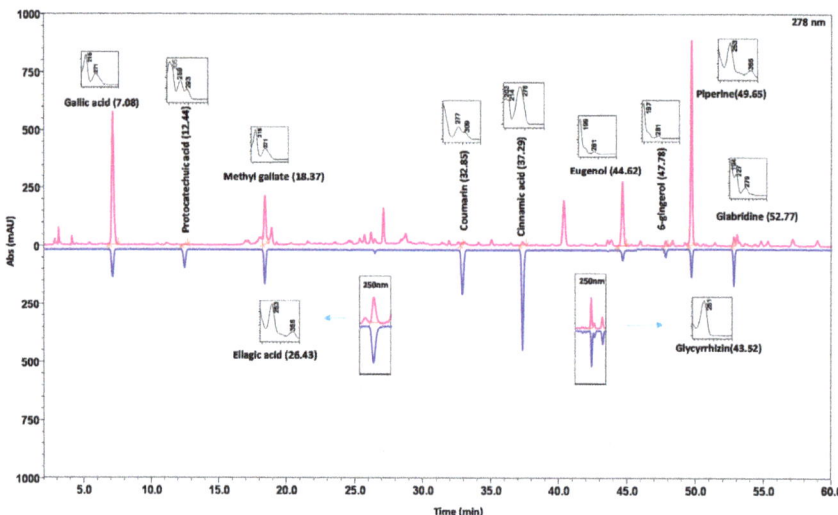

Figure 2. HPLC–DAD analysis identified and quantified the presence of 11 targeted marker components in DSV. The DSV sample (pink lines) was compared using reference standard mix (blue lines). The chromatograms were recorded at 278 nm for (methyl gallate, coumarin, cinnamic acid, eugenol, 6-gingerol, piperine and glabridin), and at 250 nm for ellagic acid and glycyrrhizin. UV-spectra of each detected analyte has been shown in the respective insets, along with HPLC retention times.

2.3.3. Robustness and Ruggedness

Deliberate variations in terms of column temperature and flow rate were taken into consideration for this method (Table 3). In all modifications, good separation of targeted analytes was achieved, and it was observed that %RSD was within the limit of not more than 20% indicating the robustness of the method. All the marker components showed %RSD less than 10% except methyl gallate which was found to be 15.63%. Ruggedness for the developed HPLC method was calculated by the %RSD of intermediate precision. The results in Table 3 show that % RSD for gallic acid, protocatechuic acid, methyl gallate, ellagic acid, coumarin, cinnamic acid, glycyrrhizin, eugenol, 6-gingerol, piperine and glabridin (NMT 10%) which indicates the ruggedness of the developed method for the analysis of the targeted analytes.

2.4. Validated HPLC–DAD Method Simultaneously Quantified Eleven Marker Analytes in Five Different Batches of DSV

The validated method was applied for the simultaneous determination of eleven marker components in five batches of DSV. The results of quantitative analysis are depicted in Figure 3. It was viewed, that the signature analytes, gallic acid, glycyrrhizin, eugenol and piperine showed marked prominence in all the batches of formulation. It is obvious from the results that detection of a single component cannot control the quality of DSV effectively. Thus simultaneous determination of multiple markers becomes imperative in this situation. Our developed HPLC method suitably detected the targeted analytes in all five DSV batches, with acceptable batch to batch variance. Gallic acid ($3438 \pm 550.7 \mu g/g$), glycyrrhizin ($4214 \pm 201.9 \mu g/g$), eugenol ($5385 \pm 980.2 \mu g/g$) and piperine ($5763 \pm 699.4 \mu g/g$) stood out in terms of showing marked prominence in DSV batches, whereas, the mean concentration of—protocatechuic acid, methyl gallate, ellagic acid, coumarin, cinnamic acid, 6-gingerol and glabridin—were found to be $65.79 \pm 9.109 \mu g/g$, $875.7 \pm 260.3 \mu g/g$, $283.3 \pm 68.82 \mu g/g$, $49.85 \pm 8.979 \mu g/g$, $40.24 \pm 2.514 \mu g/g$, $494.1 \pm 34.03 \mu g/g$, and $241.2 \pm 39.32 \mu g/g$, respectively (Figure 3).

Table 3. Validation parameters for marker components in Divya-Swasari-Vati (DSV) (batch #B SWV117) using HPLC–DAD analysis.

Parameters		Acceptance Criteria	Results Obtained										
			Gallic Acid	Protocatechuic Acid	Methyl Gallate	Ellagic Acid	Coumarin	Cinnamic Acid	Glycyrrhizin	Eugenol	6-Gingerol	Piperine	Glabridin
Specificity		No interference at retention time	In compliance										
Linearity	Correlation coefficient (r^2) NLT 0.99		0.9992	0.9991	0.9992	0.9992	0.9982	0.9995	0.9974	0.9972	0.9975	0.9974	0.9992
	Range (μg/g)		20.0–2000	20.0–2000	6.6–2000	20.0–2000	6.6–2000	3.0–2000	20.0–2000	20.0–2000	20.0–2000	6.6–2000	6.6–2000
Precision													
Intraday	%RSD NMT 2		1.13	0.32	0.34	0.67	0.96	0.49	1.55	1.16	0.13	0.86	0.93
Interday	%RSD NMT 2		1.08	0.44	1.36	1.01	1.52	0.17	0.47	1.72	0.39	1.75	0.68
Mean average recovery (%)	90–110%		96.12	95.29	93.60	94.65	95.30	95.43	97.40	97.54	94.47	92.75	100.13
Ruggedness	NMT 10		1.13	1.91	2.79	3.26	3.94	6.92	3.79	2.05	6.87	4.20	5.22
Robustness													
Flow rate	%RSD NMT 20		2.66	9.56	15.63	6.41	5.26	6.86	7.80	2.13	4.65	2.70	7.48
Column temperature	%RSD NMT 20		5.51	9.61	15.15	4.09	5.18	3.23	3.74	1.72	4.05	5.60	8.47
Limit of Detection (LOD)	%RSD of area NMT 33		1.53	1.51	0.51	1.42	0.49	0.76	3.35	0.81	6.11	0.98	0.68
	LOD (μg/g)		0.33	0.33	0.11	0.33	0.11	0.05	0.33	0.33	0.33	0.11	0.11
Limit of Quantification (LOQ)	%RSD of area NMT 10		0.60	0.93	1.10	1.48	0.99	1.64	1.02	0.52	0.38	1.28	0.48
	LOQ (μg/g)		1.0	1.0	0.33	1.0	0.33	0.15	1.0	1.0	1.0	0.33	0.33

Note: All the parameters are validated as per the ICH-Q2 (R1) guidelines. NMT: Not More Than; NLT: Not Less Than.

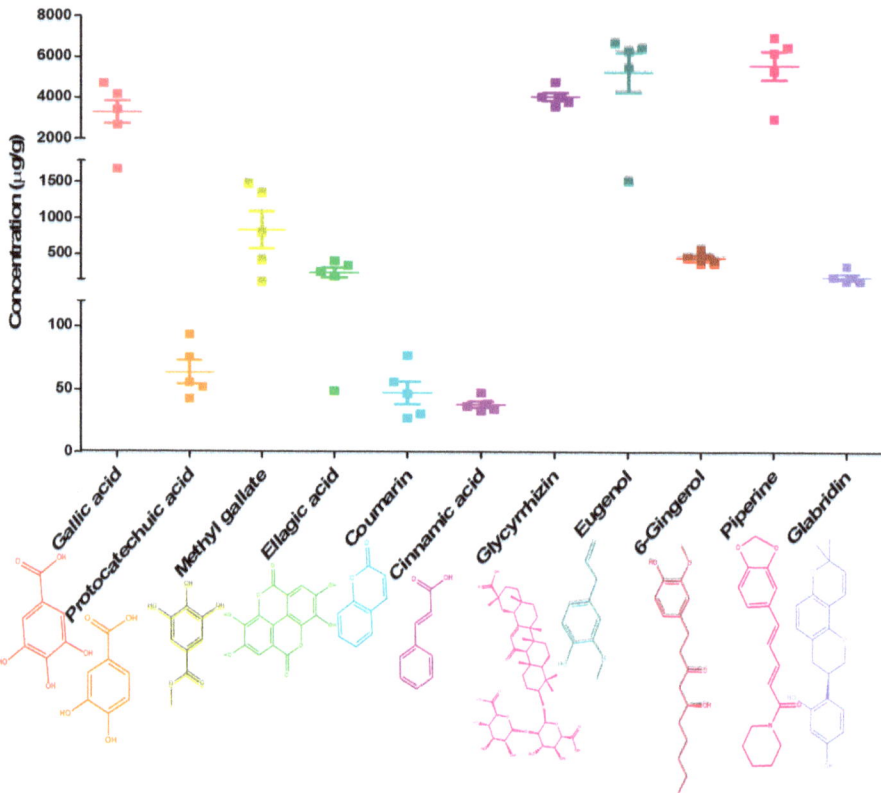

Figure 3. Quantitative analysis of gallic acid, protocatechuic acid, methyl gallate, ellagic acid, coumarin, cinnamic acid, glycyrrhzin, eugenol, 6-gingerol, piperine and glabridin using HPLC-DAD analysis in five different batches of Divya-Swasari-Vati (DSV). Scatter plot show detected concentrations of each analyte with mean and SEM (*n* = 5), in DSV formulation. Chemical structure of analytes have been sourced from www.pubchem.com (accessed on 22 March 2021).

3. Discussion

For millennia, traditional herbal medicines (THMs) have proven their value as sources of active therapeutic molecules [21]. THMs are made up of multiple herbs containing a plethora of secondary metabolites in variable concentrations. Phyto-therapeutics are complex, systematic and multi-targeted which are claimed to work synergistically [22]. The quality of THM products are usually influenced by their different plant species, growing conditions, harvest seasons, processing and other factors, which [23] have made their use more challenging. A number of attempts have been made in the academic and industrial settings, for mitigating the attrition rates of herbal drug development and their translatability to human applications. The intrinsic complexities associated with the botanicals demand the development of novel analytical procedures for reviving their lost translational capabilities [24]. The development and validation of analytical procedures plays a pivotal role in discovery, development, and manufacture of pharmaceuticals [25]. Validated test procedures further verify that the proposed analytical method is accurate and reliable for the assessment of APIs in a given drug preparation [26].

Examination of complex herbal blends bears several essential issues and significant challenges. Subsequently the identification and quantification of desired chemical markers becomes imperative, which further ensures their safety and efficacy [27]. Marker-based standardization of medicinal plants is a widely accepted and reliable technique. Ideally, the markers are selected on the basis of their therapeutic action (active constituent marker). These components must be stable and most importantly must be present consistently in the ingredients as well as in their respective formulations [28]. Another relevant criterion for their selection relies on the ease of isolation, characterization and availability. In this study, ultra-liquid chromatography coupled to quadruple time of flight (QToF) mass spectrometry was used for identification and selection of analytical markers for quality control of DSV formulation. The technique offers very high resolution and selectivity in terms of providing abundant mass information, with accurate mass measurements, and, therefore is quite useful for identifying the target compounds thoroughly [29]. Based on the existing literature [30] and the analyst's own expertise, a UPLC/QToF/MS method was developed. The developed method was utilized to identify seventy-four (74) phyto-metabolites in the DSV formulation. For example, compound number **1**, showed m/z 191.0555 in negative ionization mode, its respective mass fragmentation pattern was observed to be m/z 173.0445, m/z 149.0443, m/z 129.0184, m/z 113.0258, m/z 89.0267 which confirmed the presence of quinic acid (192.0634 Da) with [H$^-$] adduct. Compound number **3** was detected in negative ionization mode and showed m/z 169.0136, so the compound was confirmed as gallic acid (170.0215 Da), by its mass fragmentation pattern in which peaks were observed at m/z 153.0177, m/z 137.0238, m/z 125.0238 with [H$^-$] adduct. Likewise, seventy four compounds were identified and confirmed in the formulation on the basis of their accurate mass screening and fragmentation patterns as depicted in Table 2. Figures S3 and S4. Eleven markers—gallic acid, protocatechuic acid, methyl gallate, ellagic acid, coumarin, cinnamic acid, glycyrrhizin, eugenol, 6-gingerol, piperine and glabridin— were selected out of seventy four identified compounds. The strategies behind the selection of the targeted eleven markers were based on their availability, therapeutic activity and abundancy in a particular medicinal plant component. Moreover, an extensive literature search also helped in the selection of marker analytes, symbolic of a particular herb in the DSV formulation. The chief sweet-tasting triterpenoidal saponin of licorice, glycyrrhizin, represents 10% of the licorice root and glabridin, the chief isoflavone identified is found in the range of 0.08% and 0.35% [31]. Eugenol, the chief essential oil component ($\approx$ 89%) is considered to be emblematic of clove [32]. Aerial parts of *Cressa cretica* are found to be rich in coumarins [10]. Phytochemical characterization of *Anacyclus pyrethrum* showed the presence of cinnamic acid [33]. 6-Gingerol, the main bioactive component of ginger, was quantified and found to be 60.44 $\pm$ 2.53 mg/g of ginger extract [34]. Galls of *Pistacia integerrima* are reported to be rich in polyphenolics, i.e., gallic acid [35]. Chemical characterization of *Cinnamomum zeylamicum* bark revealed the presence of eugenol in appreciable amounts [36]. Besides, the herbal components, DSV formulation also contains seven different bhasma (Table 1). These are unique Ayurvedic herbo-mineral preparations, which are added to a formulation to provide optimal alkalinity, by neutralization of the harmful acids in the body. Moreover, these preparations are considered to be efficacious and non-toxic in nature [37]. Therapeutic efficacies of Tankan and Sphatika bhasma against diseases of the throat and palate are well documented [38]. Kapardak bhasma, Abhraka bhasma, Godanti bhasma and Mukta shukti bhasma are reported to have potential anti-inflammatory potential [14]. Praval pishti, processed coral calcium, is imbued with anti-inflammatory properties, moreover the preparation also confers benefits against coughs and related ailments [39]. Thus, the anti-inflammatory potentials of the herbo-mineral elements of the formulation might be beneficial to provide symptomatic relief in the current SARS-CoV-2 infectivity. It is worth mentioning that since the bhasma are inorganic compounds they exhibit poor solubility in the organic solvent methanol. Hence, these herbo-mineral preparations are not expected to hinder the current analytical strategy.

HPLC is a versatile, precise and foremost favored method among the accessible chromatographic strategies for herbal analysis [40]. HPLC frameworks hyphenated with a spectroscopic detector gives a readier data of the analytes present in a sample. [41]. Thus, chemical astuteness of DSV was investigated utilizing a validated HPLC procedure.

An analytical strategy can certainly be titled paramount which is capable of providing reliable, consistent and precise information, when performed by diverse investigators in different research environments. Optimization is much sought after for the accomplishment of consistent and repeatable outcomes. Validation plays an imperative part in fulfilling this objective [42]. Development of the HPLC method, constituted of several trial and error procedures for selection of a suitable mobile phase. Moreover, pharmacoepial and FDA requirements to achieve optimum resolution and specificity of the targeted analytes were also taken into consideration [43,44]. A few solvent compositions appeared to give longer run times, and some of them were incapable of resolving the targeted analytes at the same time. Finally, the best resolution of all the marker components was achieved using 0.1% orthophosphoric acid in water adjusted to pH 2.5 with diethylamine (solvent A) and 0.1% orthophosphoric acid in acetonitrile: water (88:12) adjusted to pH 2.5 (solvent B) with a gradient elution program. Chromatographic quality and analysis time is strongly dependent on the flow rate of the mobile phase passing through the column in unit time. The chromatograms, acquired with a flow rate of 1 mL/min appeared to give convincing partition of the analytes. Pronounced analytical outcomes are accomplished with the proper selection of wavelength. For that, it is exceptionally imperative to assess the absorption spectra of the compound intrigued. The wavelengths for the individual compounds were selected based on their λ_{max} as depicted in Figure 2. Notably, piperine shows an absorption maximum at 340 nm, but for the simplicity of the developed HPLC method we preferred to quantify the same at 278 nm. A good peak resolution relies on the choice of a suitable column. The best resolution of the targeted analytes was accomplished by employing a Shodex C18-4E (5 μm, 4.6 mm × 250 mm) column maintained at 35 °C and subjected to binary gradient elution.

Validation methods are established documented proofs that assure that the conditions selected for the strategy will reliably deliver consistent results. In addition, validation also considers the danger related with the components of a methodologically developed procedures by evaluating if the strategy is reproducible and scientifically sound [45]. These documented evidences further build certainty for the usage of the method. Thus, the developed HPLC method for the targeted analytes, gallic acid, protocatechuic acid, methyl gallate, ellagic acid, coumarin, cinnamic acid, glycyrrhizin, eugenol, 6-gingerol, piperine and glabridin were validated as per the ICH guidelines [20].

Specificity is the foremost essential parameter of any analytical procedure. It alludes to its capacity to produce a signal solely due to the analyte, in the presence of hindrances such as excipients, enantiomers and degradation products that are suspected to be present in the test framework [20]. The test should segregate the desired peak of analyte from other peaks of chromatogram. In this study, no peak was recognized near the retention times of the targeted analytes in standard solution when compared with a solvent blank. Thus, the developed HPLC method is specific for the determination of the targeted analytes in the tested DSV formulation. Limit of detection (LOD) and limit of quantification (LOQ) are the two vital performance characteristics in method validation. [20]. Signal to noise (S/N) is one of the classical methodologies for the determination of the above two important parameters. The concentration having signal to noise ratio 3:1 is referred as LOD and 10:1 as LOQ. The validation results revealed that the LOD and LOQ values for the targeted analytes were within the permissible limits, indicating the sensitivity of the developed analytical method. The linearity of an analytical method can be explained as its capability to show that the obtained test results are directly proportional to the analyte concentration within a given range. Correlation coefficient (r^2) of 0.99 is an indicative of the linearity [20]. For HPLC, the calibration curves of all the targeted analytes exhibited good linear relationship $r^2 > 0.99$. The residual analysis was performed on the individual targeted analytes (Table S1). The smaller residual sum of square (RSS) values in comparison to the regression sum of squares further confirmed that the values obtained by plotting response vs concentration are linear [46]. Thus the proposed method is in the accordance with the ICH guidelines and appropriate for the simultaneous quantification of the desired signature compounds. The precision studies were conducted at two levels, repeatability (intraday precision), which signifies the precision under the same operating conditions over a short interval of time and intermediate precision (interday precision) which represents the precision on different days. [20]. The obtained RSD values of all the targeted analytes were found to be less than 2%, confirming that the developed method is sufficiently precise. The recovery refers to the percentage of the concentration of the targeted analyte in a sample [20]. The percentage recoveries of all the targeted analytes at the three different concentrations ranged from 92.75 to 100.13% demonstrating their good recovery. The results provided evidence that established HPLC–DAD method is accurate for simultaneous estimations of gallic acid, protocatechuic acid, methyl gallate, ellagic acid, coumarin, cinnamic acid, glycyrrhizin, eugenol, 6-gingerol, piperine and glabridin in DSV. The operational components in a research area tend to vary within a realistic range. Robustness studies aim to examine the influence of the potential sources of variations such as, flow rate and column temperature in the responses of the method. The robustness of an analytical strategy is the degree of its capacity to stay unaffected by small but deliberate variations in the method parameters, likely to happen amid the routine usage [20]. %RSD of all the eighteen determinations were found to be within the prescribed limits according to the ICH guidelines indicating the robustness of the method. Rugged strategies are the one that endures minor variation in test conditions, can be run effectively by any regular chromatographer, and does not essentially requires identical HPLC system for its use. Rugged methods are essentially trouble free and transferable [20]. The results indicated that %RSD of targeted analytes were within permissible range (NMT 10%) which indicated the ruggedness of the developed HPLC method.

The developed and validated HPLC–DAD method was further applied for the simultaneous estimation of gallic acid, protocatechuic acid, methyl gallate, ellagic acid, coumarin, cinnamic acid, glycyrrhizin, eugenol, 6-gingerol, piperine and glabridin in five different batches of DSV. Differences in the climatic as well as growing conditions of herbs often leads to the variability in the detected quantity of the secondary metabolites. For this quality assessment of the herbals utilizing a single marker is considered as a very vague approach. Thus, for qualitative check of botanicals, choice of multiple markers becomes rather vital. Hence, we confirm that the proposed analytical strategy is adequate, validated and pertinent for the quality control of DSV formulation.

4. Materials and Methods

4.1. Chemicals, Reagents and Samples

The AR grade solvents, toluene, ethyl acetate, formic acid, acetic acid and methanol (HPLC grade) were procured from Merck (Darmstad, Germany), acetonitrile from Honeywell (Dusseldorf , Germany) and deionized water was obtained from a Milli Q system (Millipore, Billerica, MA, USA). Authentic standards of gallic acid (Cat No. 91215, Sigma Aldrich, St. Louis, MO, USA), protocatechuic acid (Cat No. P006, Natural Remedies, Bangalore, Karnataka, India), coumarin (Cat No. C4261, Sigma Aldrich, St. Louis, MO, USA), cinnamic acid (Cat No. 29955, Sisco Research Lab, Mumbai, Maharashtra, India), eugenol (Cat No. 35995, Sigma Aldrich, St. Louis, MO, USA), 6-gingerol (Cat No. 11707, Cayman Chemical, Ann Arbor, MI, USA), piperine (Cat No. P49007-5G, Sigma Aldrich, St. Louis, MO, USA), glabridin (Cat No. G005, Natural Remedies, Bangalore, Karnataka, India), ellagic acid (Cat No. E2250, Cayman Chemical, Ann Arbor, MI, USA) and glycyrrhizin (Cat No. G008, Natural Remedies, Bangalore, Karnataka, India) were used for the analysis. Samples from five different batches of Divya-Swasari-Vati, (#B SWV117, #B SWV084, #A SWV023, #A SWV102 and #B SWV239) were used for the chemical analysis. DSV samples were sourced from Divya Pharmacy (Haridwar, India) and were stored in airtight bottles for further use.

4.2. Analytical Investigations

4.2.1. UPLC/QToF MS Analysis

- Preparation of DSV sample solution:

10 mL of methanol:water (80:20) was added to about 100 mg of powdered DSV sample and sonicated for 15 min. The sonicated solution was then centrifuged for 5 min at 5000 rpm and filtered using 0.22 μm nylon filter. The filtered DSV solution was further used for the analysis.

- Instrumentation

Analysis was performed on a Xevo G2-XS QToF with Acquity UPLC-I Class and Unifi software (Waters Corporation, Milford, MA, USA). The main working parameters for mass spectrometry were set as follows, ionization type-ESI, mode-MS^E, acquisition time-56 min, mass range (*m/z*)—50–1200 *m/z*, low collision energy—6 eV, high collision energy—20–40 eV (ramp), cone voltage—40 V, capillary voltage—1.5 kV (for positive mode), 2 kV (for negative mode), source temperature—120 °C, desolvation temperature—500 °C, cone gas flow—50 L/h, desolvation gas flow—900 L/h. Mass was corrected during acquisition, using an external reference (Lock–Spray) consisting of 0.2 ng/mL solution of leucine enkephalin infused at a flow rate of 10 μL/min via a lock–spray interface, generating a reference ion for the positive ion mode [(M + H)$^+$ *m/z* 556.2766] and for the negative ion mode [(M − H)$^-$ *m/z* 554.2620] to ensure mass correction during the MS analysis. The lock–spray scan time was set at 0.25 s with an interval of 30 s. The elution was carried out at a flow rate of 0.3 mL/min using gradient elution of mobile phase 0.1% formic acid in water (mobile phase A) and 0.1 % formic acid in acetonitrile (mobile phase B). The volume ratio of solvent B was changed as follows, 5–10% B for 0–5 min, 10–30% B for 5–15 min, 30–55% B for 15–25 min, 55–70% B for 25–40 min, 70–80% B for 40–50 min, 80–85% B for 50–55 min, 85–5% B for 55–56 min, 5% B for 56–60 min. A total of 2 μL of the test solution was injected for the screening and the chromatograph was recorded for 56 min.

- Identification of marker components in DSV

Compounds were analyzed by their respective mass to charge ratio and fragmentation pattern. Mass/charge (*m/z*) ratio was selected based on the molecular ions of these compounds. Data acquisitions were collected under both positive (+ve) and negative (−ve) modes of ionization using full spectrum scan analysis. Further, the identified components were grouped in according to their optimum determination in each ionization mode.

4.2.2. HPLC–DAD Method Development and Optimization

- Preparation of standard solution:

Stock solutions of gallic acid, protocatechuic acid, methyl gallate, ellagic acid, coumarin, cinnamic acid, glycyrrhizin, eugenol, 6-gingerol, piperine and glabridin (1000 ppm) were prepared by dissolving accurately weighed standards in methanol. The stock solutions were mixed and diluted with methanol: water (80:20) to prepare the appropriate concentrations (50 ppm) for working standard solutions.

- Preparation of DSV sample solution

Samples of 0.5 g of powdered DSV from batches #B SWV117, #B SWV084, #A SWV023, #A SWV102 and #B SWV239 were diluted with 10 mL water:methanol (20:80) and sonicated for 30 min. The sonicated solution was centrifuged for 5 min at 10,000 rpm and filtered through 0.45 μm nylon filter (Test solution) and used for the analysis of protocatechuic acid, coumarin, cinnamic acid, 6-gingerol and glabridin. Solution A was further diluted up to 10 times with the same solvent and used for the analysis of gallic acid, methyl gallate, eugenol, piperine, ellagic acid and glycyrrhizin.

- Instrumentation and chromatographic conditions

Analysis was performed on HPLC equipment, Prominence-i LC-2030c 3D Plus (Shimadzu Corporation, Kyoto, Japan). Three different reversed phase columns, Shodex C18-4E

(5 μm, 4.6 mm × 250 mm) column, Shim pack GIST-HP C18 (3 μm, 4 mm × 150 mm) column, Shim pack GIST-HP C18 (5 μm, 4.6 mm × 250 mm) column were evaluated during chromatographic optimization. Separation was achieved using a Shodex C18-4E (5 μm, 4.6 mm × 250 mm) column. Different mobile phase, including methanol–0.1% glacial acetic acid in water, acetonitrile–0.1% acetic acid in water, methanol–0.1% orthophosphoric acid in water, acetonitrile–0.1% phosphoric acid in water, and acetonitrile–0.2% formic acid, were tried, at different pH of the mobile phase were tried. Finally, the elution was carried out using binary gradient mode using the mobile phase composed of 0.1% orthophosphoric acid in water (pH 2.5) and diethylamine (solvent A) and 0.1% orthophosphoric acid in acetonitrile: water (88:12) (solvent B) in binary gradient mode. The volume ratio of solvent B was changed as follows, 5–10% B for 0–10 min, 10–35% B for 10–30 min, 35–50% B for 30–40 min, 50–75% B for 40–50 min, 75% B for 50–55 min, 75–85% B for 55–60 min, 85–5% B for 65–66 min, 5% B for 66–70 min. The effluent from the column was detected by a diode array detector and the detection wavelength was set at 278 nm for gallic acid, methyl gallate, protocatechuic acid, coumarin, cinnamic acid, eugenol, 6-gingerol, piperine and glabridin, whereas for ellagic acid and glycyrrhizin, the detection was carried out at 250 nm. The temperature of the column was kept at 35 °C and the sample injection volume was 10 μL. The method was optimized using a suitable solvent system and monitoring suitable wavelength for separation of components with the highest sensitivity. Other parameters with optimized injection volume, flow rate and column temperature were used for maximum resolution and short analysis time.

4.3. Method Validation

Eleven marker components, namely gallic acid, protocatechuic acid, methyl gallate, ellagic acid, coumarin, cinnamic acid, glycyrrhizin, eugenol, 6-gingerol, piperine and glabridin were validated using HPLC in DSV sample as per the recommendations of International Council on Harmonization (ICH) guidelines [20]. Specificity of an analytical procedure refers to its ability to unequivocally assess an analyte in the presence of the other components which may be expected to be present [20]. The specificity of the HPLC method was evaluated to ensure that there was no interference between the solvent blank and standard solution. The specificity was studied by injecting 10 μL solutions of blank at 278 nm and 250 nm respectively. The linearity of an analytical procedure is an important parameter which signifies to its ability to produce the test results that are directly proportional to the concentration of an analyte in a given concentration range [20]. To evaluate the linearity and range of the developed method eleven different standard solutions for each of the targeted analytes were prepared in different concentration ranges (0.15–100 μg/g) by diluting the stock solutions with methanol. The calibration curves were constructed by plotting the peak area of standards versus respective concentrations. The degree of linearity was estimated by calculating correlation coefficient, using the calibration curve. The limit of detection (LOD) is described as the lowest concentration of the analyte in a sample which can be reliably detected but not necessarily quantitated by a particular analytical method. Whereas, the limit of quantification (LOQ) is considered as the lowest concentration of the analyte which can be quantitatively determined with suitable precision and accuracy [20]. LOD and LOQ of each marker component were determined based on signal-to-noise method (S/N ratio). S/N ratio for LOD was performed by injecting 6 replicates of minimum concentration at which the component was reliably detected, similarly LOQ was performed by injecting six replicates of a concentration at which the analyte can be reliably quantified. Moreover, the limit of peak area %RSD for LOD and LOQ was set at NMT 33% and NMT 10% respectively. The parameter precision expresses the degree of scatter between a series of measurements obtained from a multiple sampling of the homogeneous sample [20]. The intraday (repeatability) and interday (intermediate precision) precision ($n = 6$) was evaluated by calculating the relative standard deviation (%RSD) with accuracy in the quantification of the sample set. Accuracy of an analytical procedure refers to the closeness of the agreement between the value which is true and the experimental value [20]. The accuracy of the developed method was thoroughly evaluated by recovery studies. Analytical recovery was performed by spiking DSV sample with the reference standards at known concentration levels, such as 80%, 100% and 120% as per the area ratio method. Recoveries at three different concentrations were thus calculated. Robustness of the method provides an indication of its reliability during normal usage [20]. Robustness of method performance was verified by incorporating small intentional changes in the experimental parameters for example column temperature, and flow rate. Obtained data for each case was evaluated by calculating %RSD. Ruggedness of the current method was confirmed by testing the reproducibility of the test results under the variation in operational conditions by different analysts on different days to assure for any changes in the result. The percentage RSD for the retention area was calculated.

4.4. Quantitative Analysis of Targeted Analytes in Five Different Batches of DSV

For assuring the reliability of the developed and validated method quantitative analysis of gallic acid, protocatechuic acid, methyl gallate, ellagic acid, coumarin, cinnamic acid, glycyrrhizin, eugenol, 6-gingerol, piperine and glabridin was carried out in different batches of DSV. Quantitative analysis of particular targeted analyte was carried out against its reference standard by calculating area under the peak of analyte, in HPLC chromatogram.

4.5. Data Analysis

Statistical analyses were performed using Graph Pad Prism 7.0 (GraphPad Software, Inc., San Diego, CA, USA). Characterization of the marker analytes was performed using the Unifi software (Waters Corporation).

5. Conclusions

The analysis and quality control of traditional herbal medicines is heading in the direction of extensive and comprehensive research for uncovering their inalienable complexities. The present inventive research is an attempt to outline the applicability of two state-of-art chromatographic techniques, UPLC/QToF MS and HPLC–DAD on the quality of the calcio-herbal formulation Divya-Swasari-Vati (DSV). Seventy four phytometabolites were identified in the formulation using UPLC/QToF MS. Further, the simultaneous analysis of the selected markers—gallic acid, protocatechuic acid, methyl gallate, ellagic acid, coumarin, cinnamic acid, glycyrrhizin, eugenol, 6-gingerol, piperine and glabridin—in five different batches of DSV was carried out using the novel validated HPLC method. The established method was rapid, simple and reliable for simultaneous quantitative estimation of eleven marker components in Divya-Swasari-Vati. These outcomes may also assist in analysis of other extracts and formulations, having similar marker profiles.

Supplementary Materials: The following are available online at https://www.mdpi.com/article/10.3390/ph14040297/s1, Figure S1: Chromatograph of blank solution and standard mixture solution, Figure S2: Regression equation and correlation coefficient, Figure S3: Mass fragment pattern of the characterized fifty-nine compounds in Divya-Swasari-Vati (DSV) as observed in positive ionization mode, Figure S4: Mass fragment pattern of the characterized forty-five compounds in Divya-Swasari-Vati (DSV) as observed in negative ionization mode, Table S1: Residual sum of square (RSS) analysis of the targeted analytes.

Author Contributions: A.B., provided broad direction for the study, identified the formulations for testing, generated resources, and gave final approval for the manuscript; P.S., performed data curing, and wrote the manuscript; S.V., performed UPLC/QToF MS analysis and investigations, M.T., performed HPLC–DAD analysis and investigations; J.S., Supervised analytical chemistry experiments and reviewed the manuscript; A.V., conceptualized and supervised the overall studies, generated resources, critically reviewed, and finally approved the manuscript. All authors have read and agreed to the published version of the manuscript.

Funding: This research received no external funding. This presented work has been conducted using internal research funds from Patanjali Research Foundation Trust, Haridwar, India.

Institutional Review Board Statement: Not applicable.

Informed Consent Statement: Not applicable.

Data Availability Statement: The data presented in this study are available within the article, the associated supplementary materials, or on request from the corresponding author.

Acknowledgments: Authors thank Suman Jha and Vallabh Prakash Mulay for their relentless supports. We extend our gratitude to Priyanka Kandpal, Tarun Rajput, Gagan Kumar, and Lalit Mohan for their swift administrative supports.

Conflicts of Interest: The test articles were provided by Divya Pharmacy, Haridwar, Uttarakhand, India. Acharya Balkrishna is an honorary trustee in Divya Yog Mandir Trust. In addition, he holds an honorary managerial position in Patanjali Ayurved Ltd., Haridwar, India. Other than providing the test formulations, Divya Pharmacy was not involved in any aspect of research reported in this study. All other authors declare no conflict of interests with regards to the submitted work.

References

1. Chakraborty, I.; Maity, P. COVID-19 outbreak: Migration, effects on society, global environment and prevention. *Sci. Total Environ.* **2020**, *728*, 138882. [CrossRef]
2. Casadei, E.; Salinas, I. Comparative models for human nasal infections and immunity. *Dev. Comp. Immunol.* **2019**, *92*, 212–222. [CrossRef]
3. Jayawardena, R.; Sooriyaarachchi, P.; Chourdakis, M.; Jeewandara, C.; Ranasinghe, P. Enhancing immunity in viral infections, with special emphasis on COVID-19: A review. *Diabetes Metab. Syndr. Clin. Res. Rev.* **2020**, *14*, 367–382. [CrossRef] [PubMed]
4. Das, S.; Das, S.; Ghangrekar, M.M. The COVID-19 pandemic: Biological evolution, treatment options and consequences. *Innov. Infrastruct. Solut.* **2020**, *5*, 1–12. [CrossRef]
5. Antonio, A.D.S.; Wiedemann, L.S.M.; Veiga-Junior, V.F. Natural products' role against COVID-19. *RSC Adv.* **2020**, *10*, 23379–23393. [CrossRef]
6. Nugraha, R.V.; Ridwansyah, H.; Ghozali, M.; Khairani, A.F.; Atik, N. Traditional herbal medicine candidates as complementary treatments for COVID-19: A review of their mechanisms, pros and cons. *Evid. Based Complement Alternat. Med.* **2020**, *2020*, 1–12. [CrossRef]
7. Chen, F.; Chan, K.; Jiang, Y.; Kao, R.Y.; Lu, H.; Fan, K.; Cheng, V.C.; Tsui, W.H.; Hung, I.F.; Lee, T.S. In vitro susceptibility of 10 clinical isolates of SARS coronavirus to selected antiviral compounds. *J. Clin. Virol.* **2004**, *31*, 69–75. [CrossRef]
8. Barboza, J.N.; da Silva Maia Bezerra Filho, C.; Silva, R.O.; Medeiros, J.V.R.; de Sousa, D.P. An Overview on the Anti-inflammatory Potential and Antioxidant Profile of Eugenol. *Oxid. Med. Cell. Longev.* **2018**, *2018*, 1–9. [CrossRef]
9. Rana, S.; Shahzad, M.; Shabbir, A. Pistacia integerrima ameliorates airway inflammation by attenuation of TNF-α, IL-4, and IL-5 expression levels, and pulmonary edema by elevation of AQP1 and AQP5 expression levels in mouse model of ovalbumin-induced allergic asthma. *Phytomedicine* **2016**, *23*, 838–845. [CrossRef] [PubMed]
10. Priyashree, S.; Jha, S.; Pattanayak, S.P. Bronchodilatory and mast cell stabilising activity of Cressa cretica L.: Evaluation through in vivo and in vitro experimental models. *Asian Pac. J. Trop. Med.* **2012**, *5*, 180–186. [CrossRef]
11. Rathinavel, T.; Palanisamy, M.; Palanisamy, S.; Subramanian, A.; Thangaswamy, S. Phytochemical 6-Gingerol—A promising Drug of choice for COVID-19. *Int. J. Adv. Sci. Eng.* **2020**, *06*, 1482–1489. [CrossRef]
12. Lee, W.; Yoo, H.; Kim, J.A.; Lee, S.; Jee, J.-G.; Lee, M.Y.; Lee, Y.-M.; Bae, J.-S. Barrier protective effects of piperlonguminine in LPS-induced inflammation in vitro and in vivo. *Food Chem. Toxicol.* **2013**, *58*, 149–157. [CrossRef]
13. Bendjeddou, D.; Lalaoui, K.; Satta, D. Immunostimulating activity of the hot water-soluble polysaccharide extracts of Anacyclus pyrethrum, Alpinia galanga and Citrullus colocynthis. *J. Ethnopharmacol.* **2003**, *88*, 155–160. [CrossRef]
14. Balkrishna, A.; Solleti, S.K.; Singh, H.; Tomer, M.; Sharma, N.; Varshney, A. Calcio-herbal formulation, Divya-Swasari-Ras, alleviates chronic inflammation and suppresses airway remodelling in mouse model of allergic asthma by modulating pro-inflammatory cytokine response. *Biomed. Pharmacother.* **2020**, *126*, 110063. [CrossRef]
15. Balkrishna, A.; Verma, S.; Solleti, S.K.; Khandrika, L.; Varshney, A. Calcio-herbal medicine Divya-Swasari-Vati ameliorates SARS-CoV-2 spike protein-induced pathological features and inflammation in humanized zebrafish model by moderating IL-6 and TNF-α cytokines. *J. Inflamm. Res.* **2020**, *13*, 1219–1243. [CrossRef]
16. Altemimi, A.; Lakhssassi, N.; Baharlouei, A.; Watson, D.; Lightfoot, D. Phytochemicals: Extraction, isolation, and identification of bioactive compounds from plant extracts. *Plants* **2017**, *6*, 42. [CrossRef]
17. Cieśla, Ł. Biological fingerprinting of herbal samples by means of liquid chromatography. *Chromatogr. Res. Int.* **2012**, *2012*, 1–9. [CrossRef]
18. WHO. *General Guidelines for Methodologies on Research and Evaluation of Traditional Medicine*; World Health Organization: Geneva, Switzerland, 2000.
19. Shoko, T.; Maharaj, V.J.; Naidoo, D.; Tselanyane, M.; Nthambeleni, R.; Khorombi, E.; Apostolides, Z. Anti-aging potential of extracts from Sclerocarya birrea (A. Rich.) Hochst and its chemical profiling by UPLC-Q-TOF-MS. *BMC Complement Altern. Med.* **2018**, *18*, 54. [CrossRef] [PubMed]

20. *International Conference on Harmonization (ICH-Q2 R1). Validation of Analytical Procedures: Text and Methodology*; ICH Secretariat: Geneva, Switzerland, 2005.

21. Atanasov, A.G.; Waltenberger, B.; Pferschy-Wenzig, E.-M.; Linder, T.; Wawrosch, C.; Uhrin, P.; Temml, V.; Wang, L.; Schwaiger, S.; Heiss, E.H.; et al. Discovery and resupply of pharmacologically active plant-derived natural products: A review. *Biotechnol. Adv.* **2015**, *33*, 1582–1614. [CrossRef]

22. Pan, S.-Y.; Zhou, S.-F.; Gao, S.-H.; Yu, Z.-L.; Zhang, S.-F.; Tang, M.-K.; Sun, J.-N.; Ma, D.-L.; Han, Y.-F.; Fong, W.-F.; et al. New perspectives on how to discover drugs from herbal medicines: CAM's outstanding contribution to modern therapeutics. *Evid Based Complement Alternat Med.* **2013**, *2013*, 1–25. [CrossRef] [PubMed]

23. Lautié, E.; Russo, O.; Ducrot, P.; Boutin, J.A. Unraveling Plant Natural Chemical Diversity for Drug Discovery Purposes. *Front. Pharmacol.* **2020**, *11*, 397. [CrossRef] [PubMed]

24. Cordell, G.A. Phytochemistry and traditional medicine—The revolution continues. *Phytochem. Lett.* **2014**, *10*, 391–398. [CrossRef]

25. Harvey, A.L.; Edrada-Ebel, R.; Quinn, R.J. The re-emergence of natural products for drug discovery in the genomics era. *Nat. Rev. Drug Discov.* **2015**, *14*, 111–129. [CrossRef]

26. Betz, J.M.; Brown, P.N.; Roman, M.C. Accuracy, precision, and reliability of chemical measurements in natural products research. *Fitoterapia* **2011**, *82*, 44–52. [CrossRef] [PubMed]

27. Hou, J.-J.; Zhang, J.-Q.; Yao, C.-L.; Bauer, R.; Khan, I.A.; Wu, W.-Y.; Guo, D. Deeper chemical perceptions for better traditional chinese medicine standards. *Engineering* **2019**, *5*, 83–97. [CrossRef]

28. Bandaranayake, W.M. Quality Control, Screening, Toxicity, and Regulation of Herbal Drugs. In *Modern Phytomedicine*; Wiley-VCH Verlag GmbH & Co. KGaA: Weinheim, Germany, 2006; pp. 25–57. ISBN 3527315306.

29. Zhou, Y.; Huang, S.-X.; Pu, J.-X.; Li, J.-R.; Ding, L.-S.; Chen, D.-F.; Sun, H.-D.; Xu, H.-X. Ultra performance liquid chromatography coupled with quadrupole time-of-flight mass spectrometric procedure for qualitative and quantitative analyses of nortriterpenoids and lignans in the genus Schisandra. *J. Pharm. Biomed. Anal.* **2011**, *56*, 916–927. [CrossRef] [PubMed]

30. Vogeser, M.; Seger, C. A decade of HPLC–MS/MS in the routine clinical laboratory—Goals for further developments. *Clin. Biochem.* **2008**, *41*, 649–662. [CrossRef]

31. Pastorino, G.; Cornara, L.; Soares, S.; Rodrigues, F.; Oliveira, M.B.P. Liquorice (Glycyrrhiza glabra): A phytochemical and pharmacological review. *Phyther. Res.* **2018**, *32*, 2329–2339. [CrossRef]

32. Cortés-Rojas, D.F.; de Souza, C.R.F.; Oliveira, W.P. Clove (Syzygium aromaticum): A precious spice. *Asian Pac. J. Trop. Biomed.* **2014**, *4*, 90–96. [CrossRef]

33. Jawhari, F.Z.; Moussaoui, A.E.L.; Bourhia, M.; Imtara, H.; Saghrouchni, H.; Ammor, K.; Ouassou, H.; Elamine, Y.; Ullah, R.; Ezzeldin, E.; et al. Anacyclus pyrethrum var. pyrethrum (L.) and Anacyclus pyrethrum var. depressus (Ball) Maire: Correlation between total phenolic and flavonoid contents with antioxidant and antimicrobial activities of chemically characterized Extracts. *Plants.* **2021**, *10*, 149. [CrossRef] [PubMed]

34. Rai, S.; Mukherjee, K.; Mal, M.; Wahile, A.; Saha, B.P.; Mukherjee, P.K. Determination of 6-gingerol in ginger (Zingiber officinale) using high-performance thin-layer chromatography. *J. Sep. Sci.* **2006**, *29*, 2292–2295. [CrossRef]

35. Zahoor, M.; Zafar, R.; Rahman, N.U. Isolation and identification of phenolic antioxidants from Pistacia integerrima gall and their anticholine esterase activities. *Heliyon* **2018**, *4*, e01007. [CrossRef]

36. Sulekha, G.; Tambe, E. Identification of chemical constituents of cinnamon bark oil by GCMS and comparative study garnered from five different countries. *Glob. J. Sci. Front. Res. C Biol. Sci.* **2019**, *19*, 35–42.

37. Pal, D.; Sahu, C.; Haldar, A. Bhasma: The ancient Indian nanomedicine. *J. Adv. Pharm. Technol. Res.* **2014**, *5*, 4–12. [CrossRef]

38. Sahoo, I.; More, S.S.; Jadhav, V.; Dalai, S.; Sahoo, M. Clinical appraisal on therapeutic efficacy of tankana & sphatika bhasma with madhu pratisarana in tundikeri. *J. Drug Deliv. Ther.* **2019**, *9*, 130–134. [CrossRef]

39. Mishra, A.; Mishra, A.K.; Tiwari, O.P.; Jha, S. In-house preparation and characterization of an Ayurvedic bhasma: Praval bhasma. *J. Integr. Med.* **2014**, *12*, 52–58. [CrossRef]

40. Proestos, C.; Chorianopoulos, N.; Nychas, G.-J.E.; Komaitis, M. RP-HPLC Analysis of the phenolic compounds of plant extracts. investigation of their antioxidant capacity and antimicrobial activity. *J. Agric. Food Chem.* **2005**, *53*, 1190–1195. [CrossRef]

41. Wilson, I.; Brinkman, U.A.T. Hyphenation and hypernation: The practice and prospects of multiple hyphenation. *J. Chromatogr. A* **2003**, *1000*, 325–356. [CrossRef]

42. Shabir, G.A. Validation of high-performance liquid chromatography methods for pharmaceutical analysis. *J. Chromatogr. A* **2003**, *987*, 57–66. [CrossRef]

43. *U.S. Department of Health and Human Services, Bioanalytical Method Validation Guidance for Industry*; U.S. Department of Health and Human Services Food and Drug Administration: Rockville, MD, USA, 2018. Available online: https://www.fda.gov/files/drugs/published/Bioanalytical-Method-Validation-Guidance-for-Industry.pdf (accessed on 15 March 2021).

44. USP. <1225> Validation of Compendial Procedures. United States Pharmacopoeia XXXVII Natl. Formul. XXXII 2007. Available online: http://www.uspbpep.com/usp29/v29240/usp29nf24s0_c1225.html (accessed on 15 March 2021).

45. Seno, S.; Ohtake, S.; Kohno, H. Analytical validation in practice at a quality control laboratory in the Japanese pharmaceutical industry. In *Validation in Chemical Measurement*; Springer: Berlin/Heidelberg, Germany, 1997; pp. 56–61. ISBN 3540207880.

46. Prichard, L.; Barwick, V. *Preparation of Calibration Curves a Guide to Best Practice*; LGC Limited: Teddington, UK, 2003. [CrossRef]

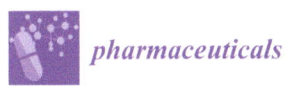

Article

Metabolite Profiling of Methanolic Extract of *Gardenia jaminoides* by LC-MS/MS and GC-MS and Its Anti-Diabetic, and Anti-Oxidant Activities

Kandasamy Saravanakumar [1,†] , SeonJu Park [2,†] , Anbazhagan Sathiyaseelan [1], Kil-Nam Kim [2] , Su-Hyeon Cho [2,3], Arokia Vijaya Anand Mariadoss [1] and Myeong-Hyeon Wang [1,*]

1 Department of Bio-Health Convergence, Kangwon National University, Chuncheon 24341, Korea; saravana732@kangwon.ac.kr (K.S.); sathiyaseelan.bio@gmail.com (A.S.); mavijaibt@gmail.com (A.V.A.M.)
2 Chuncheon Center, Korea Basic Science Institute (KBSI), Chuncheon 24341, Korea; sjp19@kbsi.re.kr (S.P.); knkim@kbsi.re.kr (K.-N.K.); chosh93@kbsi.re.kr (S.-H.C.)
3 Department of Medical Biomaterials Engineering, College of Biomedical Sciences, Kangwon National University, Chuncheon 24341, Korea
* Correspondence: mhwang@kangwon.ac.kr
† These authors contributed equally.

Citation: Saravanakumar, K.; Park, S.; Sathiyaseelan, A.; Kim, K.-N.; Cho, S.-H.; Mariadoss, A.V.A.; Wang, M.-H. Metabolite Profiling of Methanolic Extract of *Gardenia jaminoides* by LC-MS/MS and GC-MS and Its Anti-Diabetic, and Anti-Oxidant Activities. *Pharmaceuticals* **2021**, *14*, 102. https://doi.org/10.3390/ph14020102

Academic Editors: Sabina Lachowicz and Jan Oszmianski
Received: 31 December 2020
Accepted: 25 January 2021
Published: 28 January 2021

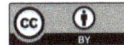

Abstract: In this study, the methanolic extract from seeds of *Gardenia jasminoides* exhibited strong antioxidant and enzyme inhibition activities with less toxicity to NIH3T3 and HepG2 cells at the concentration of 100 µg/mL. The antioxidant activities (DPPH and ABTS), α-amylase, and α-glucosidase inhibition activities were found higher in methanolic extract (MeOH-E) than H_2O extract. Besides, 9.82 ± 0.62 µg and 6.42 ± 0.26 µg of MeOH-E were equivalent to 1 µg ascorbic acid for ABTS and DPPH scavenging, respectively while 9.02 ± 0.25 µg and 6.52 ± 0.15 µg of MeOH-E were equivalent to 1 µg of acarbose for inhibition of α-amylase and α-glucosidase respectively. Moreover, the cell assay revealed that the addition of MeOH-E (12.5 µg/mL) increased about 37% of glucose uptake in insulin resistant (IR) HepG2 as compared to untreated IR HepG2 cells. The LC-MS/MS and GC-MS analysis of MeOH-E revealed a total of 54 compounds including terpenoids, glycosides, fatty acid, phenolic acid derivatives. Among the identified compounds, chlorogenic acid and jasminoside A were found promising for anti-diabetic activity revealed by molecular docking study and these molecules are deserving further purification and molecular analysis.

Keywords: *Gardenia jasminoides* Ellis; anti-diabetic activity; LC-MS/MS; GC-MS; anti-oxidant

1. Introduction

Diabetes mellitus (DM) is a commonly detected chronic disorder causing major mortality worldwide. The progression of diabetes in the global population was reported as 9.3% by 2019 and projected to increase about 10.2% by 2030 and 10.9% by 2045 [1]. Metabolic malfunctions such as high elevation of the blood sugar (glucose) levels, oxidative stress and abnormal protein and lipid metabolism all lead to DM [2]. DM is categorized into two types: insulin-dependent type-1 diabetes (T1DM) and non-insulin-dependent type-2 diabetes (T2DM) [3]. Diabetic patients who are not able to secrete insulin are characterized as T1DM [4], while patients with insulin deficiency or insulin resistance in the human metabolic system, less insulin sensitivity or signaling in the liver, skeletal muscles, and adipose tissue are characterized as T2DM [5,6]. The prolonged diabetic symptoms (hyperglycemia, polyphagia, polydipsia, and insulin resistance) trigger multiple disorders such as cardiovascular diseases, renal failure, coronary artery, neurological complications, premature death, and limb amputation [7,8]. The diabetes incidence is higher in urban areas than in rural areas. Up 50% of people do not know that they are affected by diabetes [1].

Enzymes such as α-amylase and α-glucosidase play a vital role in carbohydrate metabolism. α-Amylase catalyzes the conversion of starch into glucose, while α-glucosidase regulates the p53 signaling pathway and the cleavage of glucose from disaccharides [9,10]. Therefore, the intake of foods rich in enzyme (α-amylase and α-glucosidase) inhibitors can beneficially reduce the risk of T2DM. However, some commercially available enzyme inhibitor show side effects. For example, miglitol, voglibose, and acarbose can induce diarrhea, bowel disruption, abdominal distress, and these drugs are also not recommended to patients with gastrointestinal disorders [11]. Therefore, isolation of new α-amylase and α-glucosidase inhibitors from natural resources with less adverse effects can be considered as an alternative to existing enzyme inhibitors. α-Amylase and α-glucosidase inhibitors can be virtually screened using the molecular docking methods. That way an active imine derivative has been reported for the inhibition of these enzymes by targeting the human lysosomal acid-α-glucosidase (PDB: 5NN8) and human pancreatic α-amylase (PDB: 5E0F) [12].

Worldwide about 80% of people use herbal medicines to cure various diseases [13]. Herbal medicines have also received attention in diabetes healthcare. The investigation and isolation of novel compounds from indigenous herbal plants to cure diseases can expand the economic value of the traditional herbal industry. *G. jasminoides* is a shrub belonging to the *Rubiaceae* family and its metabolites have been proved to possess a variety of ethnopharmacological properties [14]. Traditionally *G. jasminoides* has been used as folk medicine, as a functional food and a food colorant in Asian countries [15]. The pigments produced from the ripe fruits of this plant have been used as a natural food colorant. The metabolites of *G. jasminoides* is used as a traditional natural medicine as a diuretic and to cure hemostasis, hypotension (low blood pressure) and to increase blood circulation [14]. Moreover, the pigments are not only used as a food colorant but also applied as beneficial health-promoting agents [16]. The compounds from *G. jasminoides* display promising pharmacological activities that are reviewed in earlier literature [14,17]. For instance, genipin, geniposide, crocin and crocetin isolated from *G. jasminoides* possess antidepressant, antidiabetes, antioxidant and antihypertensive activities [18–21], which has prompted additional studies to screen and identify metabolites active against T2DM. Therefore, the present study was aimed at investigating the metabolite profile of MeOH-E of *G. jasminoides* by LC-MS/MS, GC-MS and screen its anti-diabetic, and anti-oxidant effects using in vitro cytotoxicity, antioxidant, and enzyme inhibitory assays.

2. Results and Discussion

2.1. Yield, Total Phenol and Total Flavonoids Contents

The yield of different solvent extracts of seed powder of *G. jasminoides* was found to be 2.45% (*w/w*) and 1.58% (*w/w*) for methanol extract (MeOH-E) and water extract (H$_2$O-E), respectively (Table 1). The total phenol and flavonoids are major constituents in secondary metabolites of the plant extracts and they play a vital role in the biological properties of plants [22]. The bioactivities of the plant extracts are strongly correlated with the content of total flavonoids and phenolic substances. The *G. jasminoides*-derived pigments are shown to have anti-inflammatory, antioxidant, antibacterial activities with bio-health promoting properties by preventing various disorders [14]. Therefore, the content of total phenol (TPC) and total flavonoids (TFC) in MeOH-E and H$_2$O-E was determined and the results are expressed as tannic acid equivalents (TAEs) for TPC while the TFC is presented as quercetin equivalents (QEs). For TPC, 769.47 ± 3.74 μg and 632.15 ± 1.25 μg of tannic acid equivalents to one gram of MeOH-E and H$_2$O-E, where the TFC 487.54 ± 1.19 μg and 347.00 ± 2.49 μg of quercetin equivalents to one gram of MeOH-E and H$_2$O-E, respectively (Table 1).

Table 1. Total Yield, Total Phenol, and Total Flavonoids Contents in Water (H2O-E) and Methanol Extracts (MeOH-E) of Seed Powder of the *G. jasminoides* Ellis.

Samples	Yield of the Extract (%)	Total Phenol (μg of TAE/g of Extract)	Total Flavonoids (μg of QE/g of Extract
MeOH-E	2.45 [b]	769.47 ± 3.74 [b]	487.54 ± 1.19 [b]
H$_2$O-E	1.58 [a]	632.15 ± 1.25 [a]	347.00 ± 2.49 [a]

MeOH-E: Methanolic extract, H$_2$O-E: Water extract, the results presented mean ±SE, tannic acid equivalent (TAE), quercetin equivalent (QE). The different superscript values indicated the significance among the type of extracts ($p < 0.05$).

2.2. Antioxidant Activities

Oxidative stress is a major primary cause of various health disorders. Therefore, screening of antioxidants from plant extracts can be a prime way to isolate novel compound against various chronic and metabolic disorders. 1,2-Diphenyl-1-picrylhydrazyl (DPPH) is a stable free radical known to have a purple color with a strong absorption peak at 517 nm. Antioxidants can scavenge the DPPH by donating electrons [23]. (2,2′-Azino-bis(3-ethylbenzothiazoline-6-sulfonic acid) diammonium salt (ABTS$^+$) is a commonly used free radical for antioxidant assays. Mixing of ABTS and potassium persulfate produces the free radical form of the ABTS$^+$ which can be scavenged by the addition of synthetic or natural antioxidants [23]. The antioxidant activities of the DPPH and ABTS$^+$ varied significantly between the H$_2$O-E and MeOH-E ($p < 0.05$). Among the samples, the free radical scavenging activity was found higher in MeOH-E than H$_2$O-E in a dose-dependent manner. The free radical scavenging activity of these extracts was compared with a standard to obtain the ascorbic acid equivalents (AAEs). The results revealed that 9.82 ± 0.62 μg of MeOH-E and 13.20 ± 1.25 μg of H$_2$O-E were equivalent to 1 μg AAEs for ABTS scavenging. It also varied for the DPPH scavenging with the values of 6.42 ± 0.26 μg for MeOH-E and 9.22 ± 0.81 μg for H$_2$O-E, which were equivalent to 1 μg of ascorbic acid (Table 2). Further, the IC$_{50}$ concentration was found to be 120.5 ± 1.09 μg/mL and 262.5 ± 0.18 μg/mL for MeOH-E and H$_2$O-E, respectively, for the ABTS$^+$ radical scavenging (Table 2). In the case of DPPH radical scavenging, the IC$_{50}$ was found to be 274.9 ± 1.42 μg/mL and 573.1 ± 0.85 μg/mL for MeOH-E and H$_2$O-E, respectively (Table 2). Similarly, the methanol extract of *G. volkensii* reportedly shows a moderate DPPH scavenging activity [23]. Moreover, an earlier work reported that the water extract of *G. jasminoides* shows a higher DPPH and ABTS$^+$ scavenging activity than the ethanol extract. It is also observed from earlier study that the water extract of *G. jasminoides* exhibited the IC$_{50}$ values of 0.14 and 0.21 mg/mL for DPPH and ABTS $^+$ scavenging activities respectively [24]. This result indicates a variation between the present work and earlier work for IC$_{50}$ of H$_2$O-E, probably due to the differences in the extraction method and sample collection location. The present results indicated that the antioxidant activity was higher in MeOH-E than that in H$_2$O-E due to a higher total phenolic and flavonoids content [25]. The present work also found a similar relationship between antioxidant activity and total phenol content of MeOH-E and H$_2$O-E, which is in accordance with earlier works [23,25].

Table 2. Antioxidant and Diabetes-Related Enzyme Inhibitory Activities of Water (H$_2$O-E) and Methanol Extracts (MeOH-E) of Seed Powder of the *G. jasminoides*.

Samples	Inhibition Concentration (IC50:μg.mL^{-1})				Activity (μg Extract/μg AAEs)		Activity (μg Extract/μg ACEs)	
	ABTS Radical	DPPH Radical	α-Amylase Inhibition	α-Glucosidase Inhibition	ABTS Radical	DPPH Radical	α-Amylase Inhibition	α-Glucosidase Inhibition
MeOH-E	120.5 ± 1.09 [a]	274.9 ± 1.42 [a]	432.05 ± 0.51 [a]	798.25 ± 0.84 [a]	9.82 ± 0.62	6.42 ± 0.26	9.02 ± 0.25	6.52 ± 0.15
H$_2$O-E	262.5 ± 0.18 [b]	573.1 ± 0.85 [b]	784.02 ± 0.88 [b]	1052.23 ± 1.25 [b]	13.20 ± 1.25	9.22 ± 0.81	15.22 ± 0.55	12.52 ± 0.61

MeOH-E: Methanolic extract, H$_2$O-E: Water extract, the results presented mean ±SE, the different superscript in values indicated the significance among the type of extracts ($p < 0.05$). IC50 is indicated the concentration required to inhibit the 50% of free radicals or enzymes. ACEs: Acarbose equivalents, AAEs: ascorbic acid equivalents.

2.3. Enzyme Inhibitory Activities

The enzymes α-amylase and α-glucosidase are involved in carbohydrate metabolism in the conversion of simple sugars from polysaccharides or disaccharides and also in catalyzing the blood glucose level that results in T2DM hyperglycemia [26]. Therefore, inhibition of these enzymes can control the prevalence of T2DM. Moreover, several studies also reported that screening of these enzyme inhibitors is crucial for the discovery of novel diabetes drugs [27,28]. The present work showed the enzyme (α-amylase and α-glucosidase) inhibitory activity of MeOH-E and H_2O-E of seed powder of *G. jasminoides* (Table 2). Among the two samples, MeOH-E exhibited higher α-amylase and α-glucosidase inhibition activities than H_2O-E. The 9.02 ± 0.25 µg of MeOH-E and 15.22 ± 0.55 µg of H_2O-E were equivalent to 1 µg of acarbose for α-amylase inhibition activity (Table 2). In the case of α-glucosidase inhibition, 6.52 ± 0.15 µg of MeOH-E and 12.52 ± 0.61 µg of H_2O-E were found to equivalent to 1 µg of acarbose (Table 2). The IC50 of MeOH-E were found to be 432.05 ± 0.51 µg/mL and 798.25 ± 0.84 µg/mL for α-amylase and α-glucosidase inhibition activity respectively (Table 2). Among the two samples, MeOH-E showed promising activities of antioxidant and α-amylase and α-glucosidase inhibition. Therefore, MeOH-E was selected further for cell culture experiments.

2.4. Cytotoxicity

The cytotoxic effects of MeOH-E in a mouse fibroblast (NIH3T3) cell line was determined using a WST assay. The results revealed that MeOH-E at the concentration of ≤12.5 µg/mL did not show any cytotoxicity, while that at >25–100 µg/mL exhibited moderate cytotoxicity in the NIH3T3 cell line (Figure 1a). Similarly, the extract of *G. jasminoides* is reportedly non-toxic to the normal human MCF-10A cell line [29]. Another mouse model experiment confirmed that the pigments derived from *G. jasminoides* are less toxic [30]. Meanwhile, different solvent extracts of *G. jasminoides* have been reported to have promising cytotoxicity towards various cancer cells, including cervical cancer cell line (HeLa), skin malignancy cell line (A375), human non-small cell lung carcinoma cell line (H1299), and breast cancer cell line (MCF-7) [29,31]. However, to ensure the non-cytotoxicity of the MeOH-E in the NIH3T3 cell line the present study applied an acridine orange/ethidium bromide (AO/EB) fluorescent staining assay. This fluorescent method is used to determine the apoptosis-associated changes in cells based on the nucleus damage [32]. The AO/EB staining results indicated no apoptosis cells in the control group, and in the cells treated with 12.5 µg/mL; however, early stage apoptosis cells were observed at 50 µg/mL and 100 µg/mL (Figure 1b). Similarly, the early apoptosis in the osteosarcoma cells was detected by AO/EB staining as indicated by yellow-green and crescent-shaped cells [32].

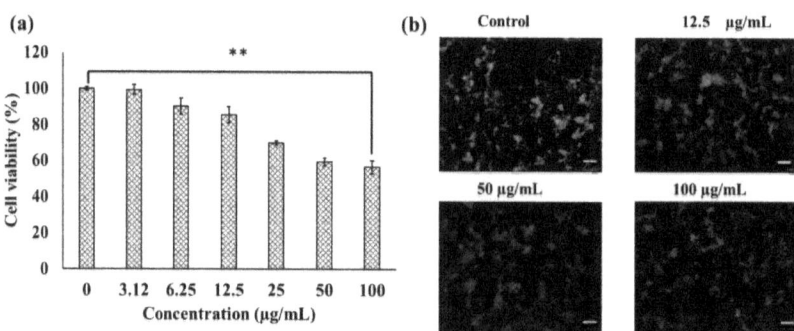

Figure 1. Cytotoxicity of the methanolic extract (MeOH-E) of *G. jasminoides* in NIH3T3 cell line (**a**), AO/EB staining assay (**b**). ** *p* < 0.01 significant. Scale bar 100 µm.

2.5. Effect of MeOH-E on Cell Viability and Glucose Uptake in HepG2 Cell Line

MeOH-E did not display significant cytotoxicity on the Hep2 cell line at the concentration of $\leq$25 µg/mL and only at 100 µg/mL was significant cytotoxicity exhibited (Figure 2a). This revealed the non-toxicity of MeOH-E in the HepG2 cell line at $\leq$25 µg/mL. Therefore, the effect of MeOH-E treatment in the glucose metabolism was tested by glucose uptake assay in non-insulin resistant and insulin resistant (IR)-HepG2 cell lines. The glucose uptake was found to be higher in the non-IR HepG2 cell line than that in the IR-HepG2 cell line. However, the addition of MeOH-E (12.5 µg/mL) increased ~37% of glucose uptake in IR-HepG2 as compared to untreated IR HepG2 cell line (Figure 2b). This experiment also led to the interesting observation that the treatment above 25 µg/mL of MeOH-E to IR-Hep2 cell line significantly decreased the glucose uptake due to toxicity of the extract (Figure 2b). This is in accordance with an earlier report on ethyl acetate extract of *Physalis alkekengi* in glucose uptake in HepG2 cells [33]. The present work revealed that the treatment of 12.5 µg/mL was optimal for the increased glucose uptake by the IR-HepG2 cell line.

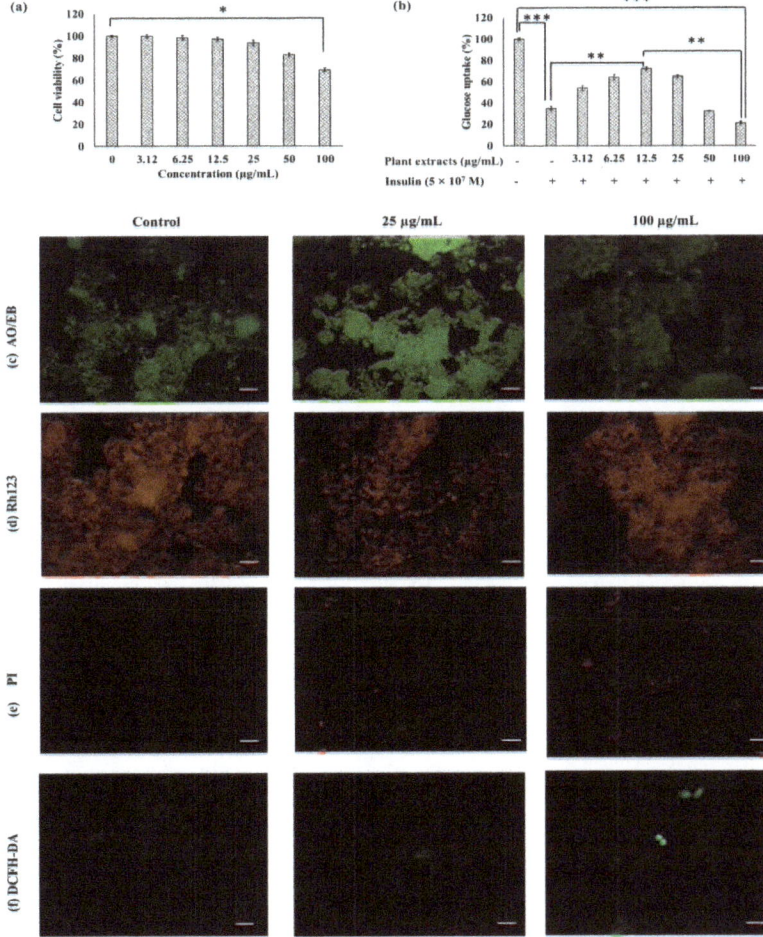

Figure 2. Cytotoxicity of the methanolic extract (MeOH-E) of *G. jasminoides* in insulin-resistant (IR) HepG2 cell line (**a**), glucose uptake (**b**), AO/EB staining assay (**c**), mitochondrial membrane potential (**d**), measurement of nucleus damage by PI (**e**), analysis of the reactive oxygen species generation (**f**). Scale bar 100 µm for C & E, and 50 µm for D & F. * $p < 0.05$, ** $p < 0.01$, *** $p < 0.001$ significant.

Fluorescent Assay

The cytotoxicity of MeOH-E in the HepG2 cell line was measured by fluorescent AO/EB, rhodamine 123 (Rh123), propidium iodide (PI), and 2'-7'dichlorofluorescin diacetate (DCFH-DA) staining assays (Figure 2c–f). The cells were grouped as live cells (light green), apoptosis cells (fluorescent or yellowish, orange), necrosis cells (red) [34]. The MeOH-E at 25 μg/mL and 100 μg/mL) caused slight cytotoxicity for IR-HepG2 cell line as evident by pyknosis and congregated chromatin emitting green or yellow and some red fluorescence while the untreated control cells emitted uniform green fluorescence (Figure 2c). Rh123 staining is adopted to measure the mitochondrial membrane potential (MMP) loss in the HepG2 cell line. Rh123 dye effectively stains with rich mmP and loss of mmP is indicated with the decrease of dye emission [35]. Similarly, the present study observed that the Rh123 was highly emitted in the HepG2 cell line treated with different concentrations of MeOH-E and it indicated less toxicity of extracts (Figure 2d). The PI is an impaired nucleic acid membrane stain used for the detection of dead cells in a cell population [36,37]. The present study observed no PI-stained cells in the untreated control group while the treatment of 25 μg/mL and 100 μg/mL of MeOH-E displayed the dead cells as red-colored (Figure 2e). DCFH-DA staining results indicated that the treatment of MeOH-E (25 μg/mL) did not cause the ROS mediated cytotoxicity while it exhibited slight cytotoxicity in the HepG2 cell line (Figure 2f).

2.6. Metabolite Profiling of the MeOH-E of G. jasminoides

To identify the components of the MeOH-E of *G. jasminoides*, we tentatively identified them using two major hyphenated techniques: gas chromatography-mass spectrometry (GC-MS) and liquid chromatography with tandem mass spectrometry (LC-MS/MS), which cover quite different subsets of metabolites. For instance, GC-MS has a preference for volatile metabolites covering primary metabolism including organic and amino acids, sugars, sugar alcohols, and phosphorylated intermediates. In contrast, LC-MS/MS covers mostly polar compounds predominant in secondary metabolites such as phenolics and terpenoids [38,39].

2.6.1. Tentative Identification of Compounds by LC-MS/MS

The compounds present in the MeOH-E were tentatively identified using LC-MS/MS and the TIC chromatogram of metabolic profile of the MeOH-E is shown in the Supplementary Figure S1. The LC-MS/MS analysis revealed the presence of 39 phytochemicals that belonging to various subclasses such as phenolic, flavonoids, terpenes, iridoid glycosides, organic acids, and gardenia carotenoids (Table 3). These compounds were identified based on the *m/z* of molecular ion [M–H]⁻ and interpretation of the MS and MS/MS spectra comparison with the MassLynx V4.1 library (Waters Corporation, Milford, MA, USA). The compounds were identified using the in-house phytochemical library (UNIFI 1.8; Waters) [40,41] and previously reported literature [14,42]. Structures of the selected compounds are presented in Figure 3.

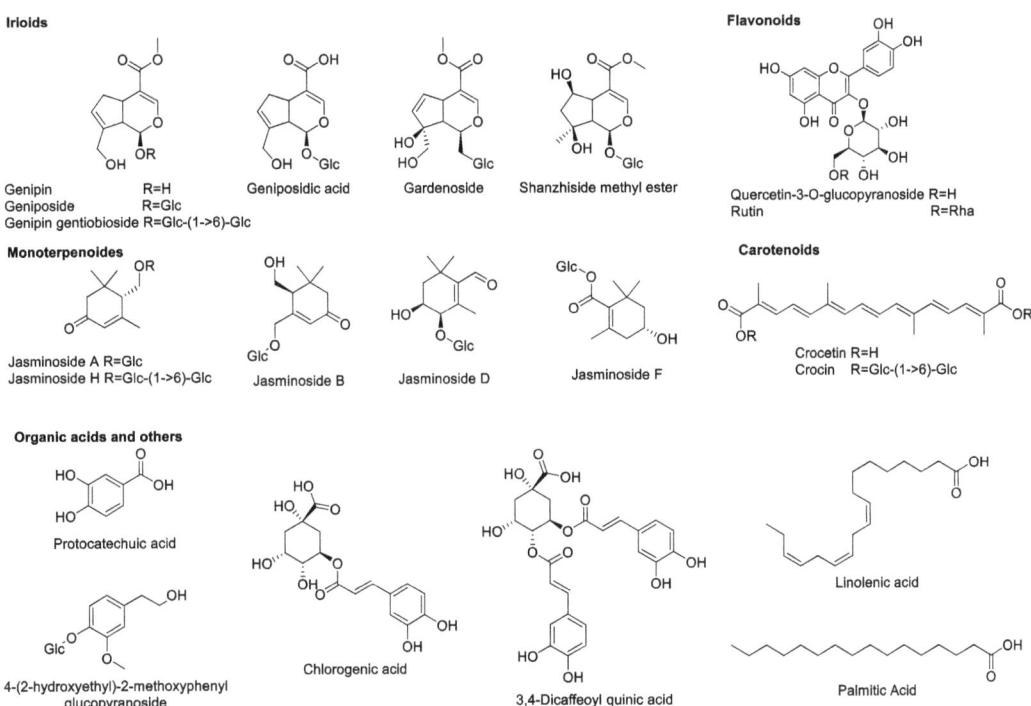

Figure 3. Structures of selected compounds identified by LC-MS/MS.

Iridoids

The iridoid glycosides are a group of phytochemicals that is commonly present in various families of the plant families including Rubaiaceae [43]. According to our LC-MS/MS analysis, MeOH-E of *G. jasminoides* (Rubiaceae) exhibited compounds such as geniposidic acid (m/z 373.11), shanzhiside methyl ester (m/z 405.14), 6β-hydroxygeniposide (m/z 403.12), gardenoside (m/z 403.12), genipin gentiobioside (m/z 549.18), genipin (m/z 225.07), geniposide (m/z 387.13), coumaroylgenipin gentiobioside (m/z 695.21), and feruloylgenipin gentiobioside (m/z 725.23). Detailed identification information of these compounds such as retention time, formula, observed m/z, mass error, response and product ion mass are listed in Table 3.

Table 3. Metabolite Profiling of Methanolic Extract (MeOH-E) of *G. jasminoides* by LC-MS/MS Analysis.

Component Name	RT (min)	Formula	Observed m/z [M–H]$^-$	Mass Error (ppm)	Response	MS/MS Fragmentation (m/z)	References
Iridoids							
Geniposidic acid	1.04	$C_{16}H_{22}O_{10}$	373.1142	0.4	6013	193.0507	[44,45]
Shanzhiside methyl ester	1.06	$C_{17}H_{26}O_{11}$	405.1402	0.0	1994	229.0722, 391.1251	[45]
6β-Hydroxygeniposide	1.43	$C_{17}H_{24}O_{11}$	403.1249	1.4	273,632	205.0511, 223.0615, 241.0721	[46]
Gardenoside	1.69	$C_{17}H_{24}O_{11}$	403.1238	0.4	1146	207.0664, 225.0770	[45]
Genipin gentiobioside	1.70	$C_{23}H_{34}O_{15}$	549.1828	0.4	464,390	207.0664, 225.0770	[45]
Genipin	2.00	$C_{11}H_{14}O_5$	225.0770	0.2	81,760	193.0506, 207.0664	[44,46]
Geniposide	2.00	$C_{17}H_{24}O_{10}$	387.1300	0.5	1,952,147	207.0664, 225.0770	[45,46]
Coumaroylgenipin gentiobioside	2.81	$C_{32}H_{40}O_{17}$	695.2191	0.2	301,727	225.0768, 469.1354	[45,46]
Feruloylgenipin gentiobioside	2.89	$C_{33}H_{42}O_{18}$	725.2300	0.2	108,903	193.0507, 225.0768	[47]

Table 3. *Cont.*

Component Name	RT (min)	Formula	Observed *m/z* [M−H]⁻	Mass Error (ppm)	Response	MS/MS Fragmentation (*m/z*)	References
Monoterpenoides							
Jasminoside F isomers	1.25	$C_{16}H_{26}O_9$	361.1506	0.5	36,284	137.0975, 181.0872, 199.0973	[45]
Jasminoside D	1.47	$C_{16}H_{26}O_8$	345.1558	1.0	171,766	165.0922, 183.1027	[48]
Jasminoside B	1.66	$C_{16}H_{26}O_8$	345.1599	0.1	37,456	151.0764, 165.0921, 169.0870	[46]
Jasminoside J	1.66	$C_{16}H_{24}O_7$	327.1446	−1.1	2058	151.0764, 165.0921	[49]
Jasminodiol	1.96	$C_{10}H_{16}O_3$	183.1029	0.2	2722	135.0817	[48]
Gardenate A	1.99	$C_{12}H_{18}O_6$	257.1033	0.3	104	225.0770	[50]
Picrocrocinic acid	2.07	$C_{16}H_{26}O_8$	345.1554	−0.1	47,270	165.0921	[45]
Jasminoside H	3.00	$C_{22}H_{36}O_{12}$	491.2123	−0.3	30,153	167.1076, 323.0976	[46]
Crocusatin C	3.64	$C_{10}H_{16}O_2$	167.1083	0.2	260	137.0973	[45,46,48]
Jasminoside A/E	3.67	$C_{16}H_{26}O_7$	329.1606	0.1	3985	167.1079	[48]
6′-Sinapoyljasminoside C	3.92	$C_{27}H_{34}O_{11}$	533.2021	−1.4	2024	165.0918, 205.0507	[48]
Methyl dihydrojasmonate	4.36	$C_{13}H_{22}O_3$	225.1495	−0.5	241	181.1596	Pubchem
2-Hydroxyethylgardenamide A	6.69	$C_{13}H_{17}NO_5$	266.1039	0.5	155	-	Pubchem
Flavonoids							
Rutin	2.28	$C_{27}H_{30}O_{16}$	609.1464	0.3	16,687	300.0278	[47]
Quercetin-3-O-β-D-glucopyranoside	2.42	$C_{21}H_{20}O_{12}$	463.0884	0.2	3003	300.027	[47]
Carotenoids							
Crocetin	2.67	$C_{20}H_{24}O_4$	327.1589	−1.3	844	283.1704	[51]
Crocin A	3.95	$C_{44}H_{64}O_{24}$	975.3707	−0.8	64,605	327.1603, 651.2661	[47,51]
Organic acids and others							
Quinic acid	0.81	$C_7H_{12}O_6$	191.0563	1.2	85,121	137.0242, 173.0459	[52]
Trimethoxy-O-glucopyranoside	1.08	$C_{15}H_{22}O_9$	391.1249	0.9	54,704	167.0716	Pubchem
4-(2-Hydroxyethyl)-2-methoxyphenyl β-D-glucopyranoside	1.37	$C_{15}H_{22}O_8$	[M+COOH]⁻ 375.1298	0.3	2140	151.0763, 167.0713	Pubchem
Caffeoylquinic acid	1.44	$C_{16}H_{18}O_9$	353.0876	−0.5	217	161.0248	[45]
Protocatechuic acid	1.51	$C_7H_6O_4$	153.0193	−0.2	11,003	109.0294	[45]
Chlorogenic acid	1.70	$C_{16}H_{18}O_9$	353.0878	0.0	4552	161.0248, 191.0562	[46,48]
Dicaffeoylquinic acid	2.79	$C_{25}H_{24}O_{12}$	515.1196	0.2	6085	179.0350, 191.0559	[47]
Linolenic acid	10.53	$C_{18}H_{30}O_2$	277.2174	0.2	1586	-	[53,54]
n-Pentadecanal	10.74	$C_{15}H_{30}O$	225.2217	−1.3	4866	-	[53]
Linoleic acid	11.60	$C_{18}H_{32}O_2$	279.233	0.2	162,838	-	[54]
Acetylursolic acid	12.71	$C_{32}H_{50}O_4$	497.3634	−0.5	3297	-	Pubchem
Palmitic acid	12.72	$C_{16}H_{32}O_2$	255.2331	0.6	10,687	-	[53,54]
Ethyl palmitate	12.96	$C_{18}H_{34}O_2$	281.2488	0.8	38,097	-	[53]

Monoterpenoids

The monoterpenes, whether linear (acyclic) or containing rings (bicyclic and monocyclic), belons to a class of terpenes that possess remarkable applications in the food and pharmaceutical industries [55]. *G. jasminoides* was reported to be a rich source of monoterpenoids and a total of 26 monoterpenoids have been reported from *G. jasminoides* [56–60]. The present study identified a total of 13 monoterpenoids from MeOH-E of *G. jasminoides* based on the deprotonated molecular ions observed in the LC-MS/MS analysis. The formulas of identified compounds were as follows: $C_{10}H_{16}O_2$ (*m/z* 167.1083), $C_{10}H_{16}O_3$ (*m/z* 183.1029), $C_{12}H_{18}O_6$ (*m/z* 257.1033), $C_{13}H_{17}NO_5$ (*m/z* 266.1039), $C_{13}H_{22}O_3$ (*m/z* 225.1495), $C_{16}H_{24}O_7$ (*m/z* 327.1446), $C_{16}H_{26}O_7$ (*m/z* 329.1606), $C_{16}H_{26}O_8$ (*m/z* 345.1599), $C_{16}H_{26}O_9$ (*m/z* 361.1506), $C_{22}H_{36}O_{12}$ (*m/z* 491.2123) and $C_{27}H_{34}O_{11}$ (*m/z* 533.2021). The compound names, MS/MS fragmentation patterns, retention times as well as response factors corresponding to each chemical are described in Table 3.

Flavonoids

Flavonoids are a major group of molecules present in the plants with rich bioactivities including antioxidant, anti-diabetes, and anticancer properties. According to the earlier literature, a total of 22 flavonoids has been reported from the various extracts of *G. jasminoides* [14]. Similarly, the present study had identified compounds such as rutin ($C_{27}H_{30}O_{16}$) and quercetin-3-O-β-D-glucopyranoside ($C_{21}H_{20}O_{12}$) with MS/MS fragmentation of quercetin, aglycone of those two previously mentioned compounds, at *m/z* 300.0278 [M–rutinoside]⁻ and 300.0275 [M–Glc]⁻, respectively (Table 3, Figure 4).

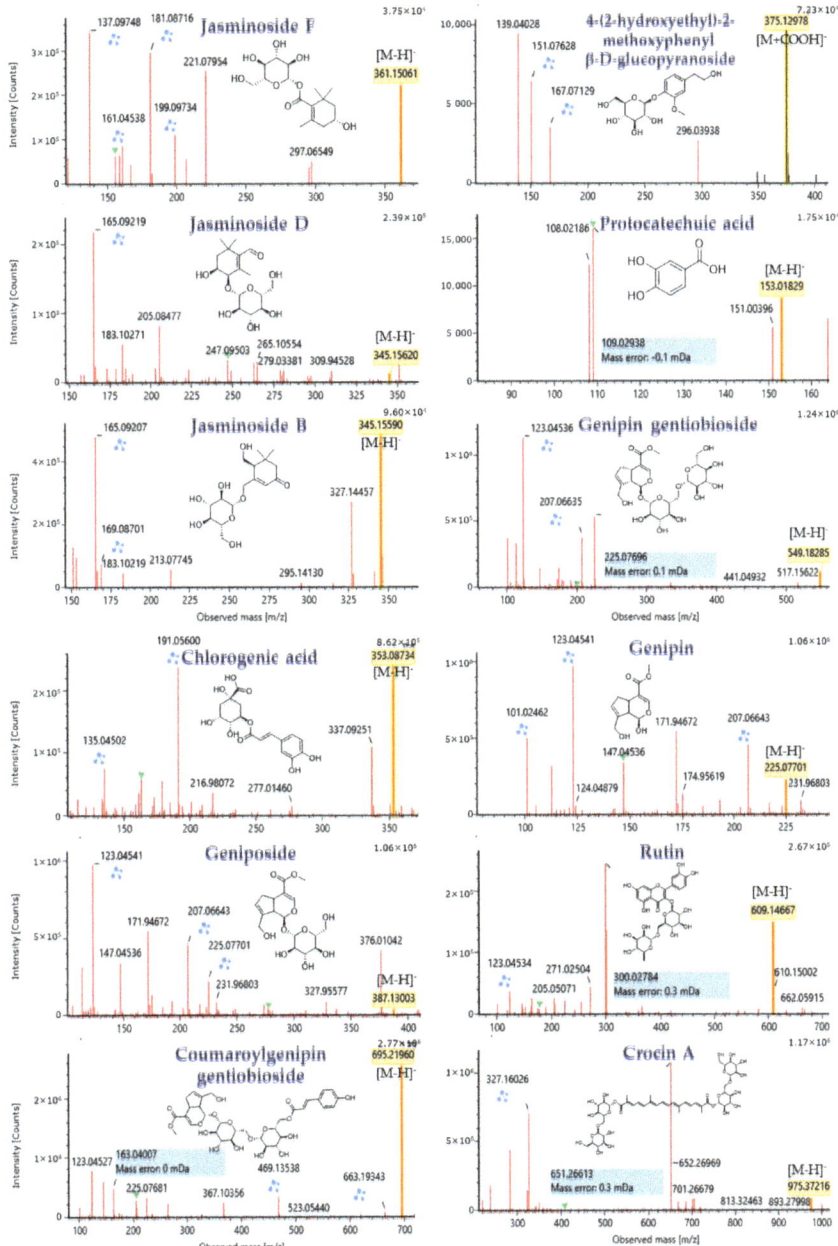

Figure 4. MS/MS spectrum of compounds identified from methanolic extract (MeOH-E) of *G. jasminoides* by LC-MS/MS analysis. Blue markings and the numbers in blue highlighter indicate the predicted MS/MS fragmentation of the compounds provided by MassFragment, an in silico fragmentation tool that uses a systematic bond disconnection approach to identify possible structures from the parent structure.

Carotenoids

The carotenoids are a major constituent of the *G. jasminoides*, which is composed of carotenoids and similar compounds [61]. These compounds are used as food colorants as well as bioactive food additives. Based on the peaks observed from the LC-QTOF MS/MS analysis of MeOH-E, crocetin and crocin A were identified by their corresponding MS/MS fragmentats at m/z 283.1704 [M–COOH]$^-$ for crocetin and 651.2661 [M–H–gentiobioside+H$_2$O]$^-$ and 327.1603 [M–H–gentiobioside * 2+H$_2$O * 2]$^-$ for crocin A (Table 3, Figure 4). Similarly, these compounds were reported from the flower and fruit of this plant [62,63].

Organic Acids and Others

According to the earlier research reports, a total of 30 organic acids with various bioactive properties, including phenolic acids and fatty acids can be isolated from *G. jasminoides* [14]. Similarly, the present study has identified a total of 13 organic acids and others from MeOH-E of *G. jasminoides* based on LC-MS/MS of deprotonated observed mass and its MS/MS fragmentation. The compounds were identified as chlorogenic acid ($C_{16}H_{18}O_9$), caffeoylquinic acid ($C_{16}H_{18}O_9$), dicaffeoylquinic acid ($C_{25}H_{24}O_{12}$), protocatechuic acid ($C_7H_6O_4$), quinic acid ($C_7H_{12}O_6$), 2,4,6-trimethoxy-1-O-glucopyranoside ($C_{15}H_{22}O_9$), 4-(2-hydroxyethyl)-2-methoxyphenyl β-D-glucopyranoside ($C_{15}H_{22}O_8$), linolenic acid ($C_{18}H_{30}O_2$), *n*-pentadecanal ($C_{15}H_{30}O$), linoleic acid ($C_{18}H_{32}O_2$), acetylursolic acid ($C_{32}H_{50}O_4$), palmitic acid ($C_{16}H_{32}O_2$), and ethyl palmitate ($C_{18}H_{34}O_2$). Further detailed identification information is shown in Table 3.

2.6.2. Tentative Identification of the Compounds by GC-MS

GC-MS analysis evidenced the presence of fifteen volatile compounds classified into organic acids and their derivatives including fatty acids and phenolic acids in MeOH-E of *G. jasminoides* based on the electronic library, W8N05ST.L (Supplementary Table S1). The major compounds were found to be (9Z,12Z)-octadeca-9,12-dienoic acid (69.43%), hexadecanoic acid (16.09%), octadecanoic acid (8.32%), thymine (0.22%), 3,5-dihydroxy-6-methyl-2,3-dihydro-4H-pyran-4-one (0.26%), 3-carene (0.89%), 2-methylphenoxyacetic acid (0.49%), 2-amino-3-hydroxybenzoic acid (0.43%), 2,6-dimethyl-3-(methoxymethyl)-*p*-benzoquinone (0.60%), tetradecanoic acid (0.08%), methyl palmitate (0.20%), methyl linoleate (1.07%), methyl elaidate (0.55%), squalene (0.78%) and vitamin E (0.36%). Some of these compounds are known for promising antioxidant, antibacterial, and anticancer activities [64,65].

2.7. In Silico Screening of Enzyme Inhibitors
2.7.1. Protein and Ligand Preparation

The protein and ligand were prepared according to the methods described earlier [12]. The protein molecular dock preparation was done using the AutoDock vina after the removal of the water molecules. Further, the ligand was selected for the molecular docking study based on Lipinski's drug-likeness rules (Supplementary Table S2). The Lipinski's indicated five rules, which is favor to select a compound as an orally active agent such as (i) the molecular weight of the compounds < 500 Da, (ii) hydrogen bond donor < 5, (iii) hydrogen bond acceptor < 10, (iv) miLogP < 5 and molar refractivity (40–130) [66]. Out of 33 unique compounds identified from MeOH-E of *G. jasminoides* by LC-MS/MS (Figure 3) and GC-MS (Supplementary Figure S2), a total of the 26 compounds were selected for the molecular docking study based on Lipinski's rules satisfactory (Supplementary Table S2).

2.7.2. Molecular Docking
Molecular Interaction with α-Amylase

Molecular docking results revealed that all the selected compounds could interact with α-amylase. Among the compounds screened, jasminoside F, chlorogenic acid, jasminoside A, and thymine showed a higher docking score against α amylase (Table 4; Figure 5). The jasminoside F exhibited the binding affinity score of −8.5 kcal/mol with two hydrogen bond interactions with amino acid residues of His 299 and Gln63 in α amylase (Figure 5a). Chlorogenic acid showed the binding affinity score of -8.7 kcal/mol by interacting with amino acid residues of Arg421, Gly403, Arg398, Ser289 through six hydrogen bond interactions in α amylase (Figure 5b). Jasminoside A displayed a strong binding affinity score of −8.7 kcal/mol on α-amylase through interacting its amino acid residues of Arg195, His299 via two hydrogen bonds (Figure 5c).

Table 4. Molecular Docking Analysis Catalytic Activity of Compounds Identified from the Methanolic Extract (MeOH-E) of *G. jasminoides* Against Diabetes Related Enzymes of α-Amylase and α-Glucosidase.

S.No	Compound	α-Amylase			α-Glucosidase		
		No. H Bonds	H Bond Interacting Amino Acids	Binding Affinity (kcal/mol)	No. H Bonds	H Bond Interacting Amino Acids	Binding Affinity (kcal/mol)
1	Quinic acid	3	Arg252	−5.7	4	His623, Leu761, Val760, Met269	−6.3
2	Jasminoside F	2	His 299, Gln63	−8.5	5	Thr473, Asn476, Arg102	−7.8
3	4-(2-Hydroxyethyl)-2-methoxyphenyl β-D-glucopyranoside	2	His299, Lys200	−6.9	2	Glu759, His490	−7.3
4	Jasminoside D	-		0	-		0
5	Protocatechuic acid	3	Arg421, Arg398	−5.5	2	Glu654, Ala655	−5.9
6	Jasminoside B	2	His299, Gln63	−7.7	6	Arg102, Tyr104,Gly241,Arg103, Asn476	−7.3
7	Jasminoside J	-	-	−8.1	2	Glu762, Leu761	−7.3
8	Chlorogenic acid	6	Arg421,Gly403,Arg398, Ser289	−8.7	5	Met269, Glu759, Val760, Tyr266	−8.2
9	Genipin	2	Arg195, His299	−6.6	1	Val760	−6.4
10	Crocusatin C	2	His305, Gln63	−5.9	3	Glu762, Met269, Leu761	−5.8
11	Jasminoside A	2	Arg195, His299	−8.7	4	Val760, Leu761, Glu762	−7.8
12	Thymine	6	Gly403, Arg398, Arg421	−5.3	3	Glu759, Ser757, Asp753	−5.1
13	3,5-Dihydroxy-6-methyl-2,3-dihydro-4*H*-pyran-4-one	4	Ala310, Gly309, Asn301, Arg346	−5.5	4	Arg317, Met314, Asn323	−5.1
14	3-Carene	-	-	−5.5	-	-	−5.3
15	2-Methylphenoxyacetic acid	1	Gln63	−5.6	3	Leu761, Val760, Glu759	−5.7
16	2-Amino-3-hydroxybenzoic acid	2	His299, Asp197	−5.6	5	Asn323, Leu311, Met314, Arg317	−5.3
17	2,6-Dimethyl-3-(methoxy-methyl)-*p*-benzoquinone	2	His185, Ala128	−5.5	2	Leu761, Met269	−5.5
18	Tetradecanoic acid	-		−5.8	-		−5.7
19	Methyl palmitate	2	His299, Asp197	−6.1	1	His301	−6.4
20	Hexadecanoic acid	-		−5.8	1	Glu759	−6.2
21	Methyl linoleate	1	Asp197	−6.5	1	Asn430	−6.3
22	Methyl elaidate	1	Asp197	−6.2	1	Asn430	−6.2
23	(9Z,12Z)-Octadeca-9,12-dienoic acid	3	Asn105, Ala106	−6.3	1	Arg491	−6.5
24	Octadecanoic acid	2	Asn105, Ala106	−6.2	1	His580	−6
25	Acarbose derived trisaccharide	11	Thr6, Arg10, Gly9, Gln7, Gly334, Arg421, Gln404	−8.3	8	Trp39, Cys40, Ala13, Pro14, Asp11, Arg237, Trp179	−8.7
26	Acarbose	3	His299, gln63, Thr163	−8.3	6	Trp39, Cys40, Pro14, Ala13, Arg237, Asp11	−8.7

The organic compound thymine showed a binding affinity score of −5.3 kcal/mol against α-amylase by interacting its residues of Gly403, Arg398, Arg421 by six hydrogen bonds (Figure 5d). Moreover, the positive control of the acarbose derived trisaccharide exhibited higher hydrogen bonds of 11 and amino acids (Thr6, Arg10, Gly9, Gln7, Gly334, Arg421, Gln404) interaction with α-amylase with binding affinity score of -8.3 kcal/mol (Figure 5e) while another control acarbose showed only three hydrogen bonds and amino acids (His299, gln63, Thr163) interactions with binding affinity score of −8.3 kcal/mol (Figure 5f). Overall, the results revealed that among the compounds tested, jasminoside A and chlorogenic acid were found to have the potential to interact with α-amylase with high binding affinity score than other molecules including positive controls. Similarly, the compound jasminoside is known for tyrosinase inhibition [56] while the phenolic compound chlorogenic acid exhibits anti-oxidative and anti-diabetic activities [67,68].

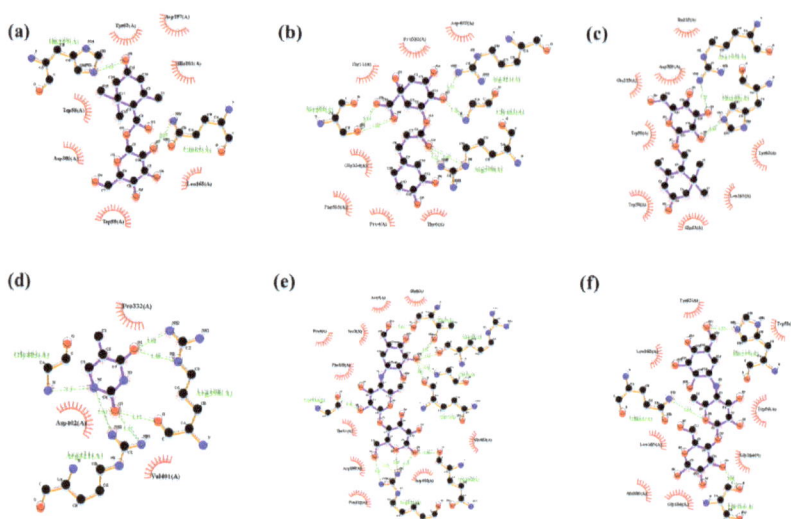

Figure 5. Molecular catalytic interaction of the compound identified from the methanolic extract (MeOH-E) of *G. jasminoides* with α amylase. Jasminoside F (**a**), chlorogenic acid (**b**), jasminoside A (**c**), thymine (**d**), acarbose derived trisaccharide (**e**), and acarbose (**f**) interacting with diabetes-related enzyme of α amylase (5E0F).

Molecular Interaction with α-Glucosidase

The in silico docking study revealed that jasminoside F, jasminoside B, chlorogenic acid and jasminoside A displayed a higher binding affinity with α-glucosidase than other compounds studied in this study (Table 4; Figure 6). The interaction between jasminoside F and α-glucosidase showed the binding affinity score of −7.8 kcal/mol through the formation of five hydrogen bonds with amino acid residues such as Thr473, Asn476, Arg102 (Figure 6a). Jasminoside B established an interaction with α-glucosidase via six hydrogen bonds interacting with amino acids residues (Arg102, Tyr104, Gly241, Arg103, Asn476) of α-glucosidase with the binding affinity of 7.3 kcal/mol (Figure 6b). The chlorogenic acid exhibited the binding affinity score of −8.2 kcal/mol with five hydrogen bond interactions with amino acid residues of Met269, Glu759, Val760, Tyr266 in α-glucosidase (Figure 6c). The molecular interaction between jasminoside A and α-glucosidase exhibited a binding affinity of 7.8 kcal/mol by forming four hydrogen bonds with the amino acid residues Val760, Leu761, Glu762 (Figure 6d). However, the positive controls such as acarbose-derived trisaccharide and acarbose showed the promising dock binding affinity of 8.7 kcal/mol for interaction with α-glucosidase (Table 4). The acarbose-derived trisaccharide was found to establish an interaction with α-glucosidase through eight hydrogen bonds with amino acid residues of Trp39, Cys40, Ala13, Pro14, Asp11, Arg237, Trp179 (Figure 6e) while the acarbose established the interaction with α-glucosidase through six hydrogen bonds with amino acid residues of Trp39, Cys40, Pro14, Ala13, Arg237, Asp11 (Figure 6f). Overall, the docking study revealed that interactions with α-glucosidase of chlorogenic acid and jasminoside A were promising as compared to other compounds screened, and we hypothesize that these interactions might inhibit the activity of α-glucosidase. This finds the support of earlier works on the antidiabetic and enzyme inhibitory activities of these compounds [56,67,68].

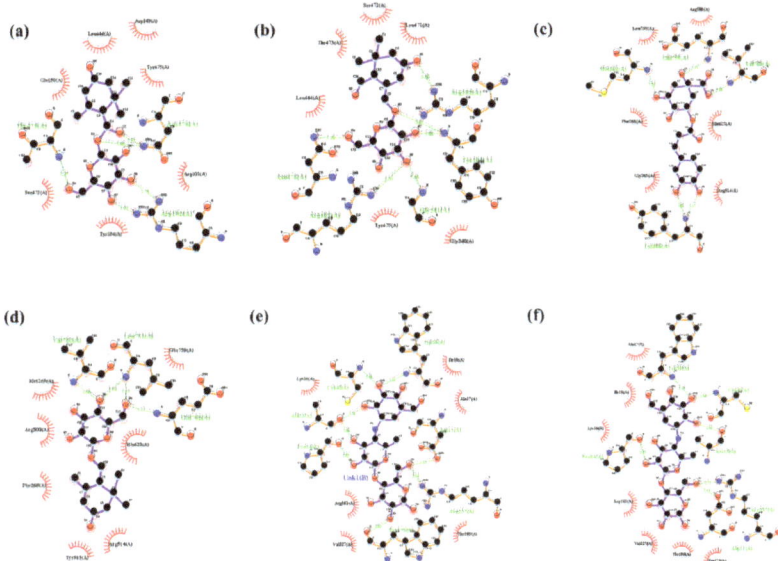

Figure 6. Molecular catalytic interaction of the compound identified from the methanolic extract (MeOH-E) of *G. jasminoides* with α glucosidase (5NN8). Jasminoside F (**a**), jasminoside B (**b**), chlorogenic acid (**c**), jasminoside A (**d**), acarbose derived trisaccharide (**e**), and acarbose (**f**) interacting with diabetes-related enzyme α glucosidase (5NN8).

3. Materials and Methods

3.1. Chemicals, Cell Line, and Maintenance

Ethidium bromide (EB), rhodamine 123 (Rh123), $2'$-$7'$ dichlorofluorescein diacetate (DCFH-DA), acridine orange (AO), $2,2'$-azinobis (3-ethylbenzothiazoline-6-sulfonic acid) diammonium salt (ABTS), 1,2-diphenyl-1-picrylhydrazyl (DPPH), α-glucosidase, and α-amylase were purchased from Sigma-Aldrich (Seoul, Korea). The seed powder of *G. jasminoides* Ellis was procured from a local herbal company in South Korea, and authenticated by Professor M.H. Wang (Kangwon National University). Fetal bovine serum (FBS), penicillin and streptomycin, Dulbecco's Modified Eagle Medium (DMEM), Roswell Park Memorial Institute Medium (RPMI) were obtained from ThermoFisher Scientific (Seoul, Korea). The cytotoxicity assay kit (WST-CELLO MAX™) was purchased from MediFab (Seoul, Korea), while the cell line human hepatic HepG2 cells and mouse fibroblast NIH3T3 cells were received from Korean Cell Line Bank, (KCLB, Seoul, Korea).

3.2. Preparation of Desiccative Ripe Fruits Extract

One hundred gram of seed powder (desiccative ripe fruits) of the *G. jasminoides* was extracted with methanol (1:5 ratio) for 24 h agitation in a magnetic stirrer. The methanol extract (MeOH-E) was filtered through Whatman no 1 filter paper and then concentrated using a rotary evaporator at 40 °C. Besides the water extraction was done according to the protocols described earlier [23]. The yield of MeOH-E and H2O-E was quantified using a weighing balance and then stored at 4 °C for further analytical experiments. The contents of total phenol and total flavonoids in MeOH-E were measured according to methods described earlier [69–71].

3.3. Antioxidant Activities

MeOH-E was analyzed for free radicals (DPPH and ABTS) scavenging activity according to the protocols reported earlier [72,73]. For DPPH inhibition assay, 100 μL of MeOH-E (1.95–1000 μg/mL) and 100 μL of DPPH (100 μM) were mixed and incubated at 27 °C for

10 min. Later the reaction mixture was observed at 517 nm using a UV spectrophotometer. The percentage of the DPPH scavenging was determined by adopting the formula reported earlier [74]. For the ABTS inhibition assay, firstly, the oxidative form of the ABTS$^+$ was generated by mixing the potassium persulfate (2.45 mm) and ABTS (7 mm) at the ratio of the 0.5:1 ratio in dark conditions at 27 °C for 24 h. For the reaction, the 100 μL of ABTS$^+$ and 100 μL of MeOH-E (1.95–1000 μg/mL) were mixed and incubated at 27 °C for 10 min. Afterward, the reaction mixture was measured at 734 nm using a UV spectrophotometer. The percentage of ABTS scavenging = ((Control-sample)/control) × 100). The control is ABTS+solution alone.

3.4. Enzyme Inhibition Activities

The inhibition of α-glucosidase and α-amylase was measured according to previously reported methods [75–77]. Acarbose was used as a positive control for this experiment. For the α-glucosidase inhibition assay, 50 μL of MeOH-E (1.95–1000 μg/mL) was added to 20 μL of α-glucosidase (1 U) and this, 25 μL of *p*-nitrophenyl glucopyranoside (pNPG; 5 M) was added and incubated at 37 °C for 30 min. Later, the 100 μL of Na$_2$ CO$_3$ (0.1 M) was added to stop the reaction and measured at 405 nm using a UV spectrophotometer. For the α-amylase inhibition assay, 50 μL of MeOH-E (1.95–1000 μg/mL), 150 μL of starch (0.5%), 10 μL of α-amylase (2 U) were mixed and incubated at 37 °C for 30 min. Later 20 μL of NaOH (2 M) was added to stop the reaction. Then 20 μL DNS of (3,5-dinitrosalicylic acid) was added to the reaction solution and boiled for 20 min at 100 °C. Finally, the reaction mixture was cooled at room temperature and read at 540 nm using a UV spectrophotometer. The percentage of enzyme inhibition was determined by following the formula reported elsewhere [74].

3.5. Cell Culture Experiments

3.5.1. Cytotoxicity

The cytotoxicity of MeOH-E was tested in the normal NIH3T3 cells and HepG2 cells (1 × 10^4 cells/well) cultured in DMEM composed of FBS (10%), antibiotic solution (1%) for 24 h at 37 °C in 5% of a CO$_2$ incubator. Later, the cells were treated with MeOH-E (0–100 μg/mL) for 24 h. After the treatment period, WST reagent (10 μL) was added, kept in a CO$_2$ incubator for 1 h, and then OD was measured at 450 nm using UV spectrophotometer (SpectraMax® Plus Microplate Reader, Molecular Devices, San Jose, CA, USA). The percentage of cell toxicity was calculated by adopting the formula reported previously [78].

3.5.2. Determination of Glucose Uptake

To assess the MeOH-E induced glucose uptake in the HepG2 cells, an insulin-resistant model cell line (IR-HepG2) was firstly generated according to the protocol reported elsewhere [79,80]. The well-established IR-HepG2 cells (1 × 10^4 cells/well) were cultured in high glucose DMEM incorporated with FBS (10%) and antibiotic solution (1%) in a 5% CO$_2$ incubator for 24 h. For the treatment, various concentrations of MeOH-E (0–100 μg/mL) were added to cells and incubated for 24 h in the above-mentioned conditions. Besides, the positive control (HepG2) cells were maintained. After the incubation, the cells including the culture media were harvested and centrifuged at 440 g for 5 min, and the supernatant was used for glucose assay by DNS method. Glucose uptake (%) was estimated using the formula:(OD of high glucose DMEM media-IR-HepG2 cultured supernatant´OD)/OD of high glucose DMEM media) × 100. Followed by the prevention of oxidative stress, mitochondrial membrane loss, and nucleus damage in IR-HepG2 by treatment of MeOH-E was observed using various staining assay as reported in earlier studies [81–83].

3.6. UHPLC-QTOF-MS/MS Analysis

For the UHPLC-QTOF-MS/MS analysis, MeOH-E was dissolved in 70% methanol, filtered with PTFE syringe filter (0.2 μm), and finalized in 20 ppm of MeOH-E. The LC/MS systems consisted of a Waters Acquity UPLC I-Class system (Waters Corp., Milford, MA,

USA) coupled to Waters Xevo G2 QTOF mass spectrometer (Waters MS Technologies, Manchester, UK) equipped with an electrospray ionization (ESI) interface. The chromatographic separation was done with LC/MS equipped Waters Acquity UPLC BEH C18 (150 mm × 2.1 mm, 1.7 μm) (Waters Corp.). For the UHPLC, 2 μL of the sample was injected with a flow rate of 300 μL/min with a temperature of auto-sampler (10 °C) and column oven (40 °C). The mobile phases were 0.1% formic acid in H_2O (A) and 0.1% formic acid in acetonitrile (B), and the following gradient was used: 10–90% B (0–12 min) and 100% B (12.1–16.0 min). The MS/MS data were obtained using a collision energy ramp from 15 to 45 eV in MS^E mode. The ESI parameters were set as follows: in negative ion mode in Continuum format, a capillary voltage of 2.5 kV, cone voltage of 45 V, source temperature of 120 °C, desolvation temperature of 350 °C, cone gas flow of 50 L/h, and desolvation gas flow of 800 L/h. The ion acquisition rate was 0.25 s with the mass range from m/z 100 to 1600. The instrument was calibrated using a sodium formate solution as the calibration standard. Leucine enkephalin (m/z 554.2615 in negative mode) was used as the reference lock mass at a concentration of 200 pg/μL and a flow rate of 5 μL/min and was sprayed into the MS instrument every 10 s to ensure accuracy and reproducibility. The data acquisition was measured by MassLynx V4.1 (Waters Corp.). The compounds were identified using the in-house phytochemical library (UNIFI 1.8; Waters Corp.) [40,41].

3.7. Gas Chromatography Analysis

The organic compounds present in MeOH-E was determined using a gas chromatography (Agilent 789A, Agilent, Santa Clara, CA, USA) mass spectrophotometry (Agilent 5975C; GC-MSD) system in the scan range of m/z 50–500 according to the detailed operation conditions described elsewhere [64,84]. The GS-MS used in this study was equipped with DB-5MS (30 m length × 0.25 mm inner diameter × 0.25 μm thickness of film) column and performed under operation condition as the flow rate of 1 mL/min, injection mode (5:1) with an inlet temperature of 250 °C, interface temperature of 280 °C, ion source of EI, 70 eV, with the temperature of 280 °C. The compounds present in the MeOH-E were tentatively identified by matching the GC-MS data with the electronic library of W8N05ST.L.

3.8. Molecular Docking

The compounds with enzyme inhibitory activity identified from MeOH-E were virtually analyzed against human lysosomal acid-α-glucosidase (PDB: 5NN8) and human pancreatic α-amylase (PDB: 5E0F) by molecular docking. The structure files of ligands were prepared using ChemBioDraw 15.0 (PerkinElmer, Waltham, MA, USA) and then saved as mol. These mol files of ligands were used for energy minimization according to the principle of gasteiger [85]. The 3D structure of PDB of 5NN8 and 5E0F were retrieved from RSCB (https://www.rcsb.org/) and before the docking experiment the water residue was removed and the binding packet size was prepared as reported earlier [12]. Finally, the molecular docking between various ligand and targeted protein was carried out using Autodock Vina 1.1.2. Finally, the interactions between the protein and compounds were observed using LIGPLOT+(v.2.2).

3.9. Statistical Analysis

All the experiments were executed in triplicate and the results are presented with mean ± standard error (SE). The descriptive statistics, student '*t*' test, and analysis of various (ANOVA), line diagrams, Duncan's multiple range test (DMRT) were made using excel. 2010 and SPSS (Ver 2016, IBM, Armonk, NY, USA). The difference at $p < 0.05$ was considered as significant among the factors.

4. Conclusions

In summary, this work analyzed the enzyme inhibition, anti-diabetic activities and metabolites present in the MeOH-E of *G. jasminoides* by using LC-MS/MS and GC-MS. The MeOH-E showed higher enzyme inhibition, antioxidant and anti-diabetic activities in

IR-HepG2 cells. Metabolic profiling studies tentatively identified a total of 54 compounds including iridoids, terpenoids, fatty acid, phenolic acid derivatives from MeOH-E of *G. jasminoides* based on the observed m/z molecular ions in LC-MS/MS and GC-MS. The compounds identified were nine iridoid glycosides, 13 monoterpenoides, two each of flavonoids and carotenoids. Among the compounds identified chlorogenic acid and jasminoside A were found promising in interacting with α-glucosidase and α- amylase, as evidenced by molecular docking studies. Therefore, the present work concluded that bioactivity of the MeOH-E of *G. jasminoides* was the synergistic effect of various compounds present in the extract. According to the molecular screening, it is recommended that chlorogenic acid and jasminoside A be considered as candidate molecules for anti-diabetic activity. However, further studies are required for the purification and characterization of these two molecules and to determine their molecular mechanism of anti-diabetic activity for the development of future therapeutics.

Supplementary Materials: The following are available online at https://www.mdpi.com/1424-824 7/14/2/102/s1, Supplementary Figure S1. TIC chromatogram of metabolites profiling of methanolic extract (MeOH-E) of *G. jasminoides* by UHPLC-ESI-qTOF-MS/MS analysis. (a) Overall TIC chromatogram of MeOH-E of retention time (14 min) and (b) magnification of the TIC chromatogram from 1–5 min of retention time. Supplementary Figure S2. Low molecular weight and alkaloids identified from the methanolic extract(MeOH-E) of *G. jasminoides* by GCMS. Supplementary Table S1. GC-MS based analysis of alkaloids and low molecular weight molecules from methanolic extract (MeOH-E) of *G. jasminoides*. Supplementary Table S2. Assessment of the Drug-likeness through Lipinski's strategies for methanolic extract (MeOH-E) of *G. jasminoides* by web tool (SwissADME).

Author Contributions: K.S.: Conceptualization, Formal analysis, Investigation, Methodology, Software, Writing—original draft, Writing—review & editing. S.P.: Investigation, Methodology, Validation, Writing—review & editing. A.S.: Methodology, Validation, Data curation. K.-N.K.: Formal analysis, Validation, S.-H.C.: Formal analysis, Validation, A.V.A.M.: Data curation, Validation. M.-H.W.: Funding acquisition, Project administration, Supervision, Writing—review & editing. All authors have read and agreed to the published version of the manuscript.

Funding: This work was supported by Korea Research Fellowship Program through the National Research Foundation of Korea (NRF) funded by the Ministry of Science, ICT and Future Planning (2017H1D3A1A01052610) and National Research Foundation of Korea (2019R1A1055452).

Institutional Review Board Statement: Not Applicable.

Informed Consent Statement: Not Applicable.

Data Availability Statement: The data presented in this study are available on request.

Conflicts of Interest: The authors declare no conflict of interest.

References

1. Saeedi, P.; Petersohn, I.; Salpea, P.; Malanda, B.; Karuranga, S.; Unwin, N.; Colagiuri, S.; Guariguata, L.; Motala, A.A.; Ogurtsova, K.; et al. Global and regional diabetes prevalence estimates for 2019 and projections for 2030 and 2045: Results from the International Diabetes Federation Diabetes Atlas, 9th edition. *Diabetes Res. Clin. Pract.* **2019**, *157*, 107843. [CrossRef] [PubMed]
2. Behl, T.; Kotwani, A. Anti-hyperglycemic effect of *Terminalia catappa* fruit extract in streptozotocin-induced diabetic rats. *Int. J. Pharm. Pharm. Sci.* **2017**, *9*, 212. [CrossRef]
3. Apoorva, S.M.; Sridhar, N.; Suchetha, A. Prevalence and severity of periodontal disease in type 2 diabetes mellitus (non-insulin-dependent diabetes mellitus) patients in Bangalore city: An epidemiological study. *J. Indian Soc. Periodontol.* **2013**, *17*, 25–29. [CrossRef] [PubMed]
4. Ram Niwas, J.; Gyan Chand, J. Evaluation of Antidiabetic Activity of Hydroalcoholic Extract of *Cassia fistula* Linn. pod in Streptozotocin-Induced Diabetic Rats. *Pharmacogn. J.* **2017**, *9*, 599–606.
5. Fargion, S.; Dongiovanni, P.; Guzzo, A.; Colombo, S.; Valenti, L.; Fracanzani, A.L. Iron and insulin resistance. *Aliment. Pharmacol. Ther.* **2005**, *22*, 61–63. [CrossRef]
6. Teng, H.; Yuan, B.; Gothai, S.; Arulselvan, P.; Song, X.; Chen, L. Dietary triterpenes in the treatment of type 2 diabetes: To date. *Trends Food Sci. Technol.* **2018**, *72*, 34–44. [CrossRef]
7. Cade, W.T. Diabetes-Related Microvascular and Macrovascular Diseases in the Physical Therapy Setting. *Phys. Ther.* **2008**, *88*, 1322–1335. [CrossRef]

8. Chawla, R.; Chawla, A.; Jaggi, S. Microvasular and macrovascular complications in diabetes mellitus: Distinct or continuum? *Indian J. Endocrinol. Metab.* **2016**, *20*, 546–551. [CrossRef]
9. Yu, Z.; Yin, Y.; Zhao, W.; Liu, J.; Chen, F. Anti-diabetic activity peptides from albumin against α-glucosidase and α-amylase. *Food Chem.* **2012**, *135*, 2078–2085. [CrossRef]
10. Khanal, P.; Patil, B.M. α-Glucosidase inhibitors from *Duranta repens* modulate p53 signaling pathway in diabetes mellitus. *Adv. Tradit. Med.* **2020**, *20*, 1–12. [CrossRef]
11. Wang, P.-C.; Zhao, S.; Yang, B.-Y.; Wang, Q.; Kuang, H. Anti-diabetic polysaccharides from natural sources: A review. *Carbohydr. Polym.* **2016**, *148*, 86–97. [CrossRef] [PubMed]
12. Aispuro-Pérez, A.; López-Ávalos, J.; García-Páez, F.; Montes-Avila, J.; Picos-Corrales, L.A.; Ochoa-Terán, A.; Bastidas, P.; Montaño, S.; Calderón-Zamora, L.; Osuna-Martínez, U.; et al. Synthesis and molecular docking studies of imines as α-glucosidase and α-amylase inhibitors. *Bioorganic Chem.* **2020**, *94*, 103491. [CrossRef] [PubMed]
13. WHO. *Global Report on Traditional and Complementary Medicine*; WHO: Geneva, Switzerland, 2019; ISBN 978-92-4-151543-6.
14. Chen, L.; Li, M.; Yang, Z.; Tao, W.; Wang, P.; Tian, X.; Li, X.; Wang, W. *Gardenia jasminoides* Ellis: Ethnopharmacology, phytochemistry, and pharmacological and industrial applications of an important traditional Chinese medicine. *J. Ethnopharmacol.* **2020**, *257*, 112829. [CrossRef] [PubMed]
15. Wang, L.; Yang, C.; Song, F.; Liu, Z.; Liu, S. The therapeutic effectiveness of *Gardenia jasminoides* on type 2 diabetes rats: Mass spectrometry-based metabolomics approach. *J. Agric. Food Chem.* **2020**, *68*, 9673–9682. [CrossRef] [PubMed]
16. Stasiak, N.; Kukuła-Koch, W.; Głowniak, K. Modern industrial and pharmacological applications of indigo dye and its derivatives—A review. *Acta Pol. Pharm. Drug Res.* **2014**, *71*, 215–221.
17. Xiao, W.; Li, S.; Wang, S.; Ho, C.-T. Chemistry and bioactivity of *Gardenia jasminoides*. *J. Food Drug Anal.* **2017**, *25*, 43–61. [CrossRef]
18. Chen, J.-L.; Shi, B.-Y.; Xiang, H.; Hou, W.-J.; Qin, X.-M.; Tian, J.-S.; Du, G. 1H nmR-based metabolic profiling of liver in chronic unpredictable mild stress rats with genipin treatment. *J. Pharm. Biomed. Anal.* **2015**, *115*, 150–158. [CrossRef]
19. Wang, G.-F.; Wu, S.-Y.; Xu, W.; Jin, H.; Zhu, Z.-G.; Li, Z.-H.; Tian, Y.; Zhang, J.-J.; Rao, J.-J.; Wu, S.-G. Geniposide inhibits high glucose-induced cell adhesion through the NF-κB signaling pathway in human umbilical vein endothelial cells. *Acta Pharmacol. Sin.* **2010**, *31*, 953–962. [CrossRef]
20. Pham, T.Q.; Cormier, F.; Farnworth, E.; Tong, A.V.H.; Van Calsteren, M.-R. Antioxidant Properties of Crocin from *Gardenia jasminoides* Ellis and Study of the Reactions of Crocin with Linoleic Acid and Crocin with Oxygen. *J. Agric. Food Chem.* **2000**, *48*, 1455–1461. [CrossRef]
21. Higashino, S.; Sasaki, Y.; Giddings, J.C.; Hyodo, K.; Sakata, S.F.; Matsuda, K.; Horikawa, Y.; Yamamoto, J. Crocetin, a Carotenoid from *Gardenia jasminoides* Ellis, Protects against Hypertension and Cerebral Thrombogenesis in Stroke-prone Spontaneously Hypertensive Rats. *Phytother. Res.* **2014**, *28*, 1315–1319. [CrossRef]
22. Dorman, H.; Peltoketo, A.; Hiltunen, R.; Tikkanen, M. Characterisation of the antioxidant properties of de-odourised aqueous extracts from selected *Lamiaceae* herbs. *Food Chem.* **2003**, *83*, 255–262. [CrossRef]
23. Juma, B.F.; Majinda, R.R.T. Constituents of *Gardenia volkensii*: Their brine shrimp lethality and DPPH radical scavenging properties. *Nat. Prod. Res.* **2007**, *21*, 121–125. [CrossRef] [PubMed]
24. Debnath, T.; Park, P.-J.; Nath, N.C.D.; Samad, N.B.; Park, H.W.; Lim, B. Antioxidant activity of *Gardenia jasminoides* Ellis fruit extracts. *Food Chem.* **2011**, *128*, 697–703. [CrossRef]
25. Sayd, S.S.; Hanan, A.A.; Taie, H.A.A.; Taha, L.S. Micropropagation, antioxidant activity, total phenolics and flavonoids con-tent of *Gardenia jasminoides* Ellis as affected by growth regulators. *Int. J. Acad. Res.* **2010**, *2*, 184–191.
26. Gowd, V.; Bao, T.; Wang, L.; Huang, Y.; Chen, S.; Zheng, X.; Cui, S.; Chen, W. Antioxidant and antidiabetic activity of blackberry after gastrointestinal digestion and human gut microbiota fermentation. *Food Chem.* **2018**, *269*, 618–627. [CrossRef]
27. Hua, D.; Luo, W.; Duan, J.; Jin, D.; Zhou, X.; Sun, C.; Wang, Q.; Shi, C.; Jiang, Z.; Wang, R.; et al. Screening and identification of potent α-glycosidase inhibitors from *Gardenia jasminoides* Ellis. *S. Afr. J. Bot.* **2018**, *119*, 377–382. [CrossRef]
28. Saravana, P.S.; Cho, Y.-N.; Patil, M.P.; Cho, Y.-J.; Kim, G.-D.; Park, Y.B.; Woo, H.-C.; Chun, B.-S. Hydrothermal degradation of seaweed polysaccharide: Characterization and biological activities. *Food Chem.* **2018**, *268*, 179–187. [CrossRef]
29. Hao, S.; Wang, J.; Li, S.; Shang, F.; Qin, Y.; Wu, T.; Bao, X.; Cao, Q.; Wang, C.; Sun, B. Preparation of *Gardenia* red pigment and its antineoplastic activity in multiple tumor cells. *Food Biosci.* **2020**, *35*, 100582. [CrossRef]
30. Moritome, N.; Kishi, Y.; Fujii, S. Properties of red pigments prepared from geniposidic acid and amino acids. *J. Sci. Food Agric.* **1999**, *79*, 810–814. [CrossRef]
31. Saravanakumar, K.; Chelliah, R.; Shanmugam, S.; Varukattu, N.B.; Oh, D.-H.; Kathiresan, K.; Wang, M.-H. Green synthesis and characterization of biologically active nanosilver from seed extract of *Gardenia jasminoides* Ellis. *J. Photochem. Photobiol. B Biol.* **2018**, *185*, 126–135. [CrossRef]
32. Wu, X.; Liu, K.; Liu, P.-C.; Liu, R. Dual AO/EB Staining to Detect Apoptosis in Osteosarcoma Cells Compared with Flow Cytometry. *Med. Sci. Monit. Basic Res.* **2015**, *21*, 15–20. [CrossRef] [PubMed]
33. Zhang, Q.; Hu, X.-F.; Xin, M.-M.; Liu, H.-B.; Sun, L.; Morris-Natschke, S.L.; Chen, Y.; Lee, K.-H. Antidiabetic potential of the ethyl acetate extract of Physalis alkekengi and chemical constituents identified by HPLC-ESI-QTOF-MS. *J. Ethnopharmacol.* **2018**, *225*, 202–210. [CrossRef] [PubMed]
34. Shao, J.; Xue, J.; Dai, Y.; Liu, H.; Chen, N.; Jia, L.; Huang, J. Inhibition of human hepatocellular carcinoma HepG2 by phthalocyanine photosensitiser PHOTOCYANINE: ROS production, apoptosis, cell cycle arrest. *Eur. J. Cancer* **2012**, *48*, 2086–2096. [CrossRef]

35. Ando, T.; Nagumo, M.; Ninomiya, M.; Tanaka, K.; Linhardt, R.J.; Koketsu, M. Synthesis of coumarin derivatives and their cytoprotective effects on t -BHP-induced oxidative damage in HepG2 cells. *Bioorganic Med. Chem. Lett.* **2018**, *28*, 2422–2425. [CrossRef] [PubMed]

36. Song, G.; Sun, Y.; Liu, Y.; Wang, X.; Chen, M.; Miao, F.; Zhang, W.; Yu, X.; Jin, J. Low molecular weight fluorescent probes with good photostability for imaging RNA-rich nucleolus and RNA in cytoplasm in living cells. *Biomaterials* **2014**, *35*, 2103–2112. [CrossRef]

37. Zhang, L.; Mizumoto, K.; Sato, N.; Ogawa, T.; Kusumoto, M.; Niiyama, H.; Tanaka, M. Quantitative determination of apoptotic death in cultured human pancreatic cancer cells by propidium iodide and digitonin. *Cancer Lett.* **1999**, *142*, 129–137. [CrossRef]

38. El Sayed, A.M.; Basam, S.M.; El-Naggar, E.-M.B.A.; Marzouk, H.S.; El-Hawary, S. LC–MS/MS and GC–MS profiling as well as the antimicrobial effect of leaves of selected *Yucca* species introduced to Egypt. *Sci. Rep.* **2020**, *10*, 1–15. [CrossRef]

39. Kivilompolo, M.; Obůrka, V.; Hyötyläinen, T. Comparison of GC–MS and LC–MS methods for the analysis of antioxidant phenolic acids in herbs. *Anal. Bioanal. Chem.* **2007**, *388*, 881–887. [CrossRef]

40. Yang, Z.-R.; Wang, Z.-H.; Tang, J.-F.; Yan, Y.; Yue, S.-J.; Feng, W.-W.; Shi, Z.-Y.; Meng, X.-T.; Peng, C.; Wang, C.-Y.; et al. UPLC-QTOF/MSE and Bioassay Are Available Approaches for Identifying Quality Fluctuation of Xueshuantong Lyophilized Powder in Clinic. *Front. Pharmacol.* **2018**, *9*, 633. [CrossRef]

41. Jeong, M.S.; Park, S.; Han, E.J.; Park, S.Y.; Kim, M.J.; Jung, K.; Cho, S.-H.; Kim, S.-Y.; Yoon, W.-J.; Ahn, G.; et al. *Pinus thunbergii* PARL leaf protects against alcohol-induced liver disease by enhancing antioxidant defense mechanism in BALB/c mice. *J. Funct. Foods* **2020**, *73*, 104116. [CrossRef]

42. Fu, Z.; Ling, Y.; Li, Z.; Chen, M.; Sun, Z.; Huang, C. HPLC-Q-TOF-MS/MS for analysis of major chemical constituents of Yinchen-Zhizi herb pair extract. *Biomed. Chromatogr.* **2014**, *28*, 475–485. [CrossRef] [PubMed]

43. Hussain, H.; Green, I.R.; Saleem, M.; Raza, M.L.; Nazir, M. Therapeutic Potential of Iridoid Derivatives: Patent Review. *Inventions* **2019**, *4*, 29. [CrossRef]

44. Jia, J.; Liu, M.; Wen, Q.; He, M.; Ouyang, H.; Chen, L.; Li, J.; Feng, Y.; Zhong, G.; Yang, S. Screening of anti-complement active ingredients from *Eucommia ulmoides* Oliv. branches and their metabolism in vivo based on UHPLC-Q-TOF/MS/MS. *J. Chromatogr. B* **2019**, *1124*, 26–36. [CrossRef] [PubMed]

45. Zhang, S.; Li, Y.; Zhang, C.-X.; Huang, W.-Z.; Ding, G.; Xiao, W.; Bi, Y.-A.; Xiao, W. Research on the change of chemical composition in productive process of Re Du Ning Injections by HPLC/Q-TOF MS. *Biomed. Chromatogr.* **2015**, *30*, 131–141. [CrossRef] [PubMed]

46. Wu, H.; Li, X.; Yan, X.; An, L.; Luo, K.; Shao, M.; Jiang, Y.; Xie, R.; Feng, F. An untargeted metabolomics-driven approach based on LC–TOF/MS and LC–MS/MS for the screening of xenobiotics and metabolites of Zhi-Zi-Da-Huang decoction in rat plasma. *J. Pharm. Biomed. Anal.* **2015**, *115*, 315–322. [CrossRef] [PubMed]

47. Wang, L.; Liu, S.; Xing, J.; Liu, Z.; Song, F. Characterization of interaction property of multi-components in *Gardenia jasminoides* with aldose reductase by microdialysis combined with liquid chromatography coupled to mass spectrometry. *Rapid Commun. Mass Spectrom.* **2016**, *30*, 87–94. [CrossRef] [PubMed]

48. Wang, L.; Liu, S.; Zhang, X.; Xing, J.; Liu, Z.; Song, F. A strategy for identification and structural characterization of compounds from *Gardenia jasminoides* by integrating macroporous resin column chromatography and liquid chromatography-tandem mass spectrometry combined with ion-mobility spectrometry. *J. Chromatogr. A* **2016**, *1452*, 47–57. [CrossRef] [PubMed]

49. Feng, W.; Dong, Q.; Liu, M.; Li, S.; Liu, T.; Wang, X.-G.; Niu, L.-Y. Screening and identification of multiple constituents and their metabolites of Zhi-zi-chi decoction in rat urine and bile by ultra-high-performance liquid chromatography quadrupole time-of-flight mass spectrometry. *Biomed. Chromatogr.* **2017**, *31*, e3978. [CrossRef]

50. Wang, S.-C.; Tseng, T.-Y.; Huang, C.-M.; Tsai, T.-H. *Gardenia* herbal active constituents: Applicable separation procedures. *J. Chromatogr. B* **2004**, *812*, 193–202. [CrossRef]

51. He, W.; Liu, X.; Xu, H.; Gong, Y.; Yuan, F.; Gao, Y. On-line HPLC-ABTS screening and HPLC-DAD-MS/MS identification of free radical scavengers in *Gardenia* (*Gardenia jasminoides* Ellis) fruit extracts. *Food Chem.* **2010**, *123*, 521–528. [CrossRef]

52. Joo, Y.H.; Nam, M.H.; Chung, N.; Lee, Y.K. UPLC-QTOF-MS/MS screening and identification of bioactive compounds in fresh, aged, and browned Magnolia denudata flower extracts. *Food Res. Int.* **2020**, *133*, 109192. [CrossRef] [PubMed]

53. Wang, C.; Zhang, N.; Wang, Z.; Qi, Z.; Zhu, H.; Zheng, B.; Li, P.; Liu, J. Nontargeted Metabolomic Analysis of Four Different Parts of *Platycodon grandiflorum* Grown in Northeast China. *Molecules* **2017**, *22*, 1280. [CrossRef] [PubMed]

54. Liu, M.; He, M.; Gao, H.; Guo, S.; Jia, J.; Ouyang, H.; Feng, Y.; Yang, S. Strategy for rapid screening of antioxidant and anti-inflammatory active ingredients in *Gynura procumbens* (Lour.) Merr. based on UHPLC–Q-TOF–MS/MS and characteristic ion filtration. *Biomed. Chromatogr.* **2019**, *33*, e4635. [CrossRef] [PubMed]

55. Breitmaier, E. Hemi- and Monoterpenes. In *Terpenes: Flavors, Fragrances, Pharmaca, Pheromones*; Wiley: Hoboken, NJ, USA, 2006; pp. 10–23. [CrossRef]

56. Chen, Q.C.; Youn, U.; Min, B.-S.; Bae, K. Pyronane Monoterpenoids from the Fruit of *Gardenia jasminoides*. *J. Nat. Prod.* **2008**, *71*, 995–999. [CrossRef]

57. Yu, Y.; Xie, Z.-L.; Gao, H.; Ma, W.-W.; Dai, Y.; Wang, Y.; Zhong, Y.; Yao, X.-S. Bioactive Iridoid Glucosides from the Fruit of *Gardenia jasminoides*. *J. Nat. Prod.* **2009**, *72*, 1459–1464. [CrossRef]

58. Akihisa, T.; Watanabe, K.; Yamamoto, A.; Zhang, J.; Matsumoto, M.; Fukatsu, M. Melanogenesis Inhibitory Activity of Monoterpene Glycosides from *Gardeniae Fructus*. *Chem. Biodivers.* **2012**, *9*, 1490–1499. [CrossRef]

59. Peng, K.; Yang, L.; Zhao, S.; Chen, L.; Zhao, F.; Qiu, F. Chemical constituents from the fruit of *Gardenia jasminoides* and their inhibitory effects on nitric oxide production. *Bioorganic Med. Chem. Lett.* **2013**, *23*, 1127–1131. [CrossRef]
60. Machida, K.; Oyama, K.; Ishii, M.; Kakuda, R.; Yaoita, Y.; Kikuchi, M. Studies of the Constituents of *Gardenia* Species. II. Terpenoids from *Gardeniae* Fructus. *Chem. Pharm. Bull.* **2000**, *48*, 746–748. [CrossRef]
61. Chen, Y.; Yang, Z.L.; Zhang, L.H.; Liu, S.J.; Zhang, X.T. Determination of geniposide, crocin and crocetin in different pro-cessing products of fructus *Gardeniae* by HPLC-ELSD. *J. Chin. Med. Mater.* **2011**, *34*, 687–690.
62. Uekusa, Y.; Sugimoto, N.; Sato, K.; Yun, Y.S.; Kunugi, A.; Yamazaki, T.; Tanamoto, K.-I. Neocrocin A: A novel crocetin glycoside with a unique system for binding sugars isolated from *Gardenia* yellow. *Chem. Pharm. Bull.* **2007**, *55*, 1643–1646. [CrossRef]
63. Cai, L.; Li, R.; Tang, W.-J.; Meng, G.; Hu, X.-Y.; Wu, T.-N. Antidepressant-like effect of geniposide on chronic unpredictable mild stress-induced depressive rats by regulating the hypothalamus–pituitary–adrenal axis. *Eur. Neuropsychopharmacol.* **2015**, *25*, 1332–1341. [CrossRef] [PubMed]
64. Saravanakumar, K.; Chellia, R.; Hu, X.; Kathiresan, K.; Oh, D.-H.; Wang, M.-H. Eradication of *Helicobacter pylori* through the inhibition of urease and peptide deformylase: Computational and biological studies. *Microb. Pathog.* **2019**, *128*, 236–244. [CrossRef] [PubMed]
65. Chandrasekaran, M.; Senthilkumar, A.; Venkatesalu, V. Antibacterial and antifungal efficacy of fatty acid methyl esters from the leaves of *Sesuvium portulacastrum* L. *Eur. Rev. Med. Pharmacol. Sci.* **2011**, *15*, 775–780. [PubMed]
66. Lipinski, C.A. Lead- and drug-like compounds: The rule-of-five revolution. *Drug Discov. Today Technol.* **2004**, *1*, 337–341. [CrossRef] [PubMed]
67. Ali, N.; Rashid, S.; Nafees, S.; Hasan, S.K.; Shahid, A.; Majed, F.; Sultana, S. Protective effect of Chlorogenic acid against methotrexate induced oxidative stress, inflammation and apoptosis in rat liver: An experimental approach. *Chem. Interact.* **2017**, *272*, 80–91. [CrossRef]
68. Mccarty, M.F. A chlorogenic acid-induced increase in GLP-1 production may mediate the impact of heavy coffee consumption on diabetes risk. *Med. Hypotheses* **2005**, *64*, 848–853. [CrossRef]
69. Ardestani, A.; Yazdanparast, R. Inhibitory effects of ethyl acetate extract of Teucrium polium on in vitro protein glycoxidation. *Food Chem. Toxicol.* **2007**, *45*, 2402–2411. [CrossRef]
70. Zhishen, J.; Mengcheng, T.; Jianming, W. The determination of flavonoid contents in mulberry and their scavenging effects on superoxide radicals. *Food Chem.* **1999**, *64*, 555–559. [CrossRef]
71. Slinkard, L.; Singleton, V.L. Total phenol analyses: Automation and comparison with manual methods. *Am. J. Enol. Vitic.* **1977**, *28*, 49–55.
72. Blois, M.S. Antioxidant Determinations by the Use of a Stable Free Radical. *Nature* **1958**, *181*, 1199–1200. [CrossRef]
73. Cano, A.; Hernández-Ruíz, J.; García-Cánovas, F.; Acosta, M.; Arnao, M.B. An end-point method for estimation of the total antioxidant activity in plant material. *Phytochem. Anal.* **1998**, *9*, 196–202. [CrossRef]
74. Sathiyaseelan, A.; Saravanakumar, K.; Mariadoss, A.V.A.; Wang, M.-H. Biocompatible fungal chitosan encapsulated phytogenic silver nanoparticles enhanced antidiabetic, antioxidant and antibacterial activity. *Int. J. Biol. Macromol.* **2020**, *153*, 63–71. [CrossRef] [PubMed]
75. Kim, Y.-M.; Wang, M.-H.; Rhee, H.-I. A novel α-glucosidase inhibitor from pine bark. *Carbohydr. Res.* **2004**, *339*, 715–717. [CrossRef] [PubMed]
76. Kandra, L.; Zajácz, Á.; Remenyik, J.; Gyémánt, G. Kinetic investigation of a new inhibitor for human salivary α-amylase. *Biochem. Biophys. Res. Commun.* **2005**, *334*, 824–828. [CrossRef] [PubMed]
77. Saravanakumar, K.; Mariadoss, A.V.A.; Sathiyaseelan, A.; Wang, M.-H. Synthesis and characterization of nano-chitosan capped gold nanoparticles with multifunctional bioactive properties. *Int. J. Biol. Macromol.* **2020**, *165*, 747–757. [CrossRef] [PubMed]
78. Saravanakumar, K.; Vivek, R.; Boopathy, N.S.; Yaqian, L.; Kathiresan, K.; Chen, J. Anticancer potential of bioactive 16-methylheptadecanoic acid methyl ester derived from marine Trichoderma. *J. Appl. Biomed.* **2015**, *13*, 199–212. [CrossRef]
79. Chen, L.; Teng, H.; Cao, H. Chlorogenic acid and caffeic acid from *Sonchus oleraceus* Linn synergistically attenuate insulin resistance and modulate glucose uptake in HepG2 cells. *Food Chem. Toxicol.* **2019**, *127*, 182–187. [CrossRef]
80. Teng, H.; Chen, L.; Song, H. The potential beneficial effects of phenolic compounds isolated from *A. pilosa* Ledeb on insulin-resistant hepatic HepG2 cells. *Food Funct.* **2016**, *7*, 4400–4409. [CrossRef]
81. Saravanakumar, K.; Jeevithan, E.; Hu, X.; Chelliah, R.; Oh, D.-H.; Wang, M.-H. Enhanced anti-lung carcinoma and anti-biofilm activity of fungal molecules mediated biogenic zinc oxide nanoparticles conjugated with β-D-glucan from barley. *J. Photochem. Photobiol. B Biol.* **2020**, *203*, 111728. [CrossRef]
82. Saravanakumar, K.; Wang, M.-H. Biogenic silver embedded magnesium oxide nanoparticles induce the cytotoxicity in human prostate cancer cells. *Adv. Powder Technol.* **2019**, *30*, 786–794. [CrossRef]
83. Sakthivel, R.; Malar, D.S.; Devi, K.P. Phytol shows anti-angiogenic activity and induces apoptosis in A549 cells by depolarizing the mitochondrial membrane potential. *Biomed. Pharmacother.* **2018**, *105*, 742–752. [CrossRef] [PubMed]
84. Saravanan, M.; Senthilkumar, P.; Kalimuthu, K.; Chinnadurai, V.; Vasantharaj, S.; Ad, P. Phytochemical and pharmacological profiling of *Turnera subulata* Sm., a vital medicinal herb. *Ind. Crop. Prod.* **2018**, *124*, 822–833. [CrossRef]
85. Wang, J.; Wang, W.; Kollman, P.A.; Case, D.A. Automatic atom type and bond type perception in molecular mechanical calculations. *J. Mol. Graph. Model.* **2006**, *25*, 247–260. [CrossRef] [PubMed]

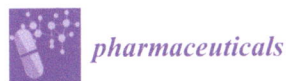

Article

Simultaneous Determination of Isothiazolinones and Parabens in Cosmetic Products Using Solid-Phase Extraction and Ultra-High Performance Liquid Chromatography/Diode Array Detector

Hazim Mohammed Ali [1,2], Ibrahim Hotan Alsohaimi [1], Mohammad Rizwan Khan [3,*] and Mohammad Azam [3]

[1] Department of Chemistry, College of Science, Jouf University, Sakaka 2014, Saudi Arabia; hmali@ju.edu.sa (H.M.A.); ehalshaimi@ju.edu.sa (I.H.A.)

[2] Forensic Chemistry Department, Forensic Medicine Authority, Cairo 11441, Egypt

[3] Department of Chemistry, College of Science, King Saud University, Riyadh 11451, Saudi Arabia; mhashim@ksu.edu.sa

*   Correspondence: mrkhan@ksu.edu.sa; Tel.: +966-114-674-198; Fax: +966-114-675-992

Received: 22 October 2020; Accepted: 20 November 2020; Published: 22 November 2020

Abstract: Isothiazolinones methylisothiazolinone (MI) and methylchloroisothiazolinone (MCI), and parabens methylparaben (MP), ethylparaben (EP), propylparaben (PP) and butylparaben (BP) are the most common synthetic preservatives. They are all known to be potential skin allergens that lead to contact dermatitis. Thus, the identification of these unsafe chemicals in cosmetic products is of high importance. In the present study, solid-phase extraction (SPE) based on HyperSep reversed-phase C8/benzene sulfonic acid ion exchanger (HyperSep C8/BSAIE) and Sep-Pak C18 sorbents, and ultra-high performance liquid chromatography/diode array detector (UHPLC/DAD) were optimized for the simultaneous determination of MI, MCI, MP, EP, PP and BP in cosmetic products. HyperSep C8/BSAIE and UHPLC/DAD with the eluting solvent mixture (acetonitrile/methanol, 2:1, v/v) and detection wavelength (255 nm) were found to be the optimal conditions, respectively. The method illustrates the excellent linearity range (0.008–20 µg/mL) with coefficient of determination (R^2, 0.997–0.999), limits of detection (LOD, 0.001–0.002 µg/mL), precision in terms of relative standard deviation (RSD < 3%, intra-day and <6%, inter-day) when examining a standard mixture at low (0.07 µg/mL), medium (3 µg/mL) and high (15 µg/mL) concentrations. A total of 31 cosmetic samples were studied, achieving concentrations (MI, not detected (nd)-0.89 µg/g), (MCI, nd-0.62 µg/g), (MP, nd-6.53 µg/g), (EP, nd-0.90 µg/g), (PP, nd-9.69 µg/g) and (BP, nd-17.80 µg/g). Recovery values ranged from 92.33 to 101.43% depending on the types of sample. To our knowledge, this is the first specific method which covers the theme and describes background amounts of such preservatives in cosmetics.

Keywords: isothiazolinones; parabens; cosmetics; SPE; UHPLC/DAD

1. Introduction

Methylisothiazolinone (MI) and methylchloroisothiazolinone (MCI) are the isothiazolinone synthetic biocide which is used as a preservative [1–3]. The combination of MI and MCI was used in numerous leave-on and rinse-off formulations comprising skin-care products, bath products, hair products, shampoos, conditioners, facial and eye makeup, face masks, suntan products and wet-wipes products [1–3]. MI is currently applied either solely or together with MCI, which comprises a proportion of MCI/MI (3:1). The final product is traded under the name of Kathon, which is sold to the cosmetics manufacturing industries as Kathon CG [4]. Kathon is also applied in the production of papers that usually come into contact with food products. Moreover, this product works as an antimicrobial agent in paper coatings and latex adhesives that interact with food as well [5]. A usual sign of sensitivity to Kathon CG is allergic-contact dermatitis. Sensitization to isothiazolinone groups preservatives was noticed in the 1980s [4,6]. In recent years, the use of isothiazolinone-based preservatives has substantially increased and reported incidence of contact allergy. [6]. In the year 2013, the isothiazolinone-based preservatives were affirmed by the American Contact Dermatitis Society as contact allergen of the year [7]. Following the same year, Cosmetics Europe [8], in coordination with the European Society of Contact Dermatitis [9], suggested to its members that the use of MI in cosmetics, which are intended to stay in long contact with the skin, and cosmetic wet wipes must be ceased. Because of high concerns relating to the potential rising rates of skin sensitivity to MI and MCI, it is highly important to study the presence of such hazardous compounds in cosmetic products available in the markets.

Parabens are frequently used as antimicrobial and antibacterial preservatives, to prevent the growth of various microbial organisms, particularly fungus and bacteria in cosmetics, drugs and foods [10]. Chemically, parabens are the esters of *p*-hydroxibenzoic acid which contain different alkyl groups, for instance, methylparaben (MP), ethylparaben (EP), propylparaben (PP), butylparaben (BP), benzylparaben (BeP), heptylparaben (HP), isobutylparaben (IBP) and isopropylparaben (IPP) [11]. Among them, MP, EP, PP and BP are the most frequently and repeatedly used in combination with others in the final products [12]. However, the antimicrobial activity increases when using them in a mixture of two or more parabens [12]. Owing to their extensive application, the potential damaging health effects ascribed to parabens could be augmented [13,14]. Although these hazardous compounds have been extensively applied for a long time, a lot of concerns about their effects on human health have remained unsolved. Many researchers have evaluated the influence of severe and persistent exposure of parabens [13,14], as a result parabens effect on the human endocrine system, potential issues in homoeostasis, metabolic syndrome, reproductive systems and breast cancer [13–16]. Because of their dreadful impact on human health, the World Health Organization and European Commission have established paraben exposure limits in cosmetics and foods [17,18]. The European Union, Health Canada and the United States Food and Drug Administration have recommended the parabens permissible limits of 0.4% (*w/w*) and 0.8% (*w/w*) in cosmetics [19,20]. Since then, the cosmetics manufacturer has started to produce cosmetics free from MI, MCI and parabens. Nonetheless, adulteration and misbranding of cosmetics takes place by still using the parabens as an ingredient in the cosmetics. Recently, Abad-Gil et al. (2021) reported the presence of isothiazolinone, paraben and alcohol-type preservatives in cosmetic products; they found PE (1800 μg/mL) and MP (590 μg/mL) in facial tonic; MI (1.20 μg/mL), PE (50 μg/mL) and MP (5.20 μg/mL) in shampoo; and PE (1500 μg/mL) and MP (710 μg/mL) in body cream [21]. Alvarez-Rivera et al. (2012) have identified isothiazolinone preservatives in cosmetic products. The products that contained MI and MCI were shampoo (0.38–4.75 and 1.12–9.34 μg/mL), face gel (1.07 and 0.35 μg/mL), hair mask (13.10 μg/mL and <limits of detection (LOD)), dental cream (0.59 μg/mL and <LOD), baby liquid soap (25.8–111 and 0.71–41.8 μg/mL), bath gel (2.05–65.70 and <LOD-3.35 μg/mL), baby shampoo (3.24 and 1.54 μg/mL), makeup (0.83 and 0.18 μg/mL), hair gel (0.72 and 0.22 μg/mL) and baby body milk (1.12–26.10 μg/mL and <LOD) [3]. In other studies, researchers have also reported the presence of isothiazolinone and paraben preservatives in cosmetic products [2,3,21–26]. Therefore, the development of sensitive methods to prohibit the adulteration and misbranding of cosmetics is highly needed. To date, there has been no earlier analytical method for the analysis of MI, MCI and parabens in cosmetics or any other matrices. However, many individual methods for MI, MCI, and parabens have been previously reported. The most frequently applied methods for the analysis of MI and MCI were ultra-high performance liquid chromatography–tandem mass spectrometry (UPLC-MS/MS) [2], high performance liquid chromatography-tandem mass spectrometry (HPLC-MS/MS) [3], gas chromatography–tandem mass spectrometry (GC-MS/MS) [27] and high-performance liquid chromatography–ultraviolet (HPLC-UV) [22]. The studied matrices

were cosmetics [2,3], shampoo [22], urine [27], milk [28], household products [3], wastewater, surface water, soil, sludge and sediment [29], hygienic consumer products [30], paints [31], food packaging materials [32], cleaning agents and pharmaceuticals [33].

Relating to the determination of parabens, different methods have been reported earlier in various matrices, for instance, HPLC-fluorescence/UV/DAD (cosmetics, toothpaste and mouthwash) [23,24,34], paper spray-MS/MS (cosmetics and drugs) [35], capillary liquid chromatography with UV detection (cosmetics, food and pharmaceuticals) [11], UHPLC-high-resolution mass spectrometry (human urine) [36], UHPLC–MS/MS (human milk) [37] HPLC-MS/MS (domestic sewage) [38] and so on. Some common methods had also been recently reported; Abad-Gil et al., (2021) optimized the simultaneous determination of MI, MCI, 4-hydroxybenzoic acid, phenoxyethanol and MP in cosmetics, using an HPLC/DAD/FL system [21]. In another study, Hefnawy et al., (2017) reported the simultaneous analysis of MI, MP, EP, PP and salicylic acid in cosmetics by monolithic HPLC–PDA [39]. In both methods, the studied compounds and applied methods were found to be different than those used in the current study. The current method (UHPLC/DAD) was found to be rapid, sensitive and economical, especially for the simultaneous determination of MI, MCI, MP, EP, PP and BP in cosmetics.

Saudi Arabia is the main marketplace for cosmetic products in the Arab and African countries, and it has one of the world's utmost cosmetics consumption rates. Recently, the Saudi Arabia personal care and beauty market was forecasted to attain $5.5 billion by 2025, rising at a compound annual growth rate of 10.49% during the forecast period (https://www.mordorintelligence.com/industry-reports/saudi-arabia-beauty-and-personal-care-marketm).

Up until now, there has been no earlier analytical system for the identification of MI, MCI and parabens (MP, EP, PP and BP) in cosmetic products by using a single extraction and determination method. Thus, our investigation aimed for the development and validation of a specific method based on solid-phase extraction (SPE) and ultra-high-performance liquid chromatography/diode array detector (UHPLC/DAD) for the simultaneous determination of MI, MCI, MP, EP, PP and BP in cosmetic products.

2. Results and Discussion

2.1. Optimization of SPE Method

At present, several extraction methods are available which deal either with MI and MCI [2,3,22] or four potential parabens (MP, EP, PP and BP) [11,23,24,34,35] determination in cosmetics. Thus, the most important aim of the current study was to develop a single extraction and determination method for MI, MCI, MP, EP, PP and BP, which usually co-occur in cosmetic samples. This is the first approach relating to the extraction and determination of these compounds in cosmetics by using a single method.

Owing to the low amounts of MI, MCI, MP, EP, PP and BP present in the cosmetic samples, the optimization of a reliable method for their analysis is of high importance, and thus, it required a very functional extraction and cleanup system which can eliminate the sample matrix interferences that typically interfere with the determination of target compounds by UHPLC/DAD system.

According to the nature of the analyzed compounds, initially, we selected two types of SPE extraction cartridges, namely HyperSep™ Verify CX Cartridges (Thermo Fisher Scientific, San Jose, CA, USA) of HyperSep C_8/BSAIE (200 mg/mL) and Sep-Pak C_{18} Classic Cartridge, 360 mg, particle size 55–105 μm (Waters (Milford, MA, USA). Preliminary studies were performed by using a 20 mL mixed solution (3 μg/mL) prepared in methanol and water of all the targeted compounds (MI, MCI, MP, EP, PP and BP). A series of experiments were carried out by the passing sample mixture solution at a controlled flow rate (1 mL/min) through two SPE cartridges separately. Once the sample solution passed completely, the targeted compounds from SPE sorbents were eluted by using different solvent mixtures (10 mL) at various proportions: water/methanol, water/acetonitrile and acetonitrile/methanol. After that, the solution was evaporated under nitrogen gas, until there remained 3 mL of the total solution volume, followed by filtration by using a polytetrafluoroethylene (PTFE) syringe filter

(0.45 μm). Finally, the filtrate was injected to UHPLC/DAD, for the determination of MI, MCI, MP, EP, PP and BP. Among them, the SPE cartridge HyperSep C$_8$/BSAIE and eluting solvent mixture (acetonitrile/methanol, 2:1, *v/v*) were found to be the optimal extraction parameters and used for the analysis of real samples. Figure 1 demonstrates the UHPLC/DAD chromatograms of MI, MCI, MP, EP, PP and BP (standard solution mixture, 3 μg/mL), obtained using different SPE cartridges and eluting solvent mixtures at proportion (2:1, *v/v*). It can be observed from Figure 1 that using (A1) water/methanol 2:1, *v/v* and Sep-Pak C18; (A2) water/acetonitrile 2:1, *v/v* and Sep-Pak C18; and (A3) acetonitrile/methanol 2:1, *v/v* and Sep-Pak C18 conditions, the compounds were either not detected or found below LOD. Nevertheless, by using (B1) water/methanol 2:1, *v/v* and HyperSep C8/BSAIE; (B2) water/acetonitrile 2:1, *v/v* and HyperSep C8/BSAIE; and (B3) acetonitrile/methanol 2:1, *v/v* and HyperSep C8/BSAIE conditions, the compounds have been identified in all cases. In B1 and B2 conditions, the compounds were identified with the poor resolution with low peak intensity. However, in B3 conditions, the compounds were identified with excellent resolution and symmetrical with high intensity.

2.2. Optimization of UHPLC/DAD Method

The most important challenge on the new UHPLC/DAD system was to separate MI, MCI, MP, EP, PP and BP in a single run, with the advantage of high peak resolution, symmetry and short analysis time. Due to differing in their polarity, many determination methods have been reported earlier which deal either with MI and MCI [2,3,22] or parabens (MP, EP, PP and BP) [11,23,24,34,35] in cosmetics. For the optimization of the UHPLC/DAD system, a standard mixture solution (3 μg/mL) was analyzed by using ACCLAIM™ 120 C$_8$ analytical column and mobile phase with different solvent proportions, such as water (0.1% formic acid) with acetonitrile/methanol; water (0.05% trifluoroacetic acid) with acetonitrile/methanol; and water (0.1% trifluoroacetic acid) with acetonitrile/methanol. During the assessment of the method parameters, the absorbance was studied in the range of 250–280 nm. The most favorable chromatographic conditions for the analysis of MI, MCI, MP, EP, PP and BP was water (0.1% trifluoroacetic acid) with acetonitrile (mobile phase) and absorbance 255 nm, selected as the final method for real sample analysis. Figure 2 displays the UHPLC/DAD chromatograms obtained at optimal chromatographic conditions. The method offers excellent peak resolution and symmetry and a total analysis time lower than 25 min. The influence of column temperature on analysis was also established in the range from room temperature, 25 °C, to 50 °C, with 5 °C variations. The analysis time was reduced with increasing column temperature beyond 35 °C, which offered a poorer compounds' separation. Consequently, the column temperature of 35 °C was selected as an optimal condition.

2.3. Performance of the Method

The performance of the proposed method was investigated in terms of linearity (R^2), limit of detection (LOD, signal-to-noise ratio 3:1) and limit of quantification (LOQ, signal-to-noise ratio 10:1), precision (intra- and inter-day) and accuracy. The achieved values have been presented in Tables 1 and 2. Linearity was determined by analyzing standard mixture at different concentrations, ranging from 0.008 to 20 μg/mL. The analysis was performed in triplicates (*n* = 3). Calibration curves were found to be linear over the broad range of concentrations with the coefficient of determination (R^2, 0.997–0.999). LOD (signal-to-noise ratio 3:1) and LOQ (signal-to-noise ratio 10:1) values were calculated from the calibration equations using formula 3*standard deviation of the response/slope. LOD and LOQ values were found in the range of 0.001 to 0.002 μg/mL and 0.004 to 0.007 μg/mL, respectively. Precision (intra- and inter-day) was estimated in terms of relative standard deviation (RSD%) and achieved < 3% for intra-day and <6% for inter-day when examining a standard mixture of targeted compounds at concentrations of low (0.07 μg/mL), medium (3 μg/mL) and high (15 μg/mL) levels. Recovery values of targeted compounds were assessed at low, medium and high levels in all of the analyzed samples, and obtained from the added and found concentrations of each compound. The recovery values were achieved between 92.33% and 101.43% depending on the types of sample. The excellent quality conditions were obtained and can be proposed for the determination of these compounds in cosmetics.

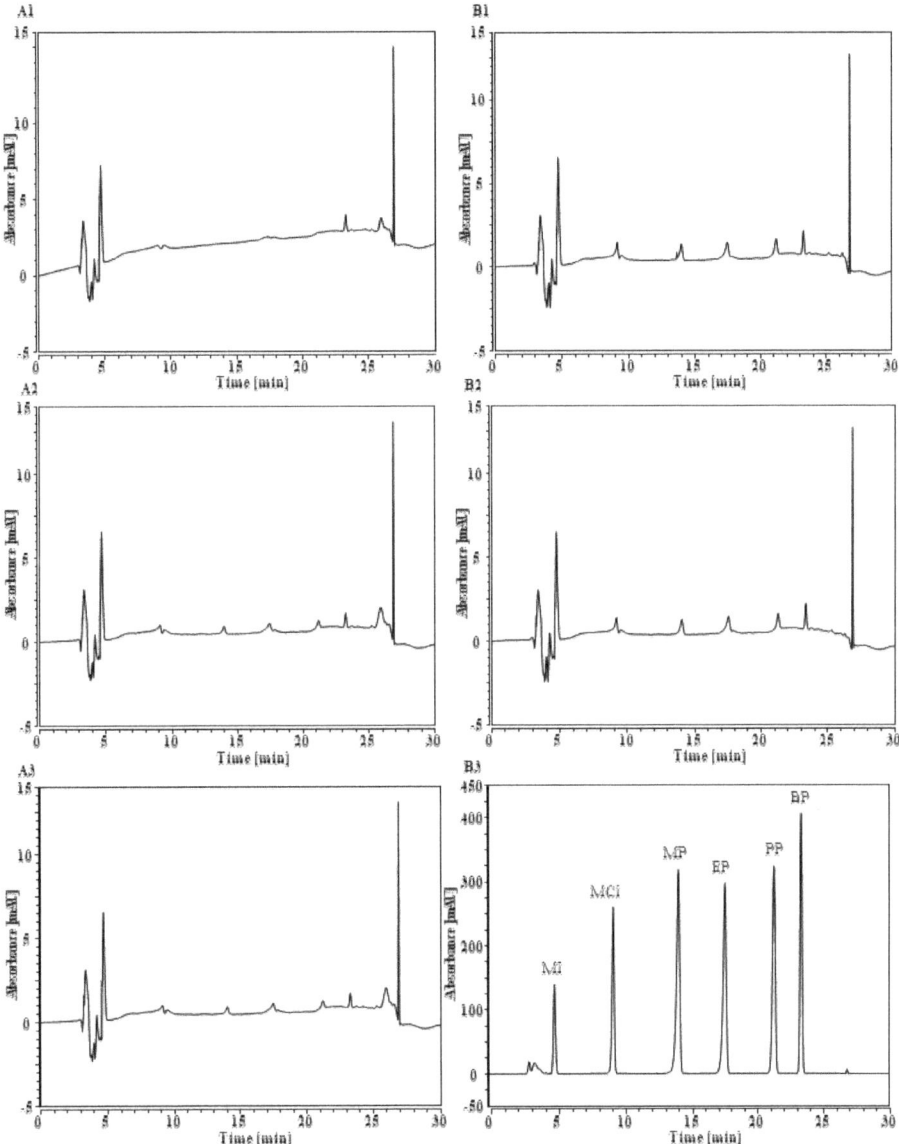

Figure 1. UHPLC/DAD chromatograms of studied compounds: (**A**) Sep-Pak C_{18} and (**B**) HyperSep C_8/BSAIE. (1) Water/methanol 2:1, *v/v*, (2) water/acetonitrile 2:1, *v/v* and (3) acetonitrile/methanol 2:1, *v/v*.

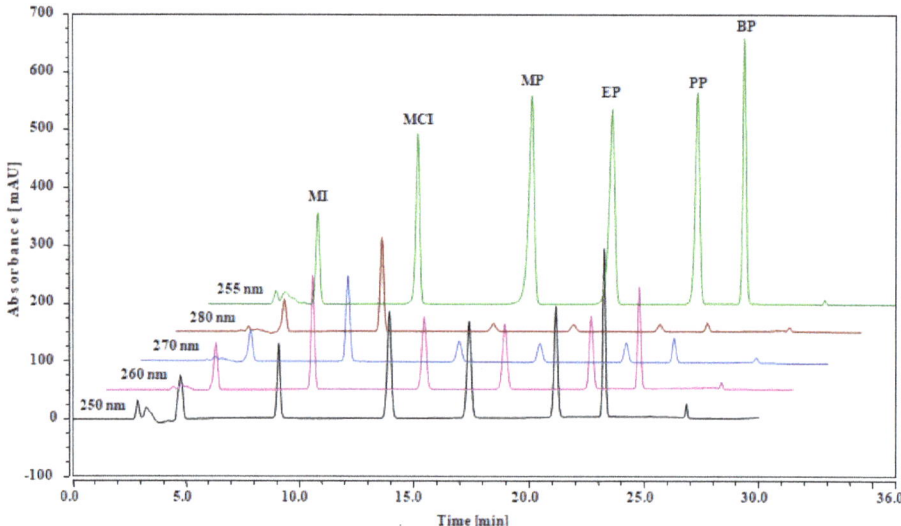

Figure 2. UHPLC/DAD chromatograms of methylisothiazolinone (MI), methylchloroisothiazolinone (MCI), methylparaben (MP), ethylparaben (EP), propylparaben (PP) and butylparaben (BP) obtained at different absorbances, ranging from 250 to 280 nm. The best separation was achieved at absorbance 255 nm.

Table 1. Results of linearity (R^2), limits of detection (LOD) and limits of quantification (LOQ).

Analyte	Linear Range (µg/mL)	R^2	LOD (µg/g) ± SD	LOQ (µg/g) ± SD
MI	0.005–10	0.997	0.002 ± 0.001	0.007 ± 0.002
MCI	0.005–10	0.998	0.002 ± 0.001	0.007 ± 0.002
MP	0.005–10	0.999	0.001 ± 0.001	0.004 ± 0.001
EP	0.005–10	0.998	0.002 ± 0.001	0.007 ± 0.002
PP	0.005–20	0.997	0.001 ± 0.001	0.004 ± 0.001
BP	0.005–20	0.999	0.001 ± 0.001	0.004 ± 0.001

LOD, signal-to-noise (s/n, 3:1); LOQ, signal-to-noise (s/n, 10:1); SD, standard deviation, obtained from three replicates.

Table 2. Accuracy and precision of the proposed (UHPLC/DAD) method.

Analyte	Concentration Added (µg/mL)	Intra-Day			Inter-Day		
		Conc. Found (µg/mL) ± SD	Recovery (%)	RSD (%)	Conc. Found (µg/mL) ± SD	Recovery (%)	RSD (%)
MI	0.07	0.07 ± 0.002	101.14	2.40	0.07 ± 0.004	99.28	5.32
	3	3.01 ± 0.003	100.17	0.11	2.95 ± 0.078	98.37	2.67
	15	14.30 ± 0.035	95.33	0.24	14.30 ± 0.035	95.33	0.24
MCI	0.07	0.07 ± 0.003	98.57	0.67	0.07 ± 0.004	97.14	2.67
	3	2.96 ± 0.003	98.67	0.70	2.95 ± 0.075	98.33	0.78
	15	14.91 ± 0.07	99.40	0.02	14.86 ± 0.02	99.07	0.41
MP	0.07	0.07 ± 0.001	100.14	1.43	0.07 ± 0.003	101.00	4.24
	3	2.99 ± 0.001	99.73	0.34	2.99 ± 0.008	99.53	0.27
	15	14.67 ± 0.003	97.78	0.02	14.66 ± 0.022	97.69	0.15
EP	0.07	0.07 ± 0.001	101.43	1.41	0.07 ± 0.004	98.57	5.80
	3	2.97 ± 0.008	98.90	0.27	2.96 ± 0.001	98.73	0.04
	15	13.9 ± 0.004	92.33	0.03	13.83 ± 0.038	92.20	0.28

Table 2. Cont.

Analyte	Concentration Added (μg/mL)	Intra-Day			Inter-Day		
		Conc. Found (μg/mL) ± SD	Recovery (%)	RSD (%)	Conc. Found (μg/mL) ± SD	Recovery (%)	RSD (%)
PP	0.07	0.07 ± 0.002	100	2.86	0.07 ± 0.003	98.57	4.35
	3	2.97 ± 0.001	99.03	0.04	2.97 ± 0.013	98.90	0.44
	15	14.34 ± 0.001	95.60	0.01	14.32 ± 0.026	95.47	0.18
BP	0.07	0.07 ± 0.001	101.43	1.41	0.07 ± 0.002	100	2.86
	3	3.01 ± 0.003	100.23	0.10	3.01 ± 0.007	100.17	0.23
	15	14.53 ± 0.013	96.87	0.09	14.53 ± 0.007	96.67	0.05

SD, standard deviation; RSD, relative standard deviation.

2.4. Comparison of Proposed Method with the Previous Works

A comparison of the proposed method with the earlier reported analytical methods is presented in Table 3. Earlier methods have individually identified MI and MCI [2] or parabens mixed with other compounds in cosmetics, environmental, biological, pharmaceuticals and personal care samples [11,23,25,33,40], but never the simultaneous identification of the MI, MCI, MP, EP, PP and BP in cosmetics by SPE/UHPLC/DAD. The reason for not identifying these two classes of compounds in a single analysis is the differing polarities, especially when applying a mass spectrometric system. In addition, the reported sample-preparation techniques for the chromatographic determination have only dealt with particular product types. In another approach, Lin et al. (2010) have optimized the UPLC–MS/MS method for the analysis of MI, MCI, 1,2-benzisothiazolinone and 2-octyl-3-isothiazolinone in paper applied for food packaging [41]. The LOD and recovery values were obtained from 0.001 to 0.010 mg/kg and 81.3%, respectively. Fei et al. (2011) studied the MP, EP, PP and BP in cosmetics, by UHPLC/DAD, and obtained LOD (0.12–0.15 mg/mL) and recovery (90.7–97.7%) [26]. Jardim et al. (2015) investigated MP, EP, PP, BP and benzyl paraben in human urine, using UPLC–MS/MS, and found LOD 0.5 ng/mL [42]. These established values [41,42] were also found in good agreement with those archived in the current study. Moreover, on the basis of the achieved outcomes from the current study, the present method could be applied for the determination of MI, MCI, MP, EP, PP and BP in various kinds of matrices. At present, there is no common method available for such kinds of determination, either in sample preparation technique or chromatographic system. The reported SPE/UHPLC/DAD method can simultaneously analyze MI, MCI and parabens (MP, EP, PP and BP) in a single chromatographic method in cosmetic products. The performance of the reported method (linearity, LOD, precision and accuracy) was found to be in good agreement with those reported in earlier works [2,11,23,25,33,40].

2.5. Application

The practical applicability of the SPE/UHPLC/DAD method was established for the simultaneous determination of MI, MCI, MP, EP, PP and BP in cosmetic products of various trademarks and origin. A total of 31 cosmetic samples (face powder, perfumed body (dusting) powder, wet wipe, shampoo, liquid hand-wash soap and shower gel) were studied (Table 4), achieving the amounts of (MI, nd-0.89 μg/g), (MCI, nd-0.62 μg/g), (MP, nd-6.53 μg/g), (EP, nd-0.90 μg/g), (PP, nd-9.69 μg/g) and (BP, nd-17.80 μg/g) (Table 4). As an example, Figure 3 demonstrates the UHPLC/DAD chromatograms identified in the perfumed body (dusting) powder (PP$_3$, Max) sample. Among 31 cosmetic samples, the BP was found in 29 samples, with higher concentrations in shampoo (17.80 μg/g, HS$_1$ Pearl touch), followed by MI (27 samples, shampoo HS$_3$, SoftCare, 0.89 μg/g), MP (14 samples, face powder FP$_7$, Nitrq beauty, 6.53 μg/g), PP (13 samples, perfumed body (dusting) powder PP$_1$ Franck Olivier, 9.69 μg/g), MCI (12 samples, face powder FP$_2$ kokuryu super summer cake, 0.62 μg/g) and EP (11 samples, perfumed body (dusting) powder PP$_3$ Max, 0.90 μg/g). The recovery values ranged from 92.33 to 101.43% depending on the types of sample. The achieved outcomes revealed that the studied cosmetic samples contained these unsafe chemicals in most of the samples even at higher amounts.

Table 3. Comparison of the proposed method with earlier developed methods.

Sample Type	Analyte	Extraction Method	Determination Method	Analysis Time (min)	Linear Range (ng/mL)	R^2	LOD (ng/mL)	Precision (RSD%)	R (%)	Reference
Cosmetics	MI, MCI	Solvent extraction	UHPLC-MS/MS	2.81	0.1-500 (MI), 0.1-1000 (MCI)	0.9997 (MI), 0.9996 (MCI)	43	<7	99-111% (MI), 93-104% (MCI)	[2]
Soil and sediments	MP, EP, PP, BP, IPP, BzP	Ultrasonic-assisted extraction	LC-MS/MS	15	0.6-0.60	0.9993-0.9987	0.04-0.17	<9	83.2-110.2	[40]
Cosmetics, cleaning agents and pharmaceuticals	MI, MCI, BA, SB, MP	Ultrasonic extraction	FLC/UV	27	330-13,330 (MI), 250-10,000 (MCI), 5000-100,000 (BA), 1000-10,000 (SB), 250-10,000 (MP)	0.9996-0.9999	60-4380	0.39-3.45	69-119	[33]
Cosmetics and personal care products	MP, EP, PP, BP, BzP	Fabric-phase sorptive extraction	HPLC/UV	25.27	50-500	0.9955	0.3-0.6	<5	88-122	[23]
Human milk	MP, EP, PP, BP	QuEChERS	HPLC-MS/MS	7.2	0.1-50	0.99	0.04	1-16	83-107	[43]
Food, cosmetics and pharmaceuticals	MP, EP, PP, BP	VA-DLLME-SFO and SA-CPE	CLC/UV	15	100-10,000	0.998	10-30 (VA-DLLME-SFO), 30 (SA-CPE)	<5	-	[11]
Saliva and toothpaste	MP, EP, PP, BP, nBP, iBP	SPE	HPLC/ UV-Vis	15	300-50,000	0.9988-0.9998	100-300	1-6.8	88-113	[25]
Cosmetics	MI, MCI, MP, EP, PP, BP	SPE	UHPLC/DAD	24.7	8-20,000	0.997-0.999	1-2	3-6	92.33-101.43	This work

IPP, isopropyl paraben; BzP, benzyl paraben; BA, benzyl alcohol; SB, sodium benzoate; FLC, fast liquid chromatography; VA-DLLME-SFO, vortex-assisted dispersive liquid–liquid microextraction based on the solidification of a floating organic drop; SA-CPE, salt-assisted cloud point extraction; CLC/UV, capillary liquid chromatography-ultraviolet; -, not described; nBP, n-butyl paraben; iBP, iso-butyl-paraben; R, recovery.

Table 4. Amounts of isothiazolinones and parabens obtained in cosmetic products of different brand and origin.

Sample *	Code	Brand	Origin	Concentration (µg/mL ± SD)					
				MI	MCI	MP	EP	PP	BP
Face powder	FP1	Max beauty compact powder	China	0.16 ± 0.04	0.23 ± 0.05	0.05 ± 0.02	0.16 ± 0.05	0.41 ± 0.06	0.56 ± 0.06
	FP2	Kokuryu super summer cake	China	0.08 ± 0.03	0.62 ± 0.08	0.08 ± 0.02	0.08 ± 0.02	0.33 ± 0.05	nd
	FP3	Diamond beauty snake oil	China	0.05 ± 0.01	nd	0.85 ± 0.09	0.13 ± 0.04	3.86 ± 0.15	0.26 ± 0.06
	FP4	Kiss beauty compact powder	China	0.07 ± 0.02	nd	nd	nd	1.23 ± 0.10	0.75 ± 0.07
	FP5	Bourjois Compact powder	China	0.11 ± 0.03	nd	nd	nd	3.51 ± 0.13	0.92 ± 0.09
	FP6	Naked moisturizing and soothing	China	0.13 ± 0.04	nd	nd	nd	0.15 ± 0.04	1.24 ± 0.10
	FP7	Nitrq beauty	China	Nd	nd	6.53 ± 0.15	0.18 ± 0.05	1.27 ± 0.11	0.76 ± 0.07
	FP8	MaXdona Compact powder	China	0.10 ± 0.03	nd	0.14 ± 0.04	nd	1.76 ± 0.14	0.66 ± 0.06
	FP9	Lilianword Compact powder	China	0.08 ± 0.03	nd	0.57 ± 0.07	0.20 ± 0.05	0.55 ± 0.06	0.45 ± 0.05
Perfumed body (Dusting) powder	PP1	Franck Olivier	France	0.06 ± 0.01	nd	6.34 ± 0.18	nd	9.69 ± 0.23	1.41 ± 0.13
	PP2	Pond's	India	0.08 ± 0.03	nd	2.02 ± 0.12	0.82 ± 0.10	0.64 ± 0.07	3.03 ± 0.20
	PP3	Max	France	0.08 ± 0.02	0.10 ± 0.04	2.16 ± 0.13	0.90 ± 0.10	0.81 ± 0.08	3.73 ± 0.22
Wet wipe	WW1	Ribbon	China	0.13 ± 0.05	0.11 ± 0.04	0.05 ± 0.02	0.08 ± 0.02	nd	0.42 ± 0.03
	WW2	Babyloy	UAE	0.10 ± 0.04	0.21 ± 0.06	nd	nd	nd	0.16 ± 0.02
	WW3	Good baby	Turkey	nd	nd	nd	0.12 ± 0.03	nd	nd
	WW4	Welziadtm	UAE	0.07 ± 0.01	0.31 ± 0.07	0.10 ± 0.03	nd	nd	0.08 ± 0.02
	WW5	Dandi	Turkey	0.26 ± 0.02	nd	0.07 ± 0.01	nd	nd	0.25 ± 0.12
	WW6	Pafilya	Turkey	0.41 ± 0.03	nd	nd	nd	nd	0.16 ± 0.03
	WW7	Omay care	Turkey	0.35 ± 0.03	nd	0.16 ± 0.05	0.07 ± 0.02	nd	0.22 ± 0.04
	WW8	Johnson's	Germany	0.52 ± 0.06	nd	0.54 ± 0.07	0.11 ± 0.03	0.21 ± 0.01	0.11 ± 0.01
	WW9	Deema	KSA	0.06 ± 0.01	nd	nd	nd	nd	0.12 ± 0.01
Shampoo	HS1	Pearl touch	UAE	0.21 ± 0.04	nd	nd	nd	nd	17.80 ± 1.32
	HS2	Perfect cosmetics	UAE	0.27 ± 0.06	nd	nd	nd	nd	13.51 ± 1.20
	HS3	SoftCare	China	0.89 ± 0.07	nd	nd	nd	nd	4.94 ± 0.86
Liquid hand wash soap	LS1	Soph	Turkey	0.22 ± 0.05	0.11 ± 0.02	nd	nd	nd	5.35 ± 0.92
	LS2	Lux	KSA	nd	nd	nd	nd	nd	1.13 ± 0.10
	LS3	Gento	KSA	nd	nd	nd	nd	nd	1.15 ± 0.10
	LS4	Mada	KSA	0.12 ± 0.04	nd	nd	nd	nd	0.62 ± 0.01
Shower gel	SG1	Amalfi	Spain	0.33 ± 0.08	0.31 ± 0.07	nd	nd	nd	0.74 ± 0.06
	SG2	Aqua vera	Turkey	0.27 ± 0.06	0.10 ± 0.02	nd	nd	nd	0.11 ± 0.01
	SG3	Gian	Turkey	0.11 ± 0.03	0.12 ± 0.02	nd	nd	nd	0.61 ± 0.05

* Samples' pH values ranged from 5 to 10; SD, standard deviation, calculated from three replicates.

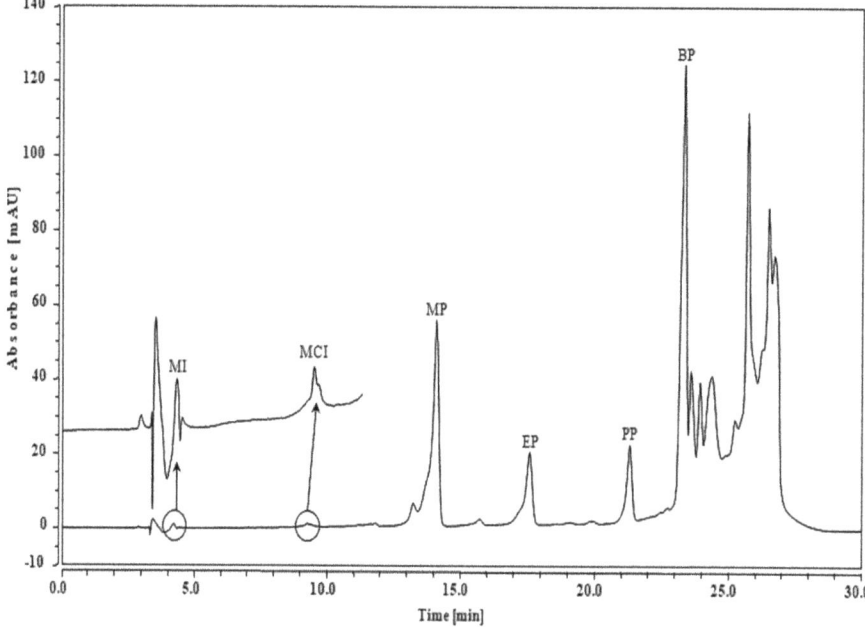

Figure 3. UHPLC/DAD chromatograms identified in perfumed body (dusting) powder (PP$_3$, Max) sample.

3. Materials and Methods

3.1. Chemical and Reagents

HPLC grade acetonitrile and methanol were purchased from Sigma-Aldrich (St. Louis, MO, USA). Trifluoroacetic acid, MI, MCI, MP, EP, PP and BP were obtained from Merck (Darmstadt, Germany). All chemicals were of high purity (>99%). The structures of the studied compounds are demonstrated in Figure 4. Ultrapure water was prepared by using a Barnstead^{TM} Smart2Pure^{TM} water purification system (Thermo Scientific, Göteborg, Sweden). Solid-phase extraction cartridges, HyperSep C$_8$/BSAIE 200 mg/mL and Sep-Pak C$_{18}$ classic cartridge, 360 mg, particle size 55–105 μm, were purchased from Thermo Fisher Scientific (San Jose, CA, USA) and Waters (Milford, MA, USA), respectively. An ARE Heating Magnetic Stirrer was obtained from VELP Scientifica (Usmate Velate (MB), Italy). Ultrasonic baths, model Bandelin Sonorex Digitec, were obtained from Bandelin electronic (Berlin, Germany). Whatman® qualitative filter paper, Grade 1 circles, diameter 90 mm, was purchased from Merck (Darmstadt, Germany). Polytetrafluoroethylene (PTFE) syringe filter (0.45 μm) was purchased from Macherey-Nagel GmbH (Düren, Germany).

The individual stock solution was prepared at a concentration of 200 mg/L, by dissolving an adequate weight in methanol, used for further dilutions. To produce the linearity range and calibration curves, standard mixtures of the studied compounds at concentrations ranging from 0.008 to 20 μg/mL were prepared. Standard solutions and cosmetic samples were filtered by a syringe PTFE filter (0.45 μm) (Macherey-Nagel GmbH, Düren, Germany) before being analyzed by the UHPLC/DAD system.

To assess the SPE efficiency and prevent the matrix influence on peak intensity, retention time and symmetry, the MI, MCI, MP, EP, PP and BP quantification was performed by a standard addition procedure (a quantitative analysis method applied to reduce matrix effects that obstruct with compound measurement signals) consisting of non-fortified (two, zero levels) and fortified (three levels, 50%, 100% and 500%) samples. The levels values demonstrated the increase of compounds in the sample after fortifying. The fortifying of samples was carried out at the start of the extraction method. Cosmetic samples were studied in triplicates (three different extractions of the same sample), and statistical data analysis of the studied samples was performed by means of ANOVA (analysis of variance).

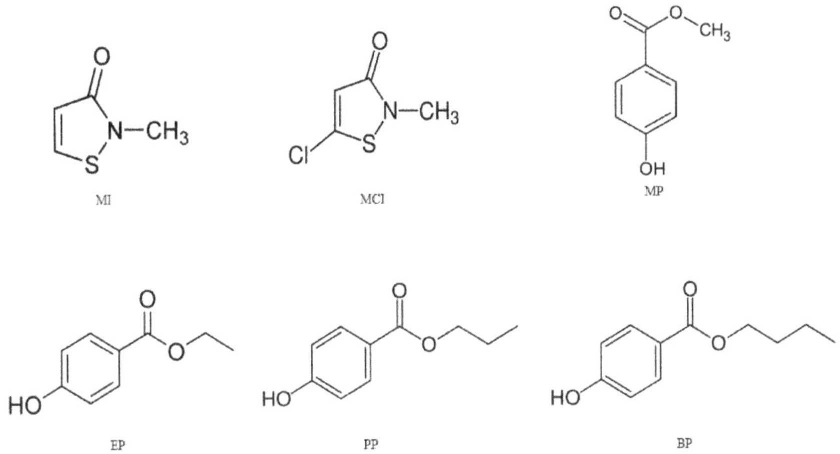

Figure 4. Structures and abbreviation of the studied compounds in cosmetic products.

LOD and LOQ were calculated from the calibration equation, i.e., 3*standard deviation of the response/slope. Recovery of MI, MCI, MP, EP, PP and BP was assessed at low, medium and high levels in all of the analyzed samples, and obtained from the added and found concentrations of each analyte.

3.2. Extraction Method

For the identification and quantification of MI and MCI, and four potential parabens, comprising MP, EP, PP and BP, cosmetics of diverse trademark and country of origin were obtained from cosmetic and pharmacy retail superstore based in Al-Jouf and Riyadh, Saudi Arabia. The sample description was presented in Table 4. Subsequent to purchase, cosmetic samples were immediately stored at 4 °C, and studied at the earliest time, to avoid any chemical loss or contamination. To examine the selective extraction by using SPE method, 0.5 g of cosmetic samples was added to a mixture solution of water and methanol (50:50, *v/v*, 20 mL), followed by mixing (10 min) by using a magnetic stirrer. Afterward, the sample mixture was sonicated (10 min) in ultrasonic baths, followed by filtration through Whatman® qualitative filter paper (grade 1 circles, diameter 90 mm). Then, the sample filtrate was eluted through the SPE cartridge (HyperSep C$_8$/BSAIE), at a controlled flow rate (1 mL/min). Finally, the analyte was eluted with a mixture solution of acetonitrile and methanol (2:1, *v/v*, 10 mL). The sample solution was evaporated, under nitrogen gas, to a final volume of 3 mL. Prior to the analysis by using UHPLC/DAD, the sample extract (3 mL) was filtered through a PTFE syringe filter (0.45 μm). The volume of sample injection was 10 μL. The samples were extracted in triplicates (three different extractions of the same sample). In order to verify the sample contamination and method sensitivity maintained throughout the study, quality control samples were analyzed. Besides this, the sampling steps were carried out with safety measures to reduce sample contamination.

Because of the complexity of cosmetics preparations, a precise pretreatment of the cosmetic samples is typically needed prior to the identification of these compounds by using the UHPLC/DAD technique. The present SPE method using HyperSep C8/BSAIE cartridge was found to be precise and selective for the analysis of MI, MCI, MP, EP, PP and BP in cosmetics. Nevertheless, in earlier studies, the authors have reported various extraction methods based on ultrasound-assisted extraction, solid-phase microextraction, vortex-assisted dispersive liquid–liquid microextraction and liquid–liquid extraction for the analysis of preservatives in different matrices [3,44–46]. These methods were also found to be precise and selective for different types of compounds extracted from different matrices.

3.3. Instrumentation

The sample analysis was performed by using a Dionex UltiMate 3000 UHPLC system (Thermo Scientific, San Jose, CA, USA), comprising a LPG-3400SD binary pump, WPS-3000TSL thermostat autosampler, TCC-3000SD thermostat column compartment and DAD-3000 diode array detector. The data were recorded and analyzed by Chromeleon™ 7.2 Chromatography Data System Software (Thermo Scientific, San Jose, CA, USA).

The chromatographic separation of MI, MCI, MP, EP, PP and BP was achieved through an ACCLAIM™ 120 C_8 analytical column with the dimensions 150 mm × 2.1 mm and 5 µm of particles size (Thermo Scientific, San Jose, USA). The optimal separation was obtained by using binary mobile phase: water (0.1% trifluoroacetic acid, pH 2.1, solvent A) and acetonitrile (solvent B) at a flow rate of 0.5 mL/min. The gradient mobile phase elution was 0–2 min (B, 12.5%), 2–4 min (B 20–30%), 4–16 min (B, 30–50%), 16–22 min (B, 50–100%), return to its equilibrium conditions and 22–30 min. The column temperature was kept at 35 °C, and the sample injection volume was 10 µL. The column was also washed with a mixture (50:50, *v/v*) of methanol and Milli-Q water solution, for five minutes, following the analysis of every ten samples. The optimal detection wavelength was performed in the UV range at 255 nm.

4. Conclusions

A HyperSep C_8/BSAIE SPE and UHPLC/DAD method for the simultaneous identification of MI, MCI, MP, EP, PP and BP in cosmetic products was optimized and validated, using 31 cosmetic samples of various trademarks and origin. These unsafe chemicals are the most common preservatives that manufacturers frequently apply in such products. In addition, excellent method performance parameters, namely linearity (R^2, 0.997–0.999), LOD (0.001–0.002 µg/mL), precision (<6%) and accuracy as percent recovery (92.33–101.43%), were achieved. These outcomes revealed that the developed method offers an alternative method for the quality control of MI, MCI, MP, EP, PP and BP in cosmetic products. The present method can be practically used for an extensive range of cosmetic products, for the identification of MI, MCI, MP, EP, PP and BP. For instance, this procedure will be appropriate to screen the frequency of wrong labeling of such unsafe chemicals (MI, MCI, MP, EP, PP and BP) on cosmetics' ingredients lists. Ingredients labels that are incorrect or omitted can go against clients and health care experts and when seeing for a causative agent to elucidate skin reactions and demanding to evade cosmetics that comprise these potential skin allergens leading to contact dermatitis.

Author Contributions: H.M.A., design and methodology and data curation; I.H.A., investigation, funding and data curation; M.R.K., writing, original draft preparation, methodology, investigation, data curation and validation; M.A., investigation and analysis. All authors have read and agreed to the published version of the manuscript.

Funding: The authors extend their appreciation to the Deputyship for Research & Innovation, "Ministry of Education" in Saudi Arabia for funding this research work through the project number IFKSURG-1437-004.

Conflicts of Interest: The authors declare no conflict of interest.

References

1. Sukakul, T.; Kanchanapenkul, D.; Bunyavaree, M.; Limphoka, P.; Kumpangsin, T.; Boonchai, W. Methylchloroisothiazolinone and/or methylisothiazolinone in cosmetic products—A market survey. *Contact Dermat.* **2019**, *80*, 110–113. [CrossRef] [PubMed]
2. Wittenberg, J.B.; Canas, B.J.; Zhou, W.; Wang, P.G.; Rua, D.; Krynitsky, A.J. Determination of methylisothiazolinone and methylchloroisothiazolinone in cosmetic products by ultra high performance liquid chromatography with tandem mass spectrometry. *J. Sep. Sci.* **2015**, *38*, 2983–2988. [CrossRef] [PubMed]

3. Alvarez-Rivera, G.; Dagnac, T.; Lores, M.; Garcia-Jares, C.; Sanchez-Prado, L.; Lamas, J.P.; Llompart, M. Determination of isothiazolinone preservatives in cosmetics and household products by matrix solid-phase dispersion followed by high-performance liquid chromatography–tandem mass spectrometry. *J. Chromatogr. A* **2012**, *1270*, 41–50. [CrossRef] [PubMed]

4. De Groot, A.C.; Weyland, J.W. Kathon CG: A review. *J. Am. Acad. Dermatol.* **1988**, *18*, 350–358. [CrossRef]

5. Elder, R.L. Final report on the safety assessment of methylisothiazolinone and methylchloroisothiazolinone. *JACT* **1992**, *11*, 75–128.

6. Hannuksela, M. Rapid increase in contact allergy to Kathon®CG in Finland. *Contact Dermat.* **1986**, *15*, 211–214. [CrossRef]

7. Castanedo-Tardana, M.P.; Zug, K.A. Methylisothiazolinone. *Dermatitis* **2013**, *24*, 2–6. [CrossRef]

8. Recommendation on MT. Available online: https//cosmeticseurope.eu/files/3614/7634/5470/Recommendation_on_MIT.pdf (accessed on 21 November 2020).

9. European Society of Contact Dermatitis. Available online: https://www.escd.org/contact-dermatitis/allergic-contact-dermatitis (accessed on 21 November 2020).

10. Błędzka, D.; Gromadzińska, J.; Wąsowicz, W. Parabens. From environmental studies to human health. *Environ. Int.* **2014**, *67*, 27–42. [CrossRef]

11. Chen, C.-W.; Hsu, W.-C.; Lu, Y.-C.; Weng, J.-R.; Feng, C.-H. Determination of parabens using two microextraction methods coupled with capillary liquid chromatography-UV detection. *Food Chem.* **2018**, *241*, 411–418. [CrossRef]

12. Soni, M.G.; Taylor, S.L.; Greenberg, N.A.; Burdock, G.A. Evaluation of the health aspects of methyl paraben: A review of the published literature. *Food Chem. Toxicol.* **2002**, *40*, 1335–1373. [CrossRef]

13. Boberg, J.; Taxvig, C.; Christiansen, S.; Hass, U. Possible endocrine disrupting effects of parabens and their metabolites. *Reprod. Toxicol.* **2010**, *30*, 301–312. [CrossRef] [PubMed]

14. Boberg, J.; Axelstad, M.; Svingen, T.; Mandrup, K.; Christiansen, S.; Vinggaard, A.M.; Hass, U. Multiple endocrine disrupting effects in rats perinatally exposed to butylparaben. *Toxicol. Sci.* **2016**, *152*, 244–256. [CrossRef] [PubMed]

15. Costa, J.R.; Campos, M.S.; Lima, R.F.; Gomes, L.S.; Marques, M.R.; Taboga, S.R.; Biancardi, M.F.; Brito, P.V.A.; Santos, F.C.A. Endocrine-disrupting effects of methylparaben on the adult gerbil prostate. *Environ. Toxicol.* **2017**, *32*, 1801–1812. [CrossRef] [PubMed]

16. Giulivo, M.; de Alda, M.L.; Capri, E.; Barceló, D. Human exposure to endocrine disrupting compounds: Their role in reproductive systems, metabolic syndrome and breast cancer. A review. *Environ. Res.* **2016**, *151*, 251–264. [CrossRef]

17. World Health Organization. *Safety Evaluation of Certain Food Additives and Contaminants*; World Health Organization: Geneva, Switzerland, 2007.

18. European Commission. Commission regulation (EU) No 1004/2014 of 18 September 2014 amending annex V to regulation (EC) No 1223/2009 of the European Parliament and of the Council on cosmetic products. *Off. J. Eur. Union* **2014**, *282*, 5–8.

19. Buzek, J.; Ask, B. Regulation (EC) No 1223/2009 of the European Parliament and of the Council of 30 November 2009 on cosmetic products. *Off. J. Eur. Union* **2009**, *342*, 59–209.

20. Guo, Y.; Kannan, K. A survey of phthalates and parabens in personal care products from the United States and its implications for human exposure. *Environ. Sci. Technol.* **2013**, *47*, 14442–14449. [CrossRef]

21. Abad-Gil, L.; Lucas-Sanchez, S.; Gismera, M.J.; Sevilla, M.T.; Procopio, J.R. Determination of paraben-, isothiazolinone- and alcohol-type preservatives in personal care products by HPLC with dual (diode-array and fluorescence) detection. *Microchem. J.* **2021**, *160*, 105613. [CrossRef]

22. Le Hoa, T.H.; Hung, V.T.N.; do Trang, T.; Thu, T.N.H.; Le, D.C. Development and validation of an HPLC method for simultaneous assay of MCI and MI in shampoos containing plant extracts. *Int. J. Anal. Chem.* **2019**, *2019*, 1851796.

23. Kaur, R.; Kaur, R.; Grover, A.; Rani, S.; Malik, A.K.; Kabir, A.; Furton, K.G. Trace determination of parabens in cosmetics and personal care products using fabric-phase sorptive extraction and high-performance liquid chromatography with UV detection. *J. Sep. Sci.* **2020**, *43*, 2626–2635. [CrossRef]

24. Razavi, N.; Es' haghi, Z. Curcumin loaded magnetic graphene oxide solid-phase extraction for the determination of parabens in toothpaste and mouthwash coupled with high performance liquid chromatography. *Microchem. J.* **2019**, *148*, 616–625. [CrossRef]

25. Zotou, A.; Sakla, I.; Tzanavaras, P.D. LC-determination of five paraben preservatives in saliva and toothpaste samples using UV detection and a short monolithic column. *J. Pharm. Biomed. Anal.* **2010**, *53*, 785–789. [CrossRef] [PubMed]

26. Fei, T.; Li, H.; Ding, M.; Ito, M.; Lin, J.-M. Determination of parabens in cosmetic products by solid-phase microextraction of poly(ethylene glycol) diacrylate thin film on fibers and ultra high-speed liquid chromatography with diode array detector. *J. Sep. Sci.* **2011**, *34*, 1599–1606. [CrossRef] [PubMed]

27. Schettgen, T.; Bertram, J.; Kraus, T. Quantification of N-methylmalonamic acid in urine as metabolite of the biocides methylisothiazolinone and chloromethylisothiazolinone using gas chromatography-tandem mass spectrometry. *J. Chromatogr. B* **2017**, *1044*, 185–193. [CrossRef]

28. Chilbule, A.; Singh, R.; Mann, B.; Arora, S.; Sharma, R.; Rao, P.S. Development and validation of an analytical method for determination of bronopol and kathon preservative in milk. *J. Food Sci. Technol.* **2019**, *56*, 3170–3176. [CrossRef]

29. Chen, Z.-F.; Ying, G.-G.; Lai, H.-J.; Chen, F.; Su, H.-C.; Liu, Y.-S.; Peng, F.-Q.; Zhao, J.-L. Determination of biocides in different environmental matrices by use of ultra-high-performance liquid chromatography—Tandem mass spectrometry. *Anal. Bioanal. Chem.* **2012**, *404*, 3175–3188. [CrossRef]

30. Heo, J.J.; Kim, U.-J.; Oh, J.-E.; Heo, J.J.; Kim, U.-J.; Oh, J.-E. Simultaneous quantitative analysis of four isothiazolinones and 3-iodo-2-propynyl butyl carbamate in hygienic consumer products. *Environ. Eng. Res.* **2018**, *24*, 137–143. [CrossRef]

31. Goodier, M.C.; Siegel, P.D.; Zang, L.-Y.; Warshaw, E.M. Isothiazolinone in residential interior wall paint: A high-performance liquid chromatographic-mass spectrometry analysis. *Dermat. Contact Atopic Occup. Drug* **2018**, *29*, 332–338. [CrossRef]

32. Rosero-Moreano, M.; Canellas, E.; Nerín, C. Three-phase hollow-fiber liquid-phase microextraction combined with HPLC–UV for the determination of isothiazolinone biocides in adhesives used for food packaging materials. *J. Sep. Sci.* **2014**, *37*, 272–280. [CrossRef]

33. Baranowska, I.; Wojciechowska, I.; Solarz, N.; Krutysza, E. Determination of preservatives in cosmetics, cleaning agents and pharmaceuticals using fast liquid chromatography. *J. Chromatogr. Sci.* **2014**, *52*, 88–94. [CrossRef]

34. Zgoła-Grześkowiak, A.; Werner, J.; Jeszka-Skowron, M.; Czarczyńska-Goślińska, B. Determination of parabens in cosmetic products using high performance liquid chromatography with fluorescence detection. *Anal. Methods* **2016**, *8*, 3903–3909. [CrossRef]

35. Bartella, L.; Di Donna, L.; Napoli, A.; Sindona, G.; Mazzotti, F. Paper Spray tandem mass spectrometry: A rapid approach for the assay of parabens in cosmetics and drugs. *J. Mass Spectrom.* **2020**, *55*, e4526. [CrossRef] [PubMed]

36. Zhou, H.-T.; Chen, H.-C.; Ding, W.-H. Accurate analysis of parabens in human urine using isotope-dilution ultrahigh-performance liquid chromatography-high resolution mass spectrometry. *J. Pharm. Biomed. Anal.* **2018**, *150*, 469–473. [CrossRef] [PubMed]

37. Vela-Soria, F.; Iribarne-Durán, L.M.; Mustieles, V.; Jiménez-Díaz, I.; Fernández, M.F.; Olea, N. QuEChERS and ultra-high performance liquid chromatography–tandem mass spectrometry method for the determination of parabens and ultraviolet filters in human milk samples. *J. Chromatogr. A* **2018**, *1546*, 1–9. [CrossRef] [PubMed]

38. Che, D.; Sun, Z.; Cheng, J.; Dou, K.; Ji, Z.; Chen, G.; Li, G.; You, J. Determination of parabens in domestic sewage by isotope-coded derivatization coupled with high performance liquid chromatography-tandem mass spectrometry. *Microchem. J.* **2017**, *130*, 420–427. [CrossRef]

39. Hefnawy, M.; Al-Majed, A.; Mohammed, M.; Al-Ghusn, A.; Al-Musallam, A.; Al-Sowidan, N.; Al-Hamid, M.; Al-Homoud, A. Fast and sensitive liquid chromatography method for simultaneous determination of methylisothiazolinone, salicylic acid and parabens in cosmetic products. *Curr. Anal. Chem.* **2017**, *13*, 430–438. [CrossRef]

40. Núñez, L.; Tadeo, J.L.; García-Valcárcel, A.I.; Turiel, E. Determination of parabens in environmental solid samples by ultrasonic-assisted extraction and liquid chromatography with triple quadrupole mass spectrometry. *J. Chromatogr. A* **2008**, *1214*, 178–182. [CrossRef]

41. Lin, Q.-B.; Wang, T.-J.; Song, H.; Li, B. Analysis of isothiazolinone biocides in paper for food packaging by ultra-high-performance liquid chromatography—Tandem mass spectrometry. *Food Addit. Contam. Part A* **2010**, *27*, 1775–1781. [CrossRef]

42. Jardim, V.C.; Melo, L.d.P.; Domingues, D.S.; Queiroz, M.E.C. Determination of parabens in urine samples by microextraction usingpacked sorbent and ultra-performance liquid chromatography coupled to tandem mass spectrometry. *J. Chromatogr. B* **2015**, *974*, 35–41. [CrossRef]

43. Dualde, P.; Pardo, O.; Fernández, S.F.; Pastor, A.; Yusà, V. Determination of four parabens and bisphenols A, F and S in human breast milk using QuEChERS and liquid chromatography coupled to mass spectrometry. *J. Chromatogr. B* **2019**, *1114*, 154–166. [CrossRef]

44. Ocana-Gonzalez, J.A.; Villar-Navarro, M.; Ramos-Payan, M.; Fernandez-Torres, R.; Bello-Lopez, M.A. New developments in the extraction and determination of parabens in cosmetics and environmental samples. A review. *Anal. Chim. Acta* **2015**, *858*, 1–15. [CrossRef] [PubMed]

45. Shaaban, H.; Mostafa, A.; Alhajri, W.; Almubarak, L.; AlKhalifah, K. Development and validation of an eco-friendly SPE-HPLC-MS method for simultaneous determination of selected parabens and bisphenol A in personal care products: Evaluation of the greenness profile of the developed method. *J. Liq. Chromatogr. Rel. Technol.* **2018**, *41*, 621–628. [CrossRef]

46. Bocato, M.Z.; Cesila, C.A.; Lataro, B.F.; de Oliveira, A.R.M.; Campiglia, A.D.; Barbosa, F., Jr. A fast-multiclass method for the determination of 21 endocrine disruptors in human urine by using vortex-assisted dispersive liquid-liquid microextraction (VADLLME) and LC-MS/MS. *Environ. Res.* **2020**, *189*, 109883. [CrossRef] [PubMed]

Publisher's Note: MDPI stays neutral with regard to jurisdictional claims in published maps and institutional affiliations.

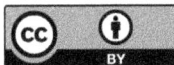

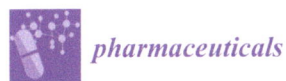

Article

Availability of Guanitoxin in Water Samples Containing *Sphaerospermopsis torques-reginae* Cells Submitted to Dissolution Tests

Kelly Afonsina Fernandes [1], Humberto Gomes Ferraz [2,*], Fanny Vereau [2] and Ernani Pinto [1,3,*]

[1] Department of Clinical and Toxicological Analyses, Faculty of Pharmaceutical Sciences, University of São Paulo, Av. Prof. Lineu Prestes, 580, Butantã CEP 05508-900, São Paulo, Brazil; kelly.af@usp.br

[2] Department of Pharmacy, Faculty of Pharmaceutical Sciences, University of São Paulo, Av. Prof. Lineu Prestes, 580, Butantã CEP 05508-900, São Paulo, Brazil; fyvereau@usp.br

[3] Centre of Nuclear Energy in Agriculture, University of São Paulo, Av. Centenário, 303, Piracicaba CEP 13416-000, Brazil

* Correspondence: sferraz@usp.br (H.G.F.); ernani@usp.br (E.P.)

Received: 8 October 2020; Accepted: 4 November 2020; Published: 19 November 2020

Abstract: Guanitoxin (GNT) is a potent neurotoxin produced by freshwater cyanobacteria that can cause the deaths of wild and domestic animals. Through reports of animal intoxication by cyanobacteria cells that produce GNT, this study aimed to investigate the bio-accessibility of GNT in simulated solutions of the gastrointestinal content in order to understand the process of toxicosis promoted by GNT in vivo. Dissolution tests were conducted with a mixture of *Sphaerospermopsis torques-reginae* (Cyanobacteria; Nostocales) cultures (30%) and gastrointestinal solutions with and without proteolytic enzymes (70%) at a temperature of 37 °C and rotation at 100 rpm for 2 h. The identification of GNT was performed by LC-QqQ-MS/MS through the transitions $[M + H]^+$ m/z 253 > 58 and $[M + H]^+$ m/z 253 > 159, which showed high concentrations of GNT in simulated gastric fluid solutions (p-value < 0.001) in comparison to simulated solutions of intestinal content. The gastric solution with pepsin promoted the stability of GNT (p-value < 0.05) compared to the simulated solution of gastric fluid at the same pH without the enzyme. However, the results showed that GNT is also available in intestinal fluids for a period of 2 h, and solutions containing the pancreatin enzyme influenced the bio-accessibility of the toxin more compared to the intestinal medium without enzyme (p-value < 0.05). Therefore, the bio-accessibility of the toxin must be considered both in the stomach and in the intestine, and may help in the diagnosis and prediction of exposure and risk in vivo through the oral ingestion of GNT-producing cyanobacteria cells.

Keywords: anatoxin-a(s); neurotoxins; cyanobacteria poisoning; bio-accessibility

1. Introduction

Guanitoxin (GNT) [1] (formerly Anatoxin-a(s)) is a potent natural neurotoxin produced by freshwater cyanobacteria [2,3]. Its mode of action is the same as synthetic organophosphates, in which the phosphate ester functional group binds to the active serine site of acetylcholinesterase (AChE), ultimately causing AChE block [3–5]. The result of the irreversible inactivation of AChE is the accumulation of acetylcholine in the synaptic clefts, thus causing cholinergic hyperstimulation that, in most cases, is lethal for organisms [6–8].

In the past, GNT has been associated with the death of domestic and wild animals that accidentally consumed water containing cyanobacterial cells [5,6,8,9]. The clinical signs observed in these animals consisted mainly of excessive salivation, muscle tremors, convulsions, fasciculation convulsions, and respiratory failure. The lethal dose (LD_{50}) of GNT was determined in mice to comprise a range from 20 µg/kg to 40 µg/kg, with a survival time of 10 to 30 min, and it is considered ten times more toxic than other cyanotoxins of the same class [3,5,10]. Other LD_{50} and inhibitory concentration (IC_{50}) values were observed in fish, Cladocera, and insects, showing symptoms of intoxication common to those observed in mammals [11–15].

There are no known variants of GNT; it is known that species of the genus *Dolichospermum* and *Sphaerospermopsis* are the main producers of this cyanotoxin [1,16]. AChE has been used as a biomarker to assess the presence of the toxin in aqueous samples [17,18]. However, enzymatic methods can generate false-positive results and can be influenced by the presence of synthetic organophosphates that are available in the environment. For this reason, analytical methodologies by LC-MS are more indicated due to the high specificity and sensitivity that they provide for the correct identification of GNT [19].

Although the presence of this toxin is less common than other cyanotoxins such as microcystins, extremely high levels of GNT have already been detected in water samples [9,20]. Furthermore, there are recent reports of the occurrence of this toxin through cases of accidental poisoning in dogs, who after drinking water with cyanobacterial cells, showed clinical signs of acute intoxication characteristic of GNT [6,21,22]. However, the monitoring of GNT in bodies of water for human use is not yet mandatory, and there are no limits for the detection of GNT established by the World Health Organization (WHO). The lack of consistent toxicological data and an analytical standard for quantifying GNT are the main factors that limit the mandatory monitoring of GNT in water bodies [18,23,24].

Environmental factors also imply a lack of data on the occurrence of GNT in water bodies, such as the instability of the toxin at high temperatures and slightly alkaline pH [7,25]. However, there are contradictory results regarding the time of degradation of the molecule, and it is not known whether GNT has resistance to other chemical substances. On the other hand, the occurrence of GNT has been reported in eutrophic environments with a slightly alkaline pH [26,27], which is associated with the predominance of species producing GNT. There is no precise information on the toxin's half-life in the environment. However, even if it prevails in the environment for a short time, it can be sufficiently lethal depending on the available concentrations; it can cause severe impacts on aquatic and terrestrial biota.

Therefore, our work aimed to investigate the availability of GNT in simulated solutions of gastric and intestinal contents with and without digestive enzymes through in vitro tests, following guidelines established by the United States Pharmacopeia [28,29]. From the dissolution tests, we expect to provide information on the bio-accessibility of GNT in the gastrointestinal system in vivo, especially for wild and domestic animals that are generally the most affected by the toxic cyanobacteria available in eutrophic environments.

2. Results

The results presented in this study came from cultures of *Sphaerospermopsis torques-reginae* (ITEP-24), with a cell concentration of 3.29×10^6. From dissolution tests, we obtained the profile of the accessibility of GNT in artificial solutions gastrointestinal content. The bio-accessibility of the toxin was measured by high-performance liquid chromatography-tandem triple-quadrupole mass spectrometry (HPLC-QqQ-MS/MS) with multiple reaction monitoring (MRM) using the transitions [M + H] + *m/z* 253 > 58 and *m/z* 253 > 159 (Scheme 1). Figure 1 refers to the total ion chromatogram and MRM for the GNT molecule, showing that the relative area of the GNT peak is greater in samples with acidic pH.

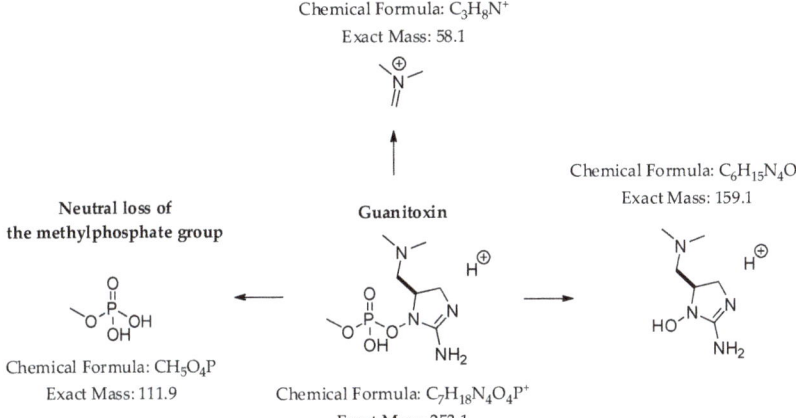

Chemical Formula: $C_3H_8N^+$
Exact Mass: 58.1

Chemical Formula: $C_6H_{15}N_4O^+$
Exact Mass: 159.1

**Neutral loss of
the methylphosphate group**

Guanitoxin

Chemical Formula: CH_5O_4P
Exact Mass: 111.9

Chemical Formula: $C_7H_{18}N_4O_4P^+$
Exact Mass: 253.1

Scheme 1. Guanitoxin fragmentation by LC-MS and product ions generated from electrospray ionization source (ESI) in positive mode, adapted from Dörr et al. (2010) [19], showing the formation of ion $[M + H]^+$ *m/z* 159 and ion $[M + H]^+$ *m/z* 58 after neutral loss of methylphosphate residue. Data presented in this study were acquired from the protonated GNT molecule and following the transitions $[M + H]^+$ *m/z* 253 > 159 and $[M + H]^+$ *m/z* 253 > 58.

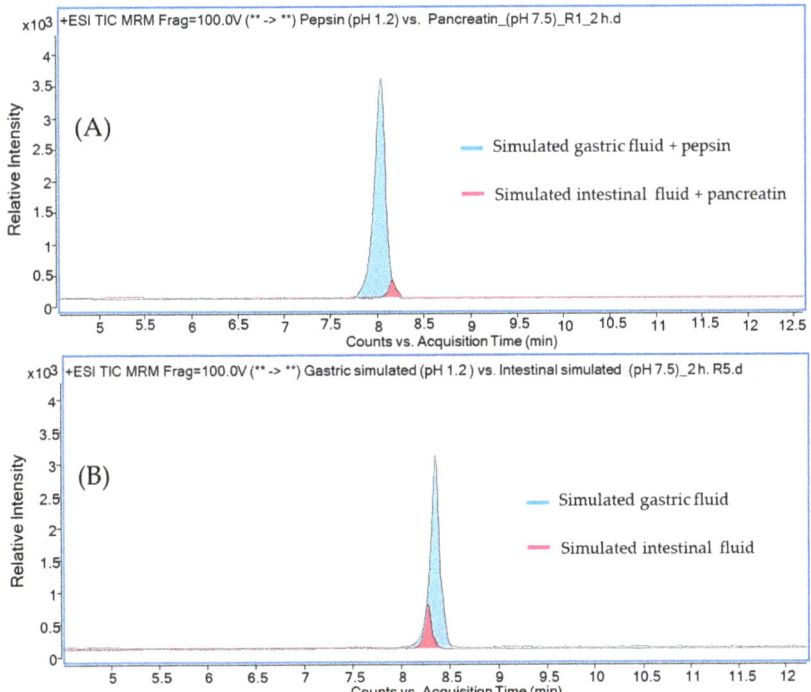

Figure 1. Total ion chromatogram (TIC) and monitoring of multiple reactions (MRM) using the transitions $[M + H]^+$ *m/z* 253 > 58 and $[M + H]^+$ *m/z* 253 > 159. Chromatograms show the peak area for the GNT content released by the cells of the *S. torques-reginae* (ITEP-24) in 2 h of experiment, showing higher values in tests using simulated gastric solutions with (**A**) and without the pepsin enzyme (**B**) compared to solutions of simulated intestinal contents with (**A**) and without the pancreatin enzyme (**B**).

The results also showed that the GNT contents were statistically higher (*p*-value < 0.001) in treatments with simulated stomach contents (with and without enzyme) compared to treatments with solutions of simulated intestinal content with enzyme and without pancreatin. Then, we compared the contents of GNT between solutions with the same pH. The graphs shown in Figure 2 show the contents (%) of GNT while the data presented in Tables S1 and S2 in the Supplementary Materials represent the raw data obtained by LC-MS.

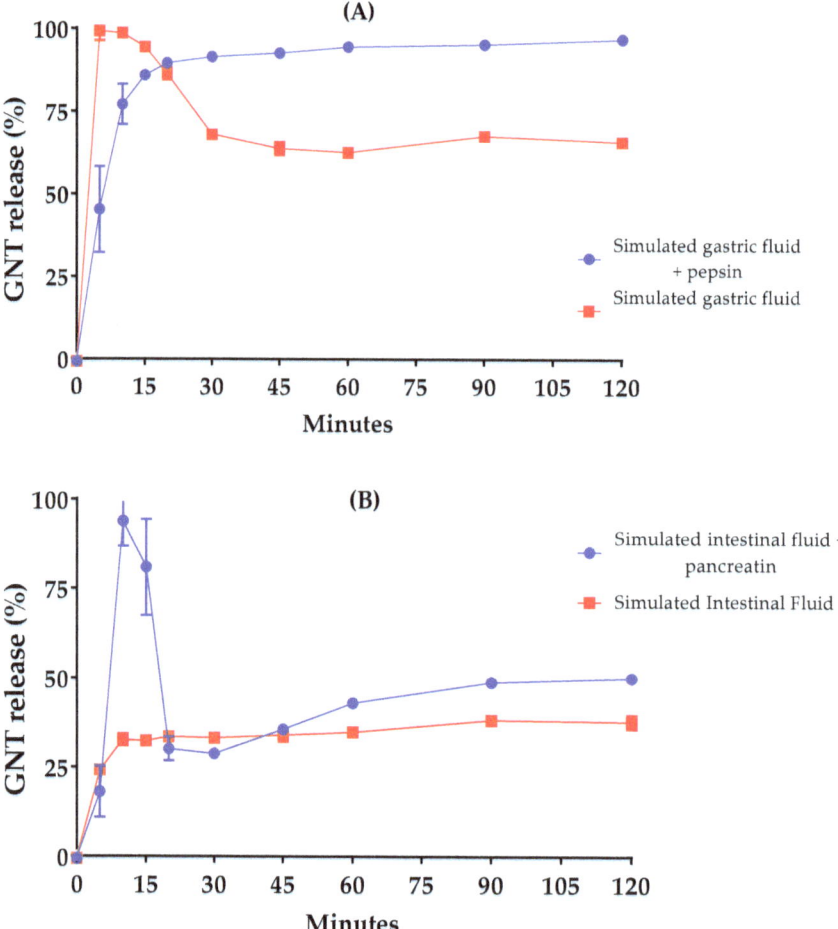

Figure 2. Dissolution profiles of *S. torques-reginae* cells (ITEP-24) producing GNT. The dissolution test was conducted for 2 h at 37 °C with rotation at 100 rpm. The graphs show the relative value of the concentration of guanitoxin released by the cells during the tests. Values for each assay are represented as the mean ± standard deviation (SD) (*n* = 3). The concentrations of GNT were higher in the tests with a simulated solution of the stomach contents (**A**) compared with simulated solutions of the intestinal content (**B**).

Treatment with the enzyme pepsin (pH 1.2) showed that the concentration of GNT increased significantly from zero to 10 min (*p*-value < 0.0001) and then continued to increase slowly, with a tendency to stabilize the concentration of the toxin until the end of the experiment. In addition, the Tukey test showed that the concentration of GNT at 10 min was statistically different from all times, except 5 and 15 min. From 0 to 15 min was the period of greatest activity of the pepsin enzyme acting on cell breakdown of the ITEP-24 strain, and consequently, availability of GNT in the extracellular medium (Figure 2A).

We compared the results obtained from the simulated fluid dissolution test of the gastric contents with the pepsin enzyme (pH 1.2) and without (pH 1.2); the statistical analysis shows that the GNT concentration at 20 min were statistically equal in the two treatments (Figure 2A). However, while the concentration of GNT begins to increase initially (0–15 min) (p-value < 0.0001) in the treatment with the enzyme, the opposite occured in treatments with gastric solution without the enzyme (p-value < 0.0001) (Figure 2A).

Figure 2B shows the results obtained in the treatments with the simulated solution of the intestinal content with and without the pancreatin enzyme. In the dissolution test performed with the simulated solution of intestinal fluid with the pancreatin enzyme, the concentration of GNT initially increased significantly between 10 to 15 min, and was statistically higher compared to all other periods (p-value < 0.0001). After 15 min, the concentration drastically decreased to 20 min, maintaining stability for up to 30 min, and from 30 min to 60 min, there was a slight increase in the concentration of the toxin, which then tended to stabilize until the end of the experiment. In treatments without the pancreatin enzyme, the toxin content released was greater 0–10 min (p-value < 0.05) and from 15 min to 120 min there was no statistical difference.

The intestinal solution treatments with the pancreatin enzyme (pH 7.5) were compared with the results obtained in the test with the simulated solution of the intestinal content without the enzyme. The statistical tests showed significant differences in the times of 10–15 min (p-value < 0.0001) and 90–120 min (p-value < 0.05). For all other times, there was no statistical difference (Figure 2B).

At the end of the experiments, measurements of the pH value were performed in all dissolution test solutions with no significant changes in the acidic (1.20 to 1.33) and alkaline (7.50 to 7.56) solutions. Microscopic analyses of the samples resulting from the dissolution tests were also performed to assess the rupture of the cell wall of the ITEP-24 strain. Microscopic analysis revealed a small number of isolated cells that appeared intact, and quite a few fragmented cells.

3. Discussion

The dissolution test was developed to study the time required for the drug to solubilize in humans and animals [29]. The dissolution method is also used to evaluate and guarantee the quality of the drugs made available for use, in which it is established that at least 80% of solid formulations are dissolved in a short period [30,31]. In general, this method aims to predict whether solid formulations will be dissolved in a simulated aqueous medium of the stomach and intestine, leaving the active ingredient available to be absorbed into the bloodstream to exert its effect on the individual [32]. In vitro dissolution tests are usually used before in vivo tests [33]; therefore, this method can be explored to assess the bio-accessibility of several active compounds of cyanobacteria of pharmaceutical and food interest [34–36].

In this sense, this study aimed to investigate the amount of intracellular GNT released in simulated media from the gastrointestinal tract when subjected to controlled experimental conditions. Based on the principles of the dissolution method, the solubility of GNT in acidic (pH 1.2) and basic (pH 7.5) media was evaluated in order to understand the bio-accessibility of GNT in the gastrointestinal tract in vivo due to cases of intoxication of animals by this cyanotoxin, as reported in the literature. The results presented here showed the relevant content and greater stability of GNT in simulated solutions of gastrointestinal content with and without enzyme action. On the other hand, the release of the toxin was more significant in solutions of stomach contents, and even greater in solutions with the presence of the enzyme pepsin.

In the simulated gastric fluid dissolution test without enzymes, although the concentration of GNT was also relevant, there was a drop in concentration after 10 min; this can be justified by the instability of the toxin in acidic solutions with pH values below 3.0. Studies carried out to evaluate the

GNT molecule's stability at different pH and temperatures showed that the toxin is stable at pH 3.0 and can be slightly degraded at acidic pH (pH 1.5 and 5.0) (unpublished results).

Dissolution tests with proteolytic enzymes are normally used for formulations coated with some gelatinous membrane that does not dissolve in an aqueous medium due to crosslinking which can interfere with the dissolution of the drug [37]. In the case of our study, GNT was protected by cyanobacterial cells. Cyanobacteria have a cell wall made up of peptidoglycan, proteins, and lipopolysaccharides, which have protective and compliance functions [38,39]. In addition, the cell wall forms a boundary between cell constituents; therefore, some stimulation is needed to break the cell wall to release intracellular components of interest [40].

According to the dissolution method's conditions, the use of the enzymes pepsin and pancreatin, together with the constant rotation promoted by the rotating blades at 100 rpm, could act in the cell lysis of cyanobacteria. In studies of extraction of secondary cyanobacteria metabolites, organic solvents and suitable equipment are usually used, such as ultrasound probes or thermal shock of cells by freezing and thawing; these methods assist in cell breakdown, promoting the release of intracellular metabolites [40].

The results of this study showed that the concentration of GNT in the dissolution test with the pepsin enzyme had an exponential growth character from 5 to 20 min; the opposite occurred in the dissolution test with simulated gastric fluid (Figure 2A). Pepsin probably acted in the breakdown of proteins present in the cyanobacterium cell wall, thus enabling the continuous release of GNT in the extracellular medium. Pepsin acts on protein metabolism by transforming them into simpler peptides; it catalyzes the hydrolysis of peptide bonds adjacent to amino acids with side chains, aromatic amino acids (phenylalanine, tryptophan and tyrosine), branched chain amino acids, and methionine [41]. Pepsin may also have had a greater role in degrading other metabolites present in the ITEP-24 strain, thus making GNT more available. However, these hypotheses require more specific studies to answer questions regarding the interaction of GNT with other molecules, especially digestive molecules.

In dissolution tests with simulated solutions of stomach fluid, usually lasting 1 h, the time was extended to 2 h to compare the tests performed with simulated solutions of intestinal content. The data show that higher GNT concentrations were more available in simulated stomach fluid solutions than simulated intestinal fluid solutions. However, although the concentration of GNT was lower in dissolution tests with simulated fluids from the intestine, the results showed that GNT was not fully degraded in the 2 h period. The fact is that some studies talk about the degradation of the toxin in alkaline solutions, but this is not entirely correct. Therefore, based on this study, we can understand that most of the toxin is available in the stomach, and can also reach the intestinal tract.

In the dissolution test performed with the pancreatin enzyme, there was an increase in the concentration of GNT from 5 to 15 min, which was statistically significant (p-value < 0.0001) compared to the results of the intestinal solution (Figure 2B). The pancreatin used in the dissolution assay comprises of a mixture of several enzymes including trypsin, amylase, lipase, ribonuclease, and protease. Pancreatic enzymes such as trypsin act mainly in the hydrolysis of lysine and arginine esters [42]. Thus, this set of pancreatic enzymes may have acted in the breakdown in the cell wall of the ITEP-24 strain, allowing the release of GNT into the extracellular environment; however, GNT is not very stable in a basic environment, so high concentrations of GNT may have been released and then hydrolyzed.

Therefore, as demonstrated in this study, the low concentration of the toxin at pH 7.5 may be associated with the low instability of the GNT at pH > 7.0. However, although its concentration was lower in tests with artificial solutions of the intestinal system, concentrations of the toxin remained in the solutions for a period of up to 2 h. The remains of cells that were still intact after 2 h indicated that gastrointestinal content solutions with and without enzymes managed to release only a part of the intracellular toxin. Depending on the morphology and metabolism of the digestive system in vivo, the presence of intact cells after 2 h can result in the continuous release of GNT in the body and cause prolonged toxic effects, even at a low concentration.

Cyanobacteria produce a variety of secondary metabolites that are toxic to many organisms [43–46], including man [47]. Most GNT-producing cyanobacteria have been identified in freshwater environments accompanied by animal poisoning. Birds and domestic mammals were the groups most affected after water consumption containing cyanobacterial cells that produce GNT [6,9,22]. The data available in the literature also show that the effect of this cyanotoxin toxicity is very rapid, affecting the nervous system to cause seizures and muscle paralysis, followed by sudden death [6,8,9,22].

In addition, laboratory tests carried out on mice and rats using intraperitoneal injections containing GNT showed that the toxic effects are more pronounced between 7 to 30 min and can cause rapid death in up to 60 min [5–7,9]. The results presented here showed higher concentrations of GNT in the dissolution tests carried out with the enzymes pepsin and pancreatin in the initial phase of the experiments (10 and 20 min), corroborating tests in vivo where the toxic signs were more severe in the same period.

Tests carried out on other animals treated with crude extracts of cyanobacteria producing GNT showed that the toxic effect of GNT can vary according to the method of exposure and the dose administered [8,11,48,49]. However, both tests with the pure toxin and tests that used cells containing the toxin showed similar clinical effects, and in many cases was followed by death of the organisms.

Despite several studies showing the negative effect of GNT on aquatic and terrestrial biota [6,8,50], the monitoring of this potent neurotoxin is not yet routinely performed in bodies of water by regulatory agencies and there is no standardization of limits for the concentration of GNT. However, there is a particular concern with aquatic organisms, which may share the same habitat with toxin-producing cyanobacterial species. In addition, cattle, domestic animals such as dogs as well as water birds can be exposure to contaminated water during bloom events. We believe that our findings can contribute substantially with information about GNT released from cyanobacterial cells after ingestion of contaminated water mainly by mammals. This in vitro released pattern can be useful for comparison in real cases of GNT poisoning and treatment of animals.

4. Materials and Methods

4.1. Reagents

The reagents employed to prepare the Artificial Seawater Medium (ASM-1) used to grow the cultures of the ITEP-24 strain were of analytical grade (Vetec, Rio de Janeiro, Brazil); the Lugol used to fix the culture of the ITEP-24 strain was purchased from Sigma-Aldrich (Sigma-Aldrich, Darmstadt, Germany). Reagents employed to prepare mobile phases used in LC-MS analyses were MS grade Acetonitrile, formic acid, and ammonium formate were all purchased from Sigma-Aldrich (Sigma-Aldrich, Darmstadt, Germany). The reagents used to prepare simulated solutions of gastric and intestinal fluids were sodium hydroxide, sodium chloride, hydrochloric acid (purity over 99%) (Sigma-Aldrich, Darmstadt, Germany), monobasic potassium phosphate, monobasic sodium phosphate, and phosphoric acid (Vetec, Rio de Janeiro, Brazil).

The enzymes used in the dissolution tests were pepsin from lyophilized powder from porcine gastric mucosa (Sigma P7000, ≥250 units/mg) and pancreatin from pig stomach and pancreatin from porcine pancreas (Sigma P-1500 4X United States Pharmacopoeia (USP) specifications) containing enzymatic components including trypsin, amylase, lipase, ribonuclease and protease, produced by the exocrine cells of the swine pancreas (Sigma-Aldrich, Darmstadt, Germany). Buffer solutions had pH values of 7.00, 4.00 and 9.00 (Millipore, Milford, MA, USA). Ultrapure water used to prepare all solutions was obtained from a Direct-Q8 water purification system (Millipore, Milford, MA, USA).

4.2. Cultivation of the Sphaerospermopsis torques-reginae (ITEP-24) Strain Producing Guanitoxin

The dissolution tests were performed with cells of the species *S. torques-reginae* (Komárek) [16], obtained from the Technological Institute of Pernambuco (ITEP). The strain ITEP-24, classified as a GNT producer [19], was isolated from water samples collected in the Tapacurá/PE/Brazil reservoir [26].

Currently, this strain is also part of the collection of cyanobacteria of the Laboratory of Toxins and Natural Products of Algae and Cyanobacteria of the Faculty of Pharmaceutical Sciences of the University of São Paulo/Brazil (FCF/USP).

The ITEP-24 strain was grown in ASM-1 medium [51] at pH 7.5–8.0 with continuous aeration for a period of approximately 20 days. During this period, the cultures were maintained at a temperature of 22.0 ± 1.0 °C and a 12:12 photoperiod (Nova Técnica, São Paulo, Brazil) under a light intensity of 40 µmol of photons m^{-2} s^{-1} measured by a quantum sensor (QSL-100, Biospherical Instruments Inc., San Diego, CA, USA).

After reaching exponential growth, the cultures were centrifuged at $15,000 \times g$ at 4 °C for 10 min, (Eppendorf 5804R centrifuge, Eppendorf AG, Hamburg, Germany). Before the dissolution experiments, 5 mL of the ITEP-24 strain culture was collected and fixed with Lugol. The samples fixed in Lugol were then inserted into a Neubauer Chamber (hemocytometer) for cell counting using a Zeiss Axiovert 135M optical microscope (Carl Zeiss, Göttingen, Germany). Cell counting was performed based on the number of cells per strand and cell density was performed according to Blakefield and Harris (1994) [52].

4.3. Preparation of Simulated Gastrointestinal Fluid Solutions with and without Digestive Enzymes

Dissolution tests were designed to understand how GNT would react after being released from *S. torques-reginae* cells (ITEP-24) in simulated solutions of gastric and enteric fluid with and without the presence of enzymes that help in the processes of metabolism of the stomach and intestine. The solutions used in the dissolution tests were prepared according to the United States Pharmacopoeia standards [28].

The simulated gastric fluid was prepared with 2.0 g of sodium chloride dissolved in ultrapure water, and 6.0 mL of hydrochloric acid was then added with ultrapure water to a volume of 1000 mL. The pH was adjusted with 1 M sodium hydroxide or 1 M hydrochloric acid until a pH of 1.2 was achieved. For the medium with the enzyme pepsin, the same solution was prepared (simulated gastric fluid), and 3.2 g of pepsin was added for a total volume of 1000 mL.

The intestinal solution was prepared with 6.81 g of monobasic potassium phosphate and 1.70 g of sodium hydroxide dissolved with ultrapure water to the volume of 1000 mL. The pH was adjusted with 1 M sodium hydroxide or 1 M phosphoric acid until a pH of 7.5 was achieved. The same medium (simulated intestinal fluid) was subsequently used to prepare the solution with the pancreatin enzyme, using 2.5 g of pancreatin for a total volume of 1000 mL of the simulated solution of the intestinal contents. The pH values were measured with a digital pH meter combined with a glass electrode (827 pH Lab/6.0224.100, Metrohm, Herisau, Switzerland). The pH meter was calibrated by standard buffer solutions with pH 7.00, 4.00 and 9.00.

4.4. Dissolution Test with the ITEP-24 Strain

The tests were carried out in a 708-DS dissolution apparatus (Agilent Technologies, Santa Clara, USA) equipped with 6 glass cylinders with a capacity of 1000 mL, using the rowing method at 100 rpm at a temperature of 37 ± 1 °C [53]. The experiments were carried out in two stages. First, experiments were performed with simulated stomach fluid solutions with and without the pepsin enzyme simultaneously, using three cylinders for each type of solution, i.e., each test was performed in triplicate. Each cylinder was composed of 700 mL of simulated gastric medium and 300 mL of culture containing cells of the ITEP-24 strain. For the simulated gastric solution with the enzyme pepsin, 2.24 g of the enzyme (560,000 U) was used; each mg of pepsin was equivalent to 250 U.

In the second stage, immediately after the tests with gastric solutions at pH 1.2, the experiments were carried out with simulated solutions of the enteric liquid with and without the pancreatic enzyme. The experimental conditions were the same mentioned in the previous experiment, i.e., the assays with simulated enteric solutions were performed together, representing three cylinders for each assay, each cylinder containing 700 mL of simulated enteric medium plus 300 mL of culture, representing a final volume of 1000 mL of medium. In the case of the pancreatin enzyme assay, a volume of 700 mL of intestinal solution with 1.75 g of the enzyme was used for each cylinder (>175,000 U of amylase activity, >14,000 U of lipase activity, and >175,000 U of protease activity). Each mg of pancreatin was equivalent to >100 U of amylase activity, >8.0 U of lipase activity, and >100 U of protease activity.

The dissolution tests lasted 2 h (120 min) and the samples were obtained through manual collections with 5 mL syringes connected to cannulas. The collections were performed after 5, 10, 15, 20, 30, 45, 60, 90, and 120 min, with total of 3 mL of solution for each time point (triplicate). After collection, the samples were filtered with a 0.45 μm Poly(vinylidene fluoride) (PVDF) membrane (Nova Analítica, São Paulo, Brazil) and stored on dry ice until the time of analysis in the LC-MS.

4.5. Liquid Chromatography-Tandem Mass Spectrometry

The samples referring to all extraction protocols were analyzed by high-performance liquid chromatographytandem coupled to a triple-quadrupole mass spectrometer (HPLC-QqQ/MS/MS) Agilent 6460 (Agilent Technologies, Santa Clara, CA, USA) with ionization by electrospray, in positive mode at 3500 V. Nitrogen was used as the gas nebulizer (45 psi) and drying gas (5 mL/min at 300 °C).

The separation of compounds was performed on a hydrophilic chromatographic column ZIC-HILIC, 150 × 2.0 mm, 5 μm (Merck, Darmstadt, Germany). The mobile phases consisted of A (water containing 10 mM ammonium formate and 0.04% formic acid) and B (acetonitrile/water (80:20 *v/v*), containing 5 mM ammonium formate and 0.01% formic acid) [19]. The injection volume was 5 μL, and the chromatographic separation was carried out in a linear gradient with a flow of 0.150 mL/min.

The toxin was identified using a linear gradient under the following conditions: from 0 to 10 min, the gradient was 90% (B). The mobile phase was then reduced to 40% (B) from 10 to 12 min, and from 12 to 12.5 min, the mobile phase was changed again to 90% (B). From 12.5 to 20 min, the mobile phase was maintained at 90% (B), finishing the analysis. The results were obtained by multiple reaction monitoring (MRM) and the identification of GNT was performed by the retention time, m/z 253 ([GNT + H]) and the quantifier and qualifier ions $[M + H]^+$ m/z 253 > 58 and $[M + H]^+$ m/z 253 > 159. Data analysis was performed using MassHunter Qualitative Analysis B06.00 software (Agilent Technologies, Santa Clara, CA, USA).

4.6. Statistical Analysis

The data obtained in this study were presented as mean ± standard deviation (SD). Significant differences were assessed by two-way ANOVA and Tukey's test for multiple comparisons (p-value < 0.05 and p-value < 0.0001). The percentages expressed in the graphs was obtained after normalizing the data. All statistical tests were performed using R Statistical software version 3.1.2 [54] and graphs were made using Prism 7 (GraphPad Software, San Diego, CA, USA).

5. Conclusions

LC-MS analyses showed that GNT was statistically more stable in simulated solutions of the stomach component, and the presence of the enzyme pepsin resulted in greater stability of the toxin in acidic solutions. Although GNT is more stable in acidic solutions, such as stomach fluid, this study showed that GNT is also available in alkaline solutions (pH 7.5), mainly in the presence of pancreatic enzymes and, therefore, its availability must be considered both in the stomach and in the intestine. Therefore, the data presented here can be useful in the diagnosis and treatment of animals or humans affected by the accidental ingestion of cyanobacterial cells that produce GNT.

Supplementary Materials: The following are available online at http://www.mdpi.com/1424-8247/13/11/402/s1, Table S1: Mean and standard deviation (SD) for cell samples of the ITEP-24 strain submitted to dissolution tests (simulated gastric with and without pepsin enzyme solutions). The absolute values presented in the table were obtained through analysis by LC-QqQ-MS/MS, Table S2: Mean and standard deviation (SD) for cell samples of the ITEP-24 strain submitted to dissolution tests (simulated intestinal with and without pancreatin enzyme solutions). The absolute values presented in the table were obtained through analysis by LC-QqQ-MS/MS.

Author Contributions: Conceptualization, K.A.F., H.G.F. and F.V.; Methodology, Experimental Design, K.A.F., F.V., H.G.F. and E.P.; Cultivation of Cyanobacteria Species, K.A.F.; Dissolution Assays, K.A.F., H.G.F. and F.V.; Mass Spectrometry Analyses, E.P. and K.A.F.; Data Processing and Software analyses, K.F and E.P.; Statistical Analyses K.A.F. and F.V.; Writing—Original Draft Preparation, K.A.F., Writing—Review and Editing: K.A.F., H.G.F., F.V., and E.P.; Acquisition of Financing: H.G.F. and E.P. All authors have read and agreed to the published version of the manuscript.

Funding: This work was supported by the São Paulo State Research Foundation–FAPESP through a grant from FAPESP (2014/50420-9), University of São Paulo Foundation (FUSP) (Project#1979), the Coordination for the Improvement of Higher Education Personnel—CAPES (Project # 23038.001401/2018-92) and the National Council for Scientific and Technological Development—CNPq (311048/2016-1 and 439065/2018-6).

Acknowledgments: We acknowledge Felipe Augusto Dörr (University of São Paulo) for his suggestions and helping with the quantification of guanitoxin.

Conflicts of Interest: The authors declare no conflict of interest.

References

1. Fiore, M.F.; de Lima, S.T.; Carmichael, W.W.; McKinnie, S.M.K.; Chekan, J.R.; Moore, B.S. Guanitoxin, re-naming a cyanobacterial organophosphate toxin. *Harmful Algae* **2020**, *92*, 101737. [CrossRef] [PubMed]

2. Carmichael, W.W.; Gorham, P.R. Anatoxins from clones of Anabaena flos-aquae isolated from lakes of western Canada: With 3 figures and 2 tables in the text. *Int. Ver. für Theor. und Angew. Limnol. Mitt.* **1978**, *21*, 285–295. [CrossRef]

3. Matsunaga, S.; Moore, R.E.; Niemczura, W.P.; Carmichael, W.W. Anatoxin-a(s), a Potent Anticholinesterase from Anabaena flos-aquae. *J. Am. Chem. Soc.* **1989**, *111*, 8021–8023. [CrossRef]

4. Carmichael, W.W. The Toxins of Cyanobacteria. *Sci. Am.* **1994**, *270*, 78–86. [CrossRef] [PubMed]

5. Mahmood, N.A.; Carmichael, W.W. The pharmacology of anatoxin-a(s), a neurotoxin produced by the freshwater cyanobacterium Anabaena flos-aquae NRC 525-17. *Toxicon* **1986**, *24*, 425–434. [CrossRef]

6. Mahmood, N.A.; Carmichael, W.W.; Pfahler, D. Anticholinesterase poisonings in dogs from a cyanobacterial (blue-green algae) bloom dominated by Anabaena flos-aquae. *Am. J. Vet. Res.* **1988**, *49*, 500–503. [PubMed]

7. Mahmood, N.A.; Carmichael, W.W. Anatoxin-a(s), an anticholinesterase from the cyanobacterium Anabaena-Flos-Aquae NRC-525-17. *Toxicon* **1987**, *25*, 1221–1227. [CrossRef]

8. Cook, W.O.; Beasley, V.R.; Lovell, R.A.; Dahlem, A.M.; Hooser, S.B.; Mahmood, N.A.; Carmichael, W.W. Consistent inhibition of peripheral cholinesterases by neurotoxins from the freshwater cyanobacterium Anabaena flos-aquae: Studies of ducks, swine, mice and a steer. *Environ. Toxicol. Chem.* **1989**, *8*, 915–922. [CrossRef]

9. Henriksen, P.; Carmichael, W.W.; An, J.; Moestrup, Ø. Detection of an anatoxin-a(s)-like anticholinesterase in natural blooms and cultures of cyanobacteria/blue-green algae from Danish lakes and in the stomach content of poisoned birds. *Toxicon* **1997**, *35*, 901–913. [CrossRef]

10. Cook, W.O.; Dellinger, J.A.; Singh, S.S.; Dahlem, A.M.; Carmichael, W.W.; Beasley, V.R. Regional brain cholinesterase activity in rats injected intraperitoneally with anatoxin-a(s) or paraoxon. *Toxicol. Lett.* **1989**, *49*, 29–34. [CrossRef]

11. Monserrat, J.M.; Yunes, J.S.; Bianchini, A. Effects of Anabaena spiroides (cyanobacteria) aqueous extracts on the acetylcholinesterase activity of aquatic species. *Environ. Toxicol. Chem.* **2001**, *20*, 1228–1235. [CrossRef]

12. Freitas, E.C.; Printes, L.B.; Rocha, O. Acute effects of Anabaena spiroides extract and paraoxon-methyl on freshwater cladocerans from tropical and temperate regions: Links between the ChE activity and survival and its implications for tropical ecotoxicological studies. *Aquat. Toxicol.* **2014**, *146*, 105–114. [CrossRef] [PubMed]

13. Santos, D.S.; Rosa, M.E.; Zanatta, A.P.; Oliveira, R.S.; de Almeida, C.G.M.; Leal, A.P.; Sanz, M.; Fernandes, K.A.; de Souza, V.Q.; de Assis, D.R. Neurotoxic effects of sublethal concentrations of cyanobacterial extract containing anatoxin-a(s) on Nauphoeta cinerea cockroaches. *Ecotoxicol. Environ. Saf.* **2019**, *171*, 138–145. [CrossRef] [PubMed]

14. Freitas, E.C.; Printes, L.B.; Rocha, O. Use of cholinesterase activity as an ecotoxicological marker to assess anatoxin-a(s) exposure: Responses of two cladoceran species belonging to contrasting geographical regions. *Harmful Algae* **2016**, *55*, 150–162. [CrossRef] [PubMed]

15. Cook, W.O.; Iwamoto, G.A.; Schaeffer, D.J.; Beasley, V.R. Effect of anatoxin-a(s) from Anabaena flos-aquae NRC-525-17 on blood pressure, heart rate, respiratory rate, tidal volume, minute volume, and phrenic nerve activity in rats. *J. Environ. Pathol. Toxicol. Oncol. Off. Organ Int. Soc. Environ. Toxicol. Cancer* **1989**, *9*, 393–400.

16. Werner, V.R.; Laughinghouse IV, H.D.; Fiore, M.F.; Sant'Anna, C.L.; Hoff, C.; de Souza Santos, K.R.; Neuhaus, E.B.; Molica, R.J.R.; Honda, R.Y.; Echenique, R.O. Morphological and molecular studies of Sphaerospermopsis torques-reginae (Cyanobacteria, Nostocales) from South American water blooms. *Phycologia* **2012**, *51*, 228–238. [CrossRef]

17. Devic, E.; Li, D.; Dauta, A.; Henriksen, P.; Codd, G.A.; Marty, J.; Fournier, D. Detection of Anatoxin-a(s) in Environmental Samples of Cyanobacteria by Using a Biosensor with Engineered Acetylcholinesterases. *Appl. Environ. Microbiol.* **2002**, *68*, 4102–4106. [CrossRef]

18. Villatte, F.; Schulze, H.; Schmid, R.; Bachmann, T. A disposable acetylcholinesterase-based electrode biosensor to detect anatoxin-a(s) in water. *Anal. Bioanal. Chem.* **2002**, *372*, 322–326. [CrossRef]

19. Dörr, F.A.; Rodríguez, V.; Molica, R.; Henriksen, P.; Krock, B.; Pinto, E. Methods for detection of anatoxin-a(s) by liquid chromatography coupled to electrospray ionization-tandem mass spectrometry. *Toxicon* **2010**, *55*, 92–99. [CrossRef]

20. Svirčev, Z.; Lalić, D.; Savić, G.B.; Tokodi, N.; Backović, D.D.; Chen, L.; Meriluoto, J.; Codd, G.A. Global geographical and historical overview of cyanotoxin distribution and cyanobacterial poisonings. *Arch. Toxicol.* **2019**, *93*, 2429–2481. [CrossRef]

21. Metcalf, J.S.; Richer, R.; Cox, P.A.; Codd, G.A. Cyanotoxins in desert environments may present a risk to human health. *Sci. Total Environ.* **2012**, *421–422*, 118–123. [CrossRef] [PubMed]

22. Chatziefthimiou, A.D.; Richer, R.; Rowles, H.; Powell, J.T.; Metcalf, J.S. Cyanotoxins as a potential cause of dog poisonings in desert environments. *Vet. Rec.* **2014**, *174*, 484–485. [CrossRef] [PubMed]

23. Ibelings, B.W.; Backer, L.C.; Kardinaal, W.E.A.; Chorus, I. Current approaches to cyanotoxin risk assessment and risk management around the globe. *Harmful Algae* **2014**, *40*, 63–74. [CrossRef] [PubMed]

24. Bartram, J.; Baum, R.; Coclanis, P.A.; Gute, D.M.; Kay, D.; McFadyen, S.; Pond, K.; Robertson, W.; Rouse, M.J. *Routledge Handbook of Water and Health*; Routledge: London, UK; New York, NY, USA, 2015; ISBN 1138910074.

25. Barros, L.P.C.; Monserrat, J.M.; Yunes, J.S. Determination of optimized protocols for the extraction of anticholinesterasic compounds in environmental samples containing cyanobacteria species. *Environ. Toxicol. Chem.* **2004**, *23*, 883–889. [CrossRef] [PubMed]

26. Molica, R.J.R.; Oliveira, E.J.A.; Carvalho, P.V.V.C.; Costa, A.N.S.F.; Cunha, M.C.C.; Melo, G.L.; Azevedo, S.M.F.O. Occurrence of saxitoxins and an anatoxin-a(s) -like anticholinesterase in a Brazilian drinking water supply. *Harmful Algae* **2005**, *4*, 743–753. [CrossRef]

27. Metcalf, J.S.; Banack, S.A.; Powell, J.T.; Tymm, F.J.M.; Murch, S.J.; Brand, L.E.; Cox, P.A. Public health responses to toxic cyanobacterial blooms: Perspectives from the 2016 Florida event. *Water Policy* **2018**, *20*, 919–932. [CrossRef]

28. Rockville, M.D. *United Pharmacopoeia/National Formulary*; USP 23/NF 18; United States Pharmacopoeil Convention, Inc.: Rockville, MD, USA, 1995; p. 1235.

29. Anand, O.; Yu, L.X.; Conner, D.P.; Davit, B.M. Dissolution Testing for Generic Drugs: An FDA Perspective. *AAPS J.* **2011**, *13*, 328. [CrossRef]

30. Qureshi, S.A.; Shabnam, J. Cause of high variability in drug dissolution testing and its impact on setting tolerances. *Eur. J. Pharm. Sci.* **2001**, *12*, 271–276. [CrossRef]

31. Tsong, Y.; Shen, M.; Shah, V.P. Three-stage sequential statistical dissolution testing rules. *J. Biopharm. Stat.* **2004**, *14*, 757–779. [CrossRef]

32. Kasim, N.A.; Whitehouse, M.; Ramachandran, C.; Bermejo, M.; Lennernäs, H.; Hussain, A.S.; Junginger, H.E.; Stavchansky, S.A.; Midha, K.K.; Shah, V.P. Molecular properties of WHO essential drugs and provisional biopharmaceutical classification. *Mol. Pharm.* **2004**, *1*, 85–96. [CrossRef]

33. Klein, S. The Use of Biorelevant Dissolution Media to Forecast the In Vivo Performance of a Drug. *AAPS J.* **2010**, *12*, 397–406. [CrossRef] [PubMed]

34. Rodrigues, M.S.; Ferreira, L.S.; Converti, A.; Sato, S.; Carvalho, J.C.M. Fed-batch cultivation of Arthrospira (Spirulina) platensis: Potassium nitrate and ammonium chloride as simultaneous nitrogen sources. *Bioresour. Technol.* **2010**, *101*, 4491–4498. [CrossRef] [PubMed]

35. Singh, R.K.; Tiwari, S.P.; Rai, A.K.; Mohapatra, T.M. Cyanobacteria: An emerging source for drug discovery. *J. Antibiot. (Tokyo)* **2011**, *64*, 401–412. [CrossRef] [PubMed]

36. Nowruzi, B.; Haghighat, S.; Fahimi, H.; Mohammadi, E. Nostoc cyanobacteria species: A new and rich source of novel bioactive compounds with pharmaceutical potential. *J. Pharm. Heal. Serv. Res.* **2018**, *9*, 5–12. [CrossRef]

37. Marques, M.R.C. Enzymes in the dissolution testing of gelatin capsules. *AAPS Pharmscitech* **2014**, *15*, 1410–1416. [CrossRef] [PubMed]

38. Stanier, R.Y.; Cohen-Bazire, G. Phototrophic prokaryotes: The cyanobacteria. *Annu. Rev. Microbiol.* **1977**, *31*, 225–274. [CrossRef]

39. Palinska, K.A.; Krumbein, W.E. Perforation patterns in the peptidoglycan wall of filamentous cyanobacteria. *J. Phycol.* **2000**, *36*, 139–145. [CrossRef]

40. Safi, C.; Ursu, A.V.; Laroche, C.; Zebib, B.; Merah, O.; Pontalier, P.-Y.; Vaca-Garcia, C. Aqueous extraction of proteins from microalgae: Effect of different cell disruption methods. *Algal Res.* **2014**, *3*, 61–65. [CrossRef]

41. Murray, R.K.; Granner, D.K.; Mayes, P.A.; Rodwell, V.W. *Illustrated Biochemistry*; McGraw-Hill: New York, NY, USA, 2003.

42. Murray, K.; Rodwell, V.; Bender, D.; Botham, K.M.; Weil, P.A.; Kennelly, P.J. *Harper's Illustrated Biochemistry*, 28th ed.; McGraw-Hill: New York, NY, USA, 2009.

43. Christoffersen, K. Ecological implications of cyanobacterial toxins in aquatic food webs. *Phycologia* **1996**, *35*, 42–50. [CrossRef]

44. Sivonen, K.; Jones, G. *Toxic Cyanobacteria in Water: A Guide to Their Public Health Consequences, Monitoring and Management*; WHO: Geneva, Switzerland, 1999.

45. Jaiswal, P.; Singh, P.K.; Prasanna, R. Cyanobacterial bioactive molecules—An overview of their toxic properties. *Can. J. Microbiol.* **2008**, *54*, 701–717. [CrossRef]

46. Fernandes, K.; Gomes, A.; Calado, L.; Yasui, G.; Assis, D.; Henry, T.; Fonseca, A.; Pinto, E. Toxicity of Cyanopeptides from Two Microcystis Strains on Larval Development of Astyanax altiparanae. *Toxins* **2019**, *11*, 220. [CrossRef] [PubMed]

47. Azevedo, S.M.F.O.; Carmichael, W.W.; Jochimsen, E.M.; Rinehart, K.L.; Lau, S.; Shaw, G.R.; Eaglesham, G.K. Human intoxication by microcystins during renal dialysis treatment in Caruaru—Brazil. *Toxicology* **2002**, *181*, 441–446. [CrossRef]

48. Rodríguez, V.; Mori, B.; Dörr, F.A.; Dal Belo, C.A.; Colepicolo, P.; Pinto, E. Effects of a cyanobacterial extract containing-anatoxin-a(s) on the cardiac rhythm of Leurolestes circunvagans. *Rev. Bras. Farmacogn.* **2012**, *22*, 775–781. [CrossRef]

49. de Abreu, F.Q.; da Ferrão-Filho, A.S. Effects of an Anatoxin-a(s)-Producing Strain of Anabaena spiroides (Cyanobacteria) on the Survivorship and Somatic Growth of Two Daphnia similis Clones. *J. Environ. Prot. (Irvine, CA)* **2013**, *4*, 12–18. [CrossRef]

50. Onodera, H.; Oshima, Y.; Henriksen, P.; Yasumoto, T. Confirmation of anatoxin-a(s), in the cyanobacterium Anabaena lemmermannii, as the cause of bird kills in Danish lakes. *Toxicon* **1997**, *35*, 1645–1648. [CrossRef]

51. Gorham, P.R.; McLachlan, J.; Hammer, U.T.; Kim, W. Isolation and culture of toxic strains of Anabaena flos-aquae (Lyngb.) Breb. *Verh. Int. Vereinigung fur Theor. und Angew. Limnol.* **1964**, *15*, 1964. [CrossRef]

52. Blakefield, M.K.; Harris, D.O. Delay of cell differentiation in Anabaena aequalis caused by UV-B radiation and the role of photoreactivation and excision repair. *Photochem. Photobiol.* **1994**, *59*, 204–208. [CrossRef]

53. Moreno, I.M.; Maraver, J.; Aguete, E.C.; Leao, M.; Gago-Martínez, A.; Cameán, A.M. Decomposition of microcystin-LR, microcystin-RR, and microcystin-YR in water samples submitted to in vitro dissolution tests. *J. Agric. Food Chem.* **2004**, *52*, 5933–5938. [CrossRef]

54. Team, R.C. *R: A Language and Environment for Statistical Computing*; R Foundation for Statistical Computing: Vienna, Austria, 2016.

Publisher's Note: MDPI stays neutral with regard to jurisdictional claims in published maps and institutional affiliations.

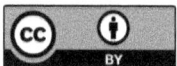

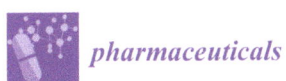

Article

Determination of Very Low Concentration of Bisphenol A in Toys and Baby Pacifiers Using Dispersive Liquid–Liquid Microextraction by In Situ Ionic Liquid Formation and High-Performance Liquid Chromatography

Yesica Vicente-Martínez[iD]**, Manuel Caravaca** *[iD] **and Antonio Soto-Meca**

Spanish Air Force Academy, University Centre of Defence, Coronel López Peña st., n/n, 30720 Murcia, Spain;
yesica.vicente@cud.upct.es (Y.V.-M.); antonio.soto@cud.upct.es (A.S.-M.)
* Correspondence: manuel.caravaca@cud.upct.es; Tel.: +34-968-189-979; Fax: +34-968-189-970

Received: 12 September 2020; Accepted: 9 October 2020; Published: 12 October 2020

Abstract: Bisphenol A (BPA) is a chemical compound used in the manufacturing of plastics and resins whose presence in the body in low concentrations can cause serious health problems. Due to this, there is a growing interest in the scientific community to develop analytical methods that allow quantifying trace concentrations of BPA in different types of samples. The determination of this compound in toys made of plastics that can be manipulated by children leads to an extra concern, because it is possible for BPA to enter the body by introducing these toys into the mouth. This work presents a novel procedure to the quickly and easily quantification of trace levels of BPA in samples of toys and pacifiers according to the current demanding regulations. The determination of very low levels of BPA was carried out by ionic liquid dispersive liquid–liquid microextraction (IL-DLLME) followed by high-performance liquid chromatography (HPLC). The formation in situ of the ionic liquid (IL) 1-octyl-3-methylimidazolium bis((trifluoromethane)sulfonyl)imide ($[C_8MIm]$ $[NTf_2]$), was achieved by mixing 1-octyl-3-methylimidazolium chloride ($[C_8MIm]Cl$) and lithium bis(trifluoromethanesulfonyl)imide ($[NTf_2]Li$) aqueous solutions, reaching an instant dispersion whose cloud of microdrops allows the total extraction of BPA in the IL from aqueous solutions. After centrifugation, BPA concentration in the sedimented phase was determined by HPLC. The optimal experimental conditions for the microextraction and determination of BPA in the IL were studied. The total extraction was achieved at pH 4, heating the sample at 30 °C for 5 min, using 100 μL of IL precursor volume, and spinning after the formation of dispersion at 3000 rpm for 10 min. The enrichment factor (EF) and detection limit (LOD) reached with the procedure were 299 and 0.19 μg L^{-1}, respectively. The relative standard deviation for ten replications at the 0.5 μg L^{-1} level was 5.2%. Recovery studies showed a mean value for BPA recovery percentage in the samples of 99%. Additionally, a hybrid model was applied to characterize the extraction kinetics. This simple, low cost and fast method simplifies traditional microextraction techniques, representing an outstanding alternative.

Keywords: bisphenol A; high-performance liquid chromatography; ionic liquid; dispersive liquid–liquid microextraction; extraction kinetic studies

---

1. Introduction

Bisphenol A (BPA) is a chemical compound widely used in the manufacturing of plastics and epoxy resins, which are later employed in toys and bottle teats production. Trace residue levels of

BPA cause serious problems in the normal function of the endocrine system [1], being a mutagenic and carcinogenic compound. Epidemiologic literature reports relationship between low BPA levels and pubertal development, fetal and childhood growth or metabolic and reproductive diseases, among others [2]. It has been stated that even extremely low doses, parts per trillion, can alter cell function [3]. Consequently, the European Union established a specific migration limit (SML) of 0.04 mg L^{-1} for BPA used in toys for children under 36 months [4]. Moreover, the European Commission established a ban on the use of BPA in the manufacturing of polycarbonate baby bottles for infants in 2011 [5].

The restrictive regulations regarding BPA content in toys and baby bottles makes necessary the development of analytical methods with high sensitivity and low detection limit (LOD) which allows to determinate trace concentrations. This high sensitivity requires preconcentration techniques during the sample preparation step. Microextraction techniques are environmentally friendly methods which have replaced classical methods last years. Nowadays, ionic liquids (IL) are very used as extractant phase to determine trace concentrations of different chemical compounds using liquid–liquid microextraction (LLME) techniques because of their suitable characteristics, such as vapor pressure, solubility, and thermal stability. However, the usual microextraction techniques often require the use of organic solvents acting as dispersing agents, or ultrasound to achieve the total extraction of the compound, also requiring long times and high temperatures for a full extraction [6–10].

Particularly, the determination of BPA has been carried out by many authors from different matrices, such as plastics by means of gas chromatography [11,12], vegetable oils using a magnetic ionic liquid [6], and a variety of foods and drinks by different analytical techniques [13–19].

In recent years, different chemical sensors have been manufactured for the determination of BPA, based on graphene-palladium nanoparticles/polyvinyl alcohol hybrids [20], using CdO nanoparticles [17], or an amperometric enzyme inhibition biosensor based on xanthine oxidase immobilised onto glassy carbon [21].

However, methods for determining traces of BPA in toys or materials used in baby bottles, such as nipples, have not been practically studied recently, since the sensitivity requirements established by European Regulations are very restrictive [4]. Notwithstanding, several interesting studies can be listed, although they present some limitations. A work carried out in 2012 to determine the content of BPA in toys by gas chromatography-mass spectrometry reached detection limits of 10 μg kg^{-1}, being necessary the sample derivatization [16]. A procedure of liquid chromatography with fluorescence detection was developed to determine BPA in toy, the LOD reached equal to 50 μg L^{-1}, not realistic in comparison to concentrations found in most toys [22]. Moreover, the concentration of BPA has been determined in toys used by dogs, reaching the quantification of concentrations of μg mL^{-1} [23].

In this work, it is introduced a procedure to simulate the migration of BPA in toys and pacifier teats. These objects were subjected to the conditions of children saliva when sucked, transferring this compound to an aqueous solution [24]. After that, the aqueous solution containing BPA is subjected to a microextraction method based on the in situ formation of IL in a straightforward ion-exchange reaction. An instantaneous dispersion is obtained after mixing the IL precursors, allowing the rapid and total extraction of BPA from aqueous solutions in the IL droplet cloud. In just a few minutes, after centrifuging the dispersion, the sedimented extract at the bottom of the tube is analyzed by HPLC to quantification of amounts of BPA present in the solution. This method allows to determine very low concentrations of BPA in a simple and cost effective-way, in comparison with other techniques requiring more expensive instrumentation. In this way, the procedure is accessible for any standard laboratory.

The experimental conditions to achieve the total extraction of BPA were studied, reached for pH = 4 and 30 °C, in just 5 min. This procedure leads to an enrichment factor (EF) and LOD of 299 and 0.19 μg L^{-1}, respectively. These values allow the determination of BPA concentrations under the very restrictive conditions of concentration that the regulations establish. The procedure was validated applying it to determination of BPA in solutions with known concentrations. Recovery, repeatability and reproducibility studies were carried out showing that it is a robust method for the established purpose, becoming a realistic and viable alternative to determine BPA in toys and baby pacifiers.

2. Results and Discussion

2.1. Optimization of the DLLME Conditions

2.1.1. Optimization of Aqueous Phase and IL Precursors Volume

The aqueous phase volume was studied with different volumes of IL precursors in order to reach the best microextractions conditions. Among them, it is important to get a constant IL sedimented volume after centrifugation, allowing to carry out the measurement by triplicate and to obtain a suitable EF. To this end, aqueous phase volumes of 5, 10, 15 and 20 mL were tested with 25, 50 and 100 μL of each IL precursor. However, regardless of the aqueous phase volume, when the volumes of IL precursors were 25 and 50 μL, the volume of the IL phase sedimented after centrifugation was so small that it was not possible to analyze it.

When a volume of aqueous phase of 5 mL and 100 μL of each IL precursors were employed, the volume of IL formed after centrifugation was 48 μL, resulting in an EF of 104. When the volume of aqueous phase was 10 mL and the volume for each IL precursor was 100 μL, the volume of IL formed after centrifugation was 33 μL, achieving an EF close to 303. A volume equal to 18 μL of IL phase was achieved when the aqueous phase volume was 15 mL and volume of precursor was 100 μL, but not allowing measurements by triplicate. Finally, when the volume of aqueous phase was equal to 20 mL and volumes of precursors were 100 μL each, the volume obtained of IL sedimented was 10 μL, also not allowing measurements by triplicate. Results are summarized in Table 1.

Table 1. IL volume and EF obtained after centrifugation for different aqueous phase volumes and a fixed IL precursors volume of 100 μL.

Aqueous Phase Volume (mL)	IL Precursors Volume (μL)	IL Volume after Centrifugation (μL)	EF
5	100	48	104
10	100	33	303
15 *	100	18	833
20 *	100	10	2000

* Measurements not achieved by triplicate.

Consequently, a volume of 10 mL of aqueous phase was chosen because for 33 μL of IL the measurements can be carried out by triplicate, still achieving a high EF, close to 300.

2.1.2. Optimization of pH Conditions

In order to determine the adequate pH to reach the maximum efficiency of the extraction of BPA in the IL, several experiments were carried out. A range of pH 1–10 was studied to obtain the best results in the extraction of BPA. Figure 1 shows that the maximum BPA extraction is achieved for a pH range between 3 and 5. For the discussion of this result, this behavior is due to a hydrophobic interaction between IL and BPA which decreases because of the deprotonation of BPA when pH increases [25]. A pH value of 4 was selected as adequate to carry out the extraction.

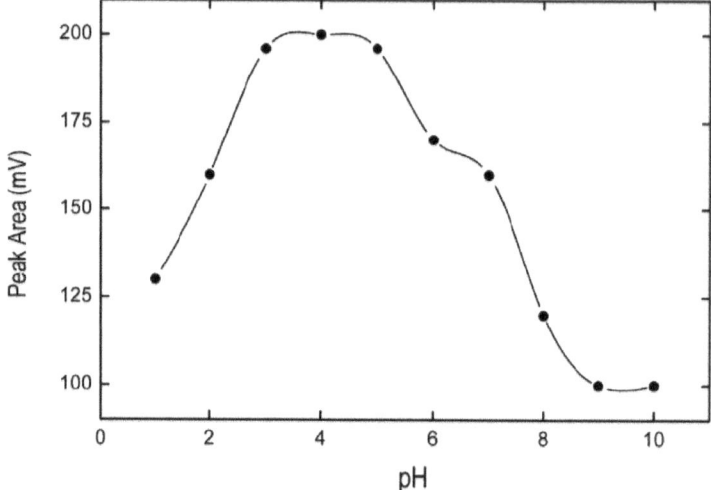

Figure 1. Effect of pH on BPA extraction. Solid line represents spline connectors. As depicted from the plot, a maximum Peak Area was achieved for pH = 4.

2.1.3. Optimization of Temperature Conditions and Incubation Time

In the extraction procedure the solution temperature plays a very important role, influencing the extraction efficiency of DLLME. Because of this, the temperature effect was studied within the range 25–60 °C. The aqueous was heated in a thermostatic bath for ten minutes, prior to the addition of the IL precursors at different temperatures belonging to the range mentioned above. As is shown in Figure 2, the best extraction efficiency was obtained at 30 °C. Accordingly, we selected this temperature as the best one for our microextraction process.

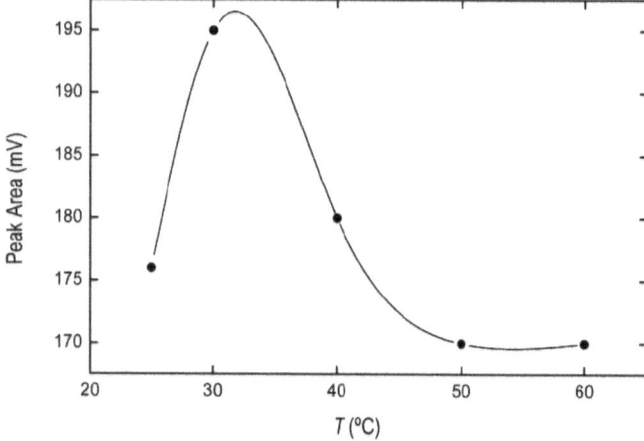

Figure 2. Effect of the temperature on the BPA signal obtained from IL phase. Solid line represents spline connectors. Maximum extraction efficiency was achieved at T = 30 °C.

Additionally, the incubation time of the samples at 30 °C was studied within the range 2–30 min. Figure 3 shows that the extraction efficiency of the BPA in the IL increased from 2 to 10 min, then remaining nearly constant until 30 min. Accordingly, five minutes was selected as the heating time for subsequent measurements. As a discussion, the extraction kinetics was characterized by an efficient hybrid kinetic model, Equation (1) (see Section 3.7), resulting in an adjusted R^2 equal to 0.974. The fit is represented by red solid line in Figure 3.

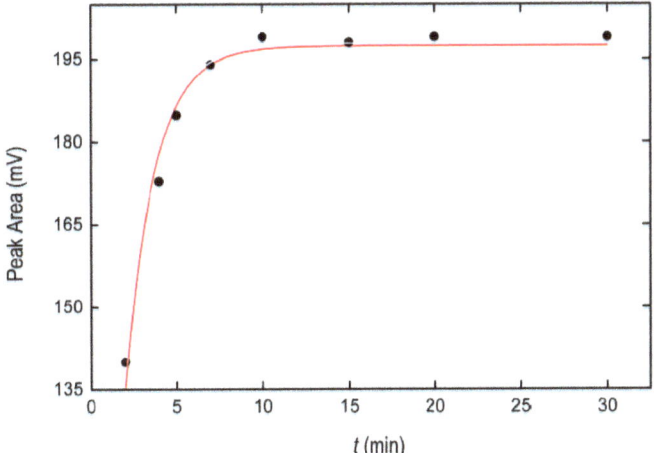

Figure 3. Effect of incubation time at 30 °C on the BPA signal obtained from the IL phase. Solid red line represents the fit to Equation (1).

2.1.4. Optimization of Centrifugation Time

The centrifugation time was studied in order to obtain the adequate IL volume after the microextraction procedure. Times equal to 2, 5, 7, 10, 15, 20 and 30 min of centrifugation were applied at 3000 rpm. Figure 4 shows that the volume of IL sedimented increased from 0 to 5 min, then remaining constant until 30 min. The choice for the adequate centrifugation time was 10 min.

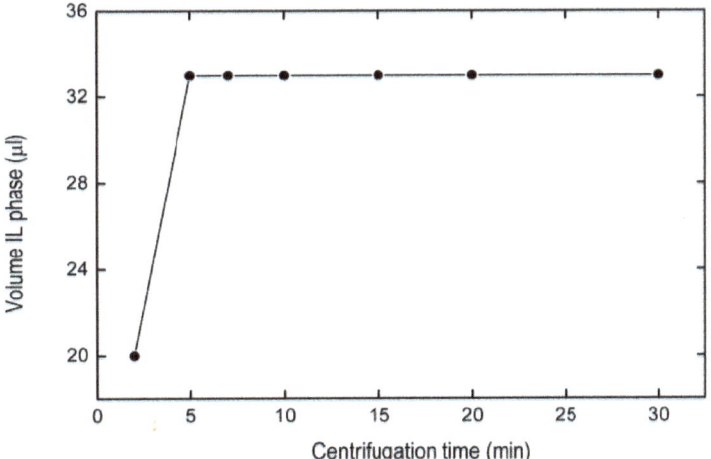

Figure 4. Effect of centrifugation time on volume IL phase. Solid line represents straight connectors.

2.2. Analytical Figures of Merit of the Proposed Method

The EF was evaluated from the quotient between the slope obtained in the calibration line, by applying the proposed preconcentration procedure in experimental section, and the slope resulting from directly measuring BPA in aqueous solution. EF achieved a value of 299. This value coincides with the quotient of the volume of the aqueous phase and the volume of the sedimented IL.

The analytes show a linear behavior within the range 0.5–0.3 µg L^{-1} (linear equation: $Y = 96.437x + 4.736$). The regression coefficient R^2 for the proposed procedure was 0.997.

Ten consecutive experiments were carried out at 0.5 µg L^{-1} level of BPA to estimate the repeatability, being the relative standard deviations (RSDs) 5.2%. The reproducibility was calculated from ten measurements obtained on five consecutive days, obtaining RSDs of 6.5%.

The LOD was calculated using the criterion that the analyte quantity is equivalent to three times the standard error of the calibration slope estimation. This results in a LOD equal to 0.19 µg L^{-1} of BPA. Additionally, the limit of quantification (LOQ) is equal to 0.63 µg L^{-1}.

To validate the proposed method, it was applied to aqueous solutions with known concentrations of BPA. Table 2 shows the results obtained. As a discussion, the concentrations obtained after applying the proposed microextraction technique are in agreement, including the standard deviations, to the concentrations of the prepared solutions.

Table 2. Results of validation of the proposed procedure in aqueous solutions presenting known concentrations of BPA.

Sample of Known Concentration	Concentration (µg L^{-1})	Content Found [a] (µg L^{-1})
blank	0.0	0.01 ± 0.00
1	0.30	0.303 ± 0.002
2	0.40	0.401 ± 0.001
3	0.50	0.500 ± 0.003

[a] Mean value ± standard deviation (*n* = 3).

2.3. Application of the Procedure to Toys and Baby Pacifier Samples

The common activity of children introducing toys into the mouth causes the possibility that some chemical compounds present in the materials for toy manufacturing are solubilized in the saliva, entering the body and causing health risk in some cases.

Regarding BPA, small doses of this chemical could cause serious health problems [1]. For this reason, the European Union established the maximum specific migration limit of BPA in baby toys at 0.04 mg L^{-1} [4]. The pacifier limit has not been established, assuming that they must contain 0% BPA in their composition. Since the elimination mechanisms in babies are not fully operating before 6 months, any exposure to this substance is not considered as safe.

Although the limit of migration of BPA in toys is established in the aforementioned concentration, it is necessary to have analytical methods that allow a safe quantification of much lower levels in materials used by babies, since it constitutes a real concerning danger.

The analytical procedure proposed in this work was applied to determination of BPA in toys and baby pacifiers. For this, it is necessary to submit these materials to a procedure that simulates the migration of chemical in the baby's saliva. The treatment is regulated by the European Union, consisting of putting 10 cm^2 of the material in continuous agitation with 100 mL of water for one hour at room temperature [4]. The aqueous solutions were later subjected to the proposed microextraction procedure by in situ formation of an IL. Regarding the toys employed in our study, we chose the samples randomly, among standard small toys from local toy stores in Murcia, Spain. Date of purchase was November 2019 for samples 1–8, and September 2020 for samples 9–11. The values found by application of the procedure under study to several toys are shown in Table 3. All values lie well below the permitted limit. Additionally, recovery studies were carried out for every sample. As can be seen in Table 3, recoveries ranged from 97% to 102%, thus confirming the reliability of the procedure.

Table 3. BPA determined from toy and pacifier samples.

Sample	Content Found [a] (μg L^{-1})	Recovery %
1—Blue ball	0.30 ± 0.02	100
2—Red ball	ND	101
3—White teat	0.23 ± 0.01	97
4—Pink teat	ND	-
5—Red teat	ND	-
6—Yellow banana	0.25 ± 0.01	102
7—Green apple	0.22 ± 0.04	101
8—Violet grape	0.30 ± 0.03	99
9—Blue ball	0.28 ± 0.02	98
10—Yellow horse	0.21 ± 0.02	101
11—Orange giraffe	0.25 ± 0.04	98

ND: Not detected; [a] Mean value $\pm$ standard deviation ($n = 3$).

To discuss the results, it is worth pointing out that trace BPA levels as those shown in Table 3 could be dangerous, even fulfilling the restrictions of the EU, as reported in the literature [2,3]. Toys and pacifiers add to other BPA sources, being food intake the primary route of human exposure [26,27]. The environment is generally considered as a secondary source and, in particular, it has been stated that it is unlikely to inhale high BPA levels from air, except maybe with the workers of BPA-based products companies [27]. The European Food Safety Authority established in 2015 [28] an average BPA dietary intake reaching 0.857 μg/kg BW/day for infants, and a non-dietary of 0.015 μg/kg BW/day. However, recent studies show that toy BPA intake can approach 246 ng/kg BW/day [29]. The EU set in 2017 a temporary tolerable daily intake (TDI) equal to 4 μg/kg BW/day, of which 10% allocates to exposure to BPA from toys [4]. Additionally, it has been reported than lower levels, such as 0.025–0.2 μg/kg BW/day can lead to severe health problems [27], so again it is emphasized that efficient detection of trace levels could be of paramount importance.

3. Materials and Methods

3.1. Chemicals and Materials

The bisphenol A standard was purchased from Sigma-Aldrich Chemie (Schnelldorf, Germany). Pure water was prepared using a water purification system formed by a delimer (CILIT MINICRONO (Cilit, SA, Barcelona, Spain) and a water purification system SETA OSMO BL-6 (Sociedad Española de Tratamiento de Agua, Madrid, Spain). Ultrapure water was employed for the preparation of 0.1 M solutions of these ILs.

Bis(trifluoromethane)sulfonamide lithium salt and 1-butyl-3-methylimidazolium chloride (Sigma-Aldrich Chemie, Schnelldorf, Germany) were used in orden to form the IL. Analytical grade acetonitrile was obtained from Applichem Panreac (Darmstadt, Germany), and water for HPLC from Macron Fine Chemicals (Gliwice, Poland). The non-ionic surfactant Triton X-114 was purchased from Sigma-Aldrich (Raleigh, NC, USA). Micro pipettes of 100–1000 μL were brought from Thermo Scientific (Wantaa, Finland).

3.2. General Procedure

Sample solution of 10 mL containing BPA in the range of 0.5–3 μg L^{-1} was heated at 30 °C for 5 min. Subsequently, 20 μL of a regulatory dissolution of pH = 4, 100 μL of the [C$_8$MIm]Cl solution, 100 μL of 0.1 mol L^{-1} Triton X-114 solution and 100 μL of the [NTf$_2$]Li were added. A turbid dispersion was instantaneously formed because of the IL formation reaction from its precursors. The mixture was centrifuged at 3000 rpm for 10 min. The IL sedimented at the bottom of the tube was collected, being 10 μL injected in HPLC using a chromatographic-type syringe. BPA concentrations were determined using the conditions described throughout the manuscript. The measurements were carried out by triplicate.

3.3. Procedure Applied to Plastic Toys and Baby Pacifiers

Eleven toy and baby pacifier samples were acquired in local stores and pharmacies, respectively in Murcia, Spain. The toy samples included one plastic blue ball (sample 1), one plastic red ball (sample 2), one plastic blue ball (sample 9), a yellow horse (sample 10), an orange giraffe (sample 11) and three different plastic fruits: one yellow banana (sample 6), one green apple (sample 7) and one purple grape (sample 8). Regarding the baby pacifiers, two samples manufactured after the modification of legislation in specific limit values for chemicals used in toys (samples 3 and 4), and one sample manufactured before legislation of BPA was enforced (sample 5).

A surface of 10 cm^2 of material from each toy and baby pacifier were contacted under mechanical agitation with 100 mL of water for 1 h with magnetic stirring at room temperature [4]. Then, 10 mL from each aqueous solution were treated with the general procedure.

3.4. Ionic Liquid as Acceptor Phase

Organic solvents as a BPA extracting medium have been extensively studied and used over the years [30–32]. In recent years, liquid–liquid microextraction techniques have been widely used to extract BPA using different organic solvents, such as benzene [33], hexane [34], ethyl acetate [35] or ethanol [36]. However, the use of IL as an extracting medium instead of the commonly used organic solvents provides a series of advantages, such as low solubility in water and low viscosity, a double condition which is not easily achieved [9,10]. Moreover, mixing water-soluble IL precursors leads to an in situ metathesis reaction, immediately giving rise to a water-immiscible IL [8]. This IL formation reaction provides a dispersed phase through a cloud of microdroplets that allows to get a large surface in contact, thus proportioning the right medium for instantaneous extraction of the analyte.

Excellent results were found when 1-octyl-3-methylimidazolium chloride ([C$_8$MIm]Cl) and bis(trifluoromethanesulfonyl)imide ([NTf$_2$]Li) were employed as IL precursors. Both precursors were mixed and a turbidity due to the formation of insoluble 1-octyl-3-methylimidazolium bis((trifluoromethane)sulfonyl)imide ([C$_8$MIm] [NTf$_2$]) was immediately observed by the metathesis reaction:

$$[C_8MIm]Cl + [NTf_2]Li \rightarrow [C_8MIm][NTf_2] + LiCl$$

This procedure greatly simplifies traditional microextraction techniques because it avoids the use of dispersing agents, organic solvents or mechanical techniques, such as ultrasound. Moreover, this method reduces the time necessary to achieve full extraction of the analytes. It has been used for the extraction of several metals and other aromatic species [8–10].

Different volumes of [C$_8$MIm]Cl and [NTf$_2$]Li were studied in order to obtain the best conditions in terms of formed IL volume and reproducibility of the process. The best results were found employing 100 µL of 1 mol L^{-1} [C$_8$MIm]Cl and 100 µL of 1 mol L^{-1} [NTf$_2$]Li, and a aqueous phase of 10 mL. After centrifugation, 33 µL of IL [C$_8$MIm][NTf$_2$] were recovered in the bottom of the tube. This volume is in agreement with the theoretical predictions, taking into account the [C$_8$MIm][NTf$_2$] density [37].

3.5. Non-Stick Agent Selection

In order to avoid that IL remains in the walls of the tube during microextraction process, thus collecting the maximum volume of IL, some authors have suggested the employment of surfactants as non-stick agents [9,10,38]. Different volumes and concentrations of surfactants were studied, achieving the best results with the use of Triton X-114. By using 200 µL of aqueous solution 0.2 mol L^{-1} of Triton X-114 at 10 mL of donor phase, the volume of sedimented IL reached a maximum, constant and reproducible value of 33 µL under the experimental conditions proposed, thereby preventing it from sticking to the walls of the container.

3.6. Instrumentation and Analytical Conditions

The measurements made in this work were carried out on an HPLC JASCO BS-4000 system (Madrid, Spain), equipped with a sample injector and an ultraviolet detector (UV-4075) operating at 230 nm.

The column used was C18 column (150 × 4.6 mm i.d., 5 μm), and the mobile phase employed consisted in a mixture of 60% acetonitrile and 40% water, at a flow rate of 0.8 mL min^{-1} and an injection volume of 10 μL.

An ultrasonic bath with a HD-5L heating system (P-Selecta S.A., Barcelona, Spain) at 40 kHz of frequency and 60W of power was used for raising the temperature up to 30 °C. An EBA 8 centrifuge (P-Selecta S.A., Barcelona, Spain) was used to disrupt sample emulsions.

3.7. Microextraction Kinetic Studies

Characterization of BPA microextraction kinetics was performed through a nonlinear fit of the experimental data, specifically the dependence of Peak Area (mV) on exposure time (min), described by the following hybrid model [39]:

$$\text{Peak Area} = (\alpha - \beta)\frac{(\beta/\alpha)e^{(\beta-\alpha)\gamma t}}{(\beta/\alpha)e^{(\beta-\alpha)\gamma t}-1}+\beta \tag{1}$$

where and α, β, γ represent characteristic parameters and t is the exposure time.

4. Conclusions

Toys and baby pacifiers are subjected to high restrictions of BPA concentrations. This fact makes it difficult in the development of analytical methods capable of quantifying very low levels of this chemical in those materials. However, very low levels of this BPA can seriously affect children's health. This work presents a novel method of determining very low concentrations of BPA in toys and baby pacifiers as an alternative to the traditional methods for its analysis.

The procedure consists of the in situ formation of an ionic liquid through a metathesis reaction of its precursors, providing a dispersed medium which allows the instantaneous extraction of BPA in IL under very mild and simple experimental conditions. After centrifuging the mixture, the IL sediments at the bottom of the tube and the BPA can be quantified by direct injection of the IL on HPLC. A high enrichment factor (EF = 299) and a low detection limit (LOD = 0.19 μg L^{-1}) were achieved. Furthermore, the proposed method presents a high reproducibility and repeatability. It was validated using aqueous solutions of known concentrations of BPA and was successfully applied to real samples of toys and pacifiers complying with the current regulations for it.

Author Contributions: Conceptualization, all authors; experimental methodology, Y.V.-M.; software, all authors; validation, Y.V.-M.; formal analysis, all authors; theoretical models, M.C. and A.S.-M.; investigation, all authors; resources, all authors; data curation, all authors; writing—original draft preparation, all authors; writing—review and editing, all authors; visualization, all authors; supervision, all authors; project administration, all authors; funding acquisition, all authors. All authors have read and agreed to the published version of the manuscript.

Funding: This research received no external funding.

Acknowledgments: The authors want to thank the University Centre of Defence at the Spanish Air Force Academy for experimental financial support.

Conflicts of Interest: The authors declare no conflict of interest.

References

1. Pan, D.D.; Gu, Y.Y.; Lan, H.Z.; Sun, Y.Y.; Gao, H.J. Functional graphene-gold nano-composite fabricated electrochemical biosensor for direct and rapid detection of bisphenol A. *Anal. Chim. Acta* **2015**, *853*, 297–302. [CrossRef] [PubMed]
2. Braun, J.M.; Hauser, R. Bisphenol A and children's health. *Curr. Opin. Pediatr.* **2011**, *23*, 233–239. [CrossRef] [PubMed]

3.   Wetherill, Y.B.; Akingbemi, B.T.; Kanno, J.; McLachlan, J.A.; Nadal, A.; Sonnenscheing, C.; Watson, C.S.; Zoeller, R.T.; Belcher, S.M. In vitro molecular mechanisms of bisphenol A action. *Reprod. Toxicol.* **2007**, *24*, 178–198. [CrossRef] [PubMed]

4.   Eurpean Union. Commision Regulation (EU) No 2017/898 of 24 May 2017 on Specific Limit Values for Certain Chemical Products Used in Toys. 2017. Available online: https://eur-lex.europa.eu/legal-content/EN/TXT/PDF/?uri=CELEX:32017L0898&from=ES (accessed on 3 October 2020).

5.   Eurpean Comissión. Commission Regulation (EU) No 10/2011 of 14 January 2011 on Plastic Materials and Articles Intended to Come into Contact with Food (OJ L 12, 15.1.2011, p.1). 2011. Available online: https://eur-lex.europa.eu/legal-content/EN/TXT/PDF/?uri=CELEX:32011R0010&from=EN (accessed on 3 October 2020).

6.   Zhu, S.Q.; Wang, L.J.; Su, A.; Zhang, H.X. Dispersive liquid-liquid microextraction of phenolic compounds from vegetable oils using a magnetic ionic liquid. *J. Sep. Sci.* **2017**, *40*, 3130–3137. [CrossRef] [PubMed]

7.   Zhong, Q.; Su, P.; Zhang, Y.; Wang, R.Y.; Yang, Y. In-situ ionic liquid-based microwave-assisted dispersive liquid-liquid microextraction of triazine herbicides. *Microchim. Acta* **2012**, *178*, 341–347. [CrossRef]

8.   Yao, C.; Anderson, J.L. Dispersive liquid-liquid microextraction using an in situ metathesis reaction to form an ionic liquid extraction phase for the preconcentration of aromatic compounds from water. *Anal. Bioanal. Chem.* **2009**, *395*, 1491–1502. [CrossRef] [PubMed]

9.   Lopez-Garcia, I.; Vicente-Martinez, Y.; Hernandez-Cordoba, M. Determination of lead and cadmium using an ionic liquid and dispersive liquid-liquid microextraction followed by electrothermal atomic absorption spectrometry. *Talanta* **2013**, *110*, 46–52. [CrossRef] [PubMed]

10. Lopez-Garcia, I.; Vicente-Martinez, Y.; Hernandez-Cordoba, M. Determination of very low amounts of chromium(III) and (VI) using dispersive liquid-liquid microextraction by in situ formation of an ionic liquid followed by electrothermal atomic absorption spectrometry. *J. Anal. At. Spectrom.* **2012**, *27*, 874–880. [CrossRef]

11. Cacho, J.I.; Campillo, N.; Vinas, P.; Hernandez-Cordoba, M. In situ ionic liquid dispersive liquid-liquid microextraction and direct microvial insert thermal desorption for gas chromatographic determination of bisphenol compounds. *Anal. Bioanal. Chem.* **2016**, *408*, 243–249. [CrossRef]

12. Cacho, J.I.; Campillo, N.; Vinas, P.; Hernandez-Cordoba, M. In situ ionic liquid dispersive liquid-liquid microextraction coupled to gas chromatography-mass spectrometry for the determination of organophosphorus pesticides. *J. Chromatogr. A* **2018**, *1559*, 95–101. [CrossRef]

13. Ye, C.L.; Liu, C.; Wang, S.; Wang, Z.K. Investigation of 1-Dodecylimidazolium Modified Filter Papers as a Thin-Film Microextraction Phase for the Preconcentration of Bisphenol A from Plant Oil Samples. *Anal. Sci.* **2017**, *33*, 229–234. [CrossRef] [PubMed]

14. Yao, C.; Li, T.H.; Twu, P.; Pitner, W.R.; Anderson, J.L. Selective extraction of emerging contaminants from water samples by dispersive liquid-liquid microextraction using functionalized ionic liquids. *J. Chromatogr. A* **2011**, *1218*, 1556–1566. [CrossRef] [PubMed]

15. Lopez-Darias, J.; Pino, V.; Ayala, J.H.; Afonso, A.M. In-situ ionic liquid-dispersive liquid-liquid microextraction method to determine endocrine disrupting phenols in seawaters and industrial effluents. *Microchim. Acta* **2011**, *174*, 213–222. [CrossRef]

16. Gao, Y.; Zhang, Y.; Gao, J.; Zhang, H.; Zheng, L.; Chen, J. Determination of bisphenol A from toys and food contact materials by derivatization and gas chromatography-mass spectrometry. *Chin. J. Chromatogr.* **2012**, *30*, 1017–1020. [CrossRef]

17. Fouladgar, M. Nanostructured Sensor for Simultaneous Determination of Trace Amounts of Bisphenol A and Vitamin B-6 in Food Samples. *Food Anal. Meth.* **2017**, *10*, 1507–1514. [CrossRef]

18. Faraji, M.; Noorani, M.; Sahneh, B.N. Quick, Easy, Cheap, Effective, Rugged, and Safe Method Followed by Ionic Liquid-Dispersive Liquid-Liquid Microextraction for the Determination of Trace Amount of Bisphenol A in Canned Foods. *Food Anal. Meth.* **2017**, *10*, 764–772. [CrossRef]

19. Fan, Y.Y.; Liu, S.H.; Xie, Q.L. Rapid determination of phthalate esters in alcoholic beverages by conventional ionic liquid dispersive liquid-liquid microextraction coupled with high performance liquid chromatography. *Talanta* **2014**, *119*, 291–298. [CrossRef]

20. Hu, Y.J.; Liu, Z.M.; Zhan, H.J.; Hu, L.Q.; Cui, L.; Wang, K. A novel electrochemiluminescence sensor for bisphenol A determination based on graphene-palladium nanoparticles/polyvinyl alcohol hybrids. *Anal. Methods* **2017**, *9*, 3870–3875. [CrossRef]

21. Ben Messaoud, N.; Ghica, M.E.; Dridi, C.; Ben Ali, M.; Brett, C.M.A. A novel amperometric enzyme inhibition biosensor based on xanthine oxidase immobilised onto glassy carbon electrodes for bisphenol A determination. *Talanta* **2018**, *184*, 388–393. [CrossRef]

22. Negev, M.; Berman, T.; Reicher, S.; Sadeh, M.; Ardi, R.; Shammai, Y. Concentrations of trace metals, phthalates, bisphenol A and flame-retardants in toys and other children's products in Israel. *Chemosphere* **2018**, *192*, 217–224. [CrossRef]

23. Wooten, K.J.; Smith, P.N. Canine toys and training devices as sources of exposure to phthalates and bisphenol A: Quantitation of chemicals in leachate and in vitro screening for endocrine activity. *Chemosphere* **2013**, *93*, 2245–2253. [CrossRef] [PubMed]

24. Eurpean Regulations. EN 71-10:2005. *Safety of Toys. Organic Chemical Compounds.* 2005. Available online: https://ilnas.services-publics.lu/ecnor/downloadPreview.action?documentReference=45158 (accessed on 4 October 2020).

25. Staples, C.A.; Dorn, P.B.; Klecka, G.M.; O'Block, S.T.; Harris, L.R. A review of the environmental fate, effects, and exposures of bisphenol A. *Chemosphere* **1998**, *36*, 2149–2173. [CrossRef]

26. Almeida, S.; Raposo, A.; Almeida-Gonzalez, M.; Carrascosa, C. Bisphenol A: Food Exposure and Impact on Human Health. *Compr. Rev. Food Sci. Food Saf.* **2018**, *17*, 1503–1517. [CrossRef]

27. Kang, J.H.; Kondo, F.; Katayama, Y. Human exposure to bisphenol A. *Toxicology* **2006**, *226*, 79–89. [CrossRef]

28. Bolognesi, C.; Castle, L.; Cravedi, J.P.; Engel, K.H.; Fowler, P.; Franz, R.; Grob, K.; Gurtler, R.; Husoy, T.; Mennes, W.; et al. Scientific Opinion on the risks to public health related to the presence of bisphenol A (BPA) in foodstuffs: Executive summary. *EFSA J.* **2015**, *13*, 3978.

29. Andaluri, G.; Manickavachagam, M.; Suri, R. Plastic toys as a source of exposure to bisphenol-A and phthalates at childcare facilities. *Environ. Monit. Assess.* **2018**, *190*, 65. [CrossRef] [PubMed]

30. Ferrer, E.; Santoni, E.; Vittori, S.; Font, G.; Manes, J.; Sagratini, G. Simultaneous determination of bisphenol A, octylphenol, and nonylphenol by pressurised liquid extraction and liquid chromatography-tandem mass spectrometry in powdered milk and infant formulas. *Food Chem.* **2011**, *126*, 360–367. [CrossRef]

31. Dorival-Garcia, N.; Zafra-Gomez, A.; Navalon, A.; Vilchez, J.L. Improved sample treatment for the determination of bisphenol A and its chlorinated derivatives in sewage sludge samples by pressurized liquid extraction and liquid chromatography-tandem mass spectrometry. *Talanta* **2012**, *101*, 1–10. [CrossRef]

32. Tu, X.J.; Wu, S.Y.; Liu, W.Y.; Gao, Z.S.; Huang, S.K.; Chen, W.B. Sugaring-Out Assisted Liquid-Liquid Extraction Combined with High-Performance Liquid Chromatography-Fluorescence Detection for the Determination of Bisphenol A and Bisphenol B in Royal Jelly. *Food Anal. Meth.* **2019**, *12*, 705–711. [CrossRef]

33. Notardonato, I.; Passarella, S.; Ianiri, G.; Di Fiore, C.; Russo, M.V.; Avino, P. Analytical Scheme for Simultaneous Determination of Phthalates and Bisphenol A in Honey Samples Based on Dispersive Liquid-Liquid Microextraction Followed by GC-IT/MS. Effect of the Thermal Stress on PAE/BP-A Levels. *Methods Protoc.* **2020**, *3*, 23. [CrossRef]

34. Amini, R.; Khandaghi, J.; Mogaddam, M.R.A. Combination of Vortex-Assisted Liquid-Liquid Extraction and Air-Assisted Liquid-Liquid Microextraction for the Extraction of Bisphenol A and Bisphenol B in Canned Doogh Samples. *Food Anal. Meth.* **2018**, *11*, 3267–3275. [CrossRef]

35. Mo, R.H.; Liu, H.X.; Lai, R.T.; Deng, G.F.; Zhang, Z.Q.; Pei, Z.Z.; Li, H.B.; Xia, E.Q. Ultrasound-Assisted Upper Liquid Microextraction Coupled to Molecular Fluorescence for Detection of Bisphenol A in Commercial Beverages. *Food Anal. Meth.* **2017**, *10*, 1575–1581. [CrossRef]

36. Nascimento, C.F.; Rocha, F.R.P. Spectrofluorimetric determination of bisphenol A in tap waters by exploiting liquid-liquid microextraction in a sequential injection system. *Microchem. J.* **2018**, *137*, 429–434. [CrossRef]

37. Freire, M.G.; Santos, L.; Fernandes, A.M.; Coutinho, J.A.P.; Marrucho, I.M. An overview of the mutual solubilities of water-imidazolium-based ionic liquids systems. *Fluid Phase Equilibria* **2007**, *261*, 449–454. [CrossRef]

38. Lopez-Garcia, I.; Vicente-Martinez, Y.; Hernandez-Cordoba, M. Cloud point extraction assisted by silver nanoparticles for the determination of traces of cadmium using electrothermal atomic absorption spectrometry. *J. Anal. At. Spectrom.* **2015**, *30*, 375–380. [CrossRef]

39. Vicente-Martínez, Y.; Caravaca, M.; Soto-Meca, A.; De Francisco-Ortiz, O.; Gimeno, F. Graphene oxide and graphene oxide functionalized with silver nanoparticles as adsorbents of phosphates in waters. A comparative study. *Sci. Total Environ.* **2020**, *709*, 136111. [CrossRef]

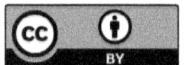

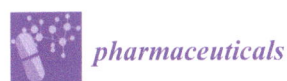

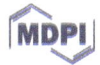

Article

Fragaria viridis Fruit Metabolites: Variation of LC-MS Profile and Antioxidant Potential during Ripening and Storage

Daniil N. Olennikov [1,*] **, Aina G. Vasilieva** [2] **and Nadezhda K. Chirikova** [2]

[1] Laboratory of Medical and Biological Research, Institute of General and Experimental Biology,
    Siberian Division, Russian Academy of Science, 6 Sakh'yanovoy Street, 670047 Ulan-Ude, Russia
[2] Department of Biology, Institute of Natural Sciences, North-Eastern Federal University, 58 Belinsky Street,
    677027 Yakutsk, Russia; aina_vasilieva@mail.ru (A.G.V.); hofnung@mail.ru (N.K.C.)
*   Correspondence: olennikovdn@mail.ru; Tel.: +7-9021-600-627

Received: 7 September 2020; Accepted: 21 September 2020; Published: 22 September 2020

Abstract: *Fragaria viridis* Weston or creamy strawberry is one of the less-known species of the *Fragaria* genus (Rosaceae family) with a wide distribution in Eurasia and is still in the shadow of more popular relatives *F. ananassa* (garden strawberry) or *F. vesca* (wild strawberry). Importantly, there is a lack of scientific knowledge on *F. viridis* compounds, their stability in the postharvest period, and bioactivity. In this study, metabolites of *F. viridis* fruits in three ripening stages were characterized with high-performance liquid chromatography with photodiode array and electrospray ionization triple quadrupole mass spectrometric detection (HPLC-PAD-ESI-tQ-MS). In total, 95 compounds of various groups including carbohydrates, organic acids, phenolics, and triterpenes, were identified for the first time. The quantitative content of the compounds varied differently during the ripening progress; some of them increased (anthocyanins, organic acids, and carbohydrates), while others demonstrated a decrease (ellagitannins, flavonols, etc.). The most abundant secondary metabolites of *F. viridis* fruits were ellagitannins (5.97–7.54 mg/g of fresh weight), with agrimoniin (1.41–2.63 mg/g) and lambertianin C (1.20–1.86 mg/g) as major components. Antioxidant properties estimated by in vitro assays (2,2-diphenyl-1-picrylhydrazyl radical (DPPH), 2,2'-azino-bis(3-ethylbenzothiazoline-6-sulfonic acid) cation radical (ABTS), ferric reducing antioxidant power (FRAP), and oxygen radical absorbance capacity (ORAC)) showed good antioxidant potential in all ripening stages of *F. viridis* fruits. The pilot human experiment on the effect of *F. viridis* fruit consumption on the serum total antioxidant capacity confirmed the effectiveness of this kind of strawberry. Postharvest storage of ripe fruits at 4 °C and 20 °C lead to declining content in the majority of compounds particularly ascorbic acid, ellagitannins, and flavonols, with the most significant loss at room temperature storage. These results suggest that *F. viridis* fruits are a prospective source of numerous metabolites that have potential health benefits.

Keywords: *Fragaria viridis*; creamy strawberry; ellagitannins; HPLC; mass spectrometry; fruit ripening; antioxidant potential

1. Introduction

Genus *Fragaria* (strawberry) of the Rosaceous family is a well-known source of dietary fruits that are popular all over the world and is widely consumed due to its unique taste and fragrance. The global production of strawberries has reached 9 million tons per year with maximal production levels in China, USA, and Mexico [1]. Such high consumption makes it necessary to examine the various aspects of biology, chemistry, cultivation, and technology of strawberry manufacturing. The most common studies devoted to the metabolic diversity of the *Fragaria* genus include many groups of compounds such as carbohydrates, organic acids, vitamins, anthocyanins, ellagitannins, flavonoids, and minerals [2]. Special attention is also paid to understanding the nature of postharvest changes in the chemical profile and physical properties of strawberry fruits in different storage conditions [3]. Despite the significance of strawberry as a food, pharmaceutical interest is also given due to the presence of various bioactive compounds including antioxidative [4], anti-inflammatory [5], antibacterial [6], anti-allergic [7], antidiabetic [8], and cancer preventive [9] properties. The antioxidative properties of various strawberries were discussed previously, and high effectiveness was revealed for *Fragaria* extracts and unprocessed fruits [10], thereby strengthening the interest to study strawberries. An age-old tradition of strawberry use resulted in the cultivation of many *Fragaria* species, not only popular species such as *F. ananassa* (garden strawberry), *F. vesca* (wild strawberry), and *F. moschata* (musk strawberry) but also exotic species like *F. chiloensis* (Chilean strawberry), *F. × bifera*, and *F. viridis* (creamy strawberry) [2]. In this regard, significant attention also needs to be focused on little-known strawberries, specifically *F. viridis* (Figure 1).

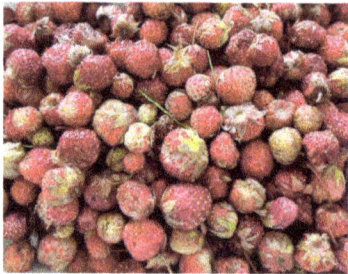

Figure 1. *Fragaria viridis* Weston (creamy strawberry).

Botanically, *F. viridis* is a green perennial herbaceous rhizomatous plant that can grow up to 25 cm tall with numerous adventitious roots. The stems are erect, and the length of the leaves are slightly longer, densely dressed with protruding trichomes. The stipules are narrow and brown, and the leaves have shaggy petioles from prominent trichomes that densely cover them. The inflorescences are small, corymbose, loose, and few-flowered and are dressed at the base with a solid or tripartite apical leaf. The pedicels are short and dressed with appressed or occasionally horizontally protruding trichomes. The flowers are relatively large, up to 2.5 cm in diameter, usually bisexual with triangular and lanceolate sepals. The petals are rounded, overlapping each other, short-clawed, and yellowish-white. The fragrant fruits are spherical, narrowed at the base, mostly yellowish-white, only reddish at the top, and rarely entirely pink or pale red, with achenes slightly immersed in the pulp, which are difficult to separate from the receptacle [11]. The fruits are separated from the stem together with sepals at inconsist density, and they are distinguished by good transportability, better that *F. vesca* and *F. ananassa*. The species is ecologically plastic. It grows in aspen-birch groves, on open grassy mountain slopes, on edges and glades of mountain forests, in meadows, and in meadow steppes in Europe, Russia, the Caucasus, and Western and Eastern Siberia. Sensory evaluation of *F. viridis* fruits demonstrated good taste and extraordinary fresh-fruity flavour [12].

The literature data about *F. viridis* are meagre and demonstrated that the essential oil of leaves consists of major components β-linalool, *n*-nonanal, tetradecanal, nerolidol, α-bisabolol, and phytol, which distinguishes it from fruit essential oil with the dominant *m/p*-xylene, isoledene, methyleugenol, α-cedrene, α-muurolene, and α-cedrol [13]. The known phenolics of *F. viridis* fruits are catechin, epicatechin, epigallocatechin gallate, cyanidin 3-*O*-glucoside, pelargonidin 3-*O*-glucoside, quercetin 3-*O*-glucoside, ellagic acid [14], quercetin 3-*O*-galactoside, quercetin 3-*O*-rutinoside, and chlorogenic acid [15], equalling the phenolic profile of *F. viridis* leaves. Both fruits and leaf extracts showed good radical-scavenging and ferric-reducing ability [14]. Despite easy cultivation, high breeding potential, and good sensory parameters, *F. viridis* remains one of the underutilized strawberry species [12]. The growing interest in new strawberries as perspective food sources obliges us to do more in-depth research, particularly in the area of *Fragaria* metabolomics using high-performance liquid chromatography-mass spectrometric techniques (nothing has been done previously with these techniques). It is, of course, of great interest in revealing specificities of metabolite changes in *F. viridis* fruits during the ripening progress as well as metabolite transformation during fruit storage.

In the present report, we realized the first detailed metabolomic profiling of *F. viridis* fruits in three stages of ripening (unripe, intermediate ripe, and fully ripe) using high-performance liquid chromatography with photodiode array and electrospray ionization triple quadrupole mass spectrometric detection (HPLC-PAD-ESI-tQ-MS), and antioxidant properties of *F. viridis* fruits were also studied in four in vitro models (scavenging capacity against 2,2-diphenyl-1-picrylhydrazyl radical and 2,2'-azino-bis(3-ethylbenzothiazoline-6-sulfonic acid) cation radical, ferric reducing antioxidant power, and oxygen radical absorbance capacity) during ripening progress and one pilot human experiment (serum total antioxidant capacity). Finally, the variation of selected compounds and antioxidant potential of ripe *F. viridis* fruits was investigated in response to cool and room temperature storage. To our knowledge, this is the first comprehensive study of *F. viridis* fruits.

2. Results and Discussion

2.1. Metabolites of F. viridis Fruits: LS-MS Profile

Chromatographic profiling of *F. viridis* fruit metabolites was completed by high-performance liquid chromatography with photodiode array and electrospray ionization mass spectrometric detection (HPLC-PAD-ESI-tQ-MS). The identification of components found in *F. viridis* was done after a precise interpretation of chromatographic (retention times) and spectral data (ultraviolet-visible spectra and mass spectral patterns) in comparison with reference standards and literature data. The extraction procedures of fresh fruits were preliminarily tested with various solvents (methanol, ethanol, isopropanol, water, and acetone), solvent–material ratios, temperatures (20–90 °C), and methods of extraction (ultrasound-, microwave-, and water-bath-assisted). The resultant protocol used was 100% methanol with a solvent–material ratio of 1:1 followed by 5 min homogenization and sonification (30 min, 45 °C). After comparison of *F. viridis* fruit extracts in three ripening stages (unripe, intermediate ripe, and fully ripe), the HPLC-ESI-tQ-MS chromatogram of fully ripe fruit extract showed the presence of the maximal amount of compounds (**95**) with interpretable data (Figure 2), details of which are provided in Table 1.

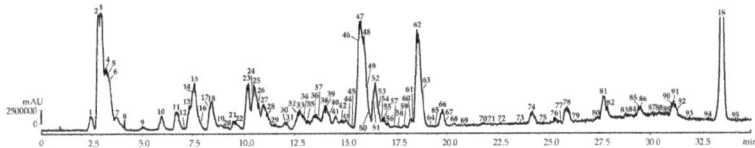

Figure 2. High-Performance Liquid Chromatography with Electrospray Ionization Triple Quadrupole Mass Spectrometric Detection (HPLC-ESI-tQ-MS) chromatogram (Total Ion Chromatogram (TIC) mode, negative ionization) of extract of *F. viridis* ripe fruits: compounds are numbered as listed in Table 1. IS—internal standard (genkwanin).

Table 1. Chromatographic (t_R) and mass-spectrometric data of compounds **1–95** found in *F. viridis* fruits.

No.	t_R, min	[M-H]−[I], [M-2H]−[II], [M-2H]2−[III], m/z	MS/MS, m/z	Group [a]	Compound [ref.] [b]	Presence in Ripening Stages [c]
1	2.51	341[I]		CR	Hexosyl-hexose [L] [16]	+/+/+
2	2.94	179[I]		CR	Hexose [L] [16]	+/+/+
3	3.08	191[I]		OA	Citric acid [S]	+/+/+
4	3.33	133[I]		OA	Malic acid [S]	+/+/+
5	3.41	149[I]		OA	Tartaric acid [S]	+/+/+
6	3.50	115[I]		OA	Fumaric acid [S]	+/+/+
7	3.82	175[I]		OA	Ascorbic acid [S]	+/+/+

Table 1. Cont.

No.	t_R, min	[M-H]$^{-}$ [I], [M-2H]$^{-}$ [II], [M-2H]$^{2-}$ [III], m/z	MS/MS, m/z	Group [a]	Compound [ref.] [b]	Presence in Ripening Stages [c]
8	4.22	89 [I]		OA	Oxalic acid [S]	+/+/+
9	5.03	331 [I]	169, 125	GA	1-O-Galloyl glucose [S] [17]	+/+/+
10	5.98	169 [I]		GA	Gallic acid [S] [17]	+/+/+
11	6.71	783 [I]; 391 [III]	633, 481, 301	ET	Pedunculagin [S] [18]	+/+/+
12	7.03	161 [I]		CO	Umbelliferone [S] [19]	+/+/+
13	7.43	353 [I]	191, 179, 173, 135	HC	4-O-Caffeoylquinic acid [S] [20]	+/+/+
14	7.50	633 [I]	481, 331, 301	ET	Strictinin [S] [18]	+/+/+
15	7.58	353 [I]	191, 165	HC	5-O-Caffeoylquinic acid [S] [20]	+/+/+ [15]
16	7.44	633 [I]	481, 331, 301	ET	Strictinin isomer [L] [18]	+/+/+
17	7.83	353 [I]	191, 179, 135	HC	3-O-Caffeoylquinic acid [S] [20]	+/+/+
18	8.01	783 [I]; 391 [III]	633, 481, 301	ET	Pedunculagin isomer [L] [18]	+/+/+
19	8.85	577 [I]	289	PC	Procyanidin B2 (catechin dimer) [S] [17]	+/+/+
20	9.15	609 [II]	447, 285	CY	Cyanidin 3-O-sophoroside [S] [21]	−/+/+
21	9.48	577 [I]	289	PC	Procyanidin B4 (catechin-epicatechin dimer) [S] [17]	+/+/+
22	9.67	593 [II]	431, 269	CY	Pelargonidin di-O-hexoside [L] [21]	−/+/+
23	10.14	289 [I]		CT	Catechin [S] [21]	+/+/+ [14]
24	10.49	325 [I]	163, 119	HC	p-Coumaric acid O-hexoside [L] [22]	+/+/+
25	10.58	325 [I]	163, 119	HC	p-Coumaric acid 4-O-glucoside [S] [22]	+/+/+
26	10.79	593 [II]	447, 285	CY	Cyanidin 3-O-rutinoside [S] [21]	−/+/+
27	11.02	447 [II]	285	CY	Cyanidin 3-O-glucoside [S] [21]	−/+/+ [14]
28	11.14	577 [II]	431, 269	CY	Pelargonidin 3-O-rutinoside [S] [21]	−/+/+
29	11.52	431 [II]	269	CY	Pelargonidin 3-O-glucoside [S] [21]	+/+/+ [14]
30	12.01	933 [I]; 466 [III]	301	ET	Castalagin [S] [18,23]	+/+/+
31	12.11	865 [I]	577, 289	PC	Procyanidin C2 (catechin trimer) [S] [17]	+/+/+
32	12.63	593 [II]	447, 285	CY	Cyanidin O-p-coumaroyl-O-hexoside [L] [21]	−/+/+
33	12.78	935 [I]; 467 [III]	633, 463, 301	ET	Casuarictin isomer [18]	+/+/+
34	12.88	933 [I]; 466 [III]	301	ET	Castalagin isomer [L] [18,23]	+/+/+
35	13.09	1103 [I]; 551 [III]	951, 933, 783, 633, 481, 301	ET	Sanguiin H2 [S] [18,24]	+/+/+
36	13.41	865 [I]	577, 289	PC	Procyanidin trimer (catechin/epicatechin trimer) [L] [17]	+/+/+
37	13.70	577 [II]	431, 269	CY	Pelargonidin O-p-coumaroyl-O-hexoside [L] [21]	−/+/+
38	13.98	489 [II]	447, 285	CY	Cyanidin O-acetyl-O-hexoside [L] [21]	−/+/+
39	14.03	625 [I]	463, 301	FG	Quercetin 3-O-sophoroside [S] [25]	+/+/+
40	14.11	935 [I]; 467 [III]	633, 463, 301	ET	Casuarictin isomer [18]	+/+/+
41	14.51	433 [I]	301	ET	Ellagic acid O-pentoside [L] [26,27]	+/+/+
42	14.88	1567 [I]; 783 [III]	933, 633, 301	ET	Sanguiin H10 [S] [18,24]	+/+/+
43	15.01	447 [I]	301	ET	Ellagic acid O-desoxyhexoside [L] [26,27]	+/+/+
44	15.11	1103 [I]; 551 [III]	933, 783, 633, 481, 301	ET	Sanguiin H2 isomer [L] [18,24]	+/+/+
45	15.34	609 [I]	463, 301	FG	Quercetin 3-O-rutinoside [S] [25]	+/+/+ [15]
46	15.53	1869 [I]; 934 [III]	1567, 1265, 935, 783, 633, 481, 301	ET	Sanguiin H6 isomer [L] [18,24]	+/+/+
47	15.72	1401 [III]	1235, 933, 783, 633, 301	ET	Lambertianin C [S] [18,24]	+/+/+

Table 1. *Cont.*

No.	t_R, min	[M-H]⁻ I, [M-2H]⁻ II, [M-2H]²⁻ III, m/z	MS/MS, m/z	Group [a]	Compound [ref.] [b]	Presence in Ripening Stages [c]
48	15.81	473 II	431, 269	CY	Pelargonidin *O*-acetyl-*O*-hexoside [L] [21]	−/+/+
49	15.94	463 I	301	FG	Quercetin 3-*O*-glucoside [S] [25]	+/+/+ [14]
50	16.02	477 I	301	FG	Quercetin 3-*O*-glucuronide [S] [25]	+/+/+
51	16.33	1103 I; 551 III	801, 783, 499, 481, 319, 301	ET	Agrimonic acid A [S] [28]	+/+/+
52	16.50	1869 I; 934 III	1701, 1567, 1265, 1085, 935, 783, 633, 481, 301	ET	Sanguiin H6 [S] [18,24]	+/+/+
53	16.71	301 I	229	ET	Ellagic acid [S] [18]	+/+/+ [14]
54	16.81	1103 I; 551 III	801, 783, 499, 481, 319, 301	ET	Agrimonic acid B [S] [28]	+/+/+
55	16.95	433	301	FG	Quercetin 3-*O*-xyloside [S] [25]	+/+/+
56	17.07	433	301	FG	Quercetin 3-*O*-arabinoside [S] [25]	+/+/+
57	17.41	593 I	447, 285	FG	Kaempferol 3-*O*-rutinoside [S] [25]	+/+/+
58	17.56	447 I	285	FG	Kaempferol 3-*O*-glucoside [S] [25]	+/+/+
59	17.92	461 I	285	FG	Kaempferol 3-*O*-glucuronide [S] [25]	+/+/+
60	18.21	609 I	463, 301	FG	Quercetin 3-*O*-(6″-*O*-*p*-coumaroyl)-glucoside [S] [25]	+/+/+
61	18.29	609 I	463, 301	FG	Quercetin *O*-*p*-coumaroyl-*O*-hexoside [L] [25]	+/+/+
62	18.50	1869 I; 934 III	1567, 1265, 1085, 935, 783, 633, 481, 301	ET	Agrimoniin [S] [23,29]	+/+/+
63	18.68	1018 III	1691, 1567, 1265, 1209, 935, 783, 633, 481, 301	ET	Fragariin A [L] [23,29]	+/+/+
64	19.06	549 I	463, 301	FG	Quercetin *O*-malonyl-*O*-hexoside [L] [30,31]	+/+/+
65	19.42	549 I	463, 301	FG	Quercetin 3-*O*-(6″-*O*-malonyl)-glucoside [S] [30,31]	+/+/+
66	19.75	593 I	447, 285	FG	Kaempferol 3-*O*-(6″-*O*-*p*-coumaroyl)-glucoside [S] [25]	+/+/+
67	19.83	939 I	787, 635, 483, 331, 169	GA	1,2,3,4,6-Penta-*O*-galloylglucose [S] [17]	+/+/+
68	20.39	533 I	447, 285	FG	Kaempferol *O*-malonyl-*O*-hexoside [L] [30,31]	+/+/+
69	20.82	533 I	447, 285	FG	Kaempferol 3-*O*-(6″-*O*-malonyl)-glucoside [S] [30,31]	+/+/+
70	21.83	505 I	463, 301	FG	Quercetin 3-*O*-(2″-*O*-acetyl)-glucoside [S] [32]	+/+/+
71	22.14	505 I	463, 301	FG	Quercetin 3-*O*-(6″-*O*-acetyl)-glucoside [S] [32]	+/+/+
72	22.67	489 I	447, 285	FG	Kaempferol *O*-acetyl-*O*-hexoside [L] [30–32]	+/+/+
73	23.52	489 I	447, 285	FG	Kaempferol *O*-acetyl-*O*-hexoside [L] [30–32]	−/+/+
74	24.21	301 I		FG	Quercetin [S] [25]	+/+/+ [14]
75	24.78	811 I	649, 487	TR	Tormentic acid di-*O*-hexoside [L] [16]	+/+/+
76	25.34	285 I		FG	Kaempferol [S] [25]	+/+/+
77	25.54	795 I	633, 471	TR	Pomolic acid di-*O*-hexoside [L] [16]	+/+/+
78	25.87	649 I	487	TR	Tormentic acid *O*-hexoside [L] [16]	+/+/+
79	26.41	547 I	505, 463, 301	FG	Quercetin 3-*O*-(2″,6″-di-*O*-acetyl)-glucoside [S] [32]	+/+/+

Table 1. *Cont.*

No.	t_R, min	[M-H]−I, [M-2H]−II, [M-2H]2−III, m/z	MS/MS, m/z	Group a	Compound [ref.] b	Presence in Ripening Stages c
80	27.52	591 I	549, 505, 463, 301	FG	Quercetin O-acetyl-O-malonyl-O-hexoside L [30–32]	+/+/+
81	27.73	487 I		TR	Tormentic acid S [16]	+/+/+
82	27.89	461 I	315, 301	ET	Ellagic acid O-methyl ester-O-desoxyhexoside L [26,27]	+/+/+
83	28.78	633 I	471	TR	Pomolic acid O-hexoside L [16]	+/+/+
84	29.14	695 I	609, 463, 301	FG	Quercetin O-malonyl-O-p-coumaroyl-O-hexoside L [30–32]	+/+/+
85	29.49	695 I	609, 463, 301	FG	Quercetin O-malonyl-O-p-coumaroyl-O-hexoside L [30–32]	+/+/+
86	29.57	475 I	329, 301	ET	Ellagic acid di-O-methyl ester-O-desoxyhexoside L [26,27]	+/+/+
87	30.08	531 I	489, 447, 285	FG	Kaempferol di-O-acetyl-O-hexoside L [30–32]	+/+/+
88	30.41	651 I	609, 463, 301	FG	Quercetin O-acetyl-O-p-coumaroyl-O-hexoside L [30–32]	+/+/+
89	30.92	575 I	533, 489, 447, 285	FG	Kaempferol O-acetyl-O-malonyl-O-hexoside L [30–32]	+/+/+
90	31.02	679 I	593, 447, 285	FG	Kaempferol O-malonyl-O-p-coumaroyl-O-hexoside L [30–32]	+/+/+
91	31.22	471 I		TR	Pomolic acid S [16]	+/+/+
92	31.38	679 I	593, 447, 285	FG	Kaempferol O-malonyl-O-p-coumaroyl-O-hexoside L [30–32]	+/+/+
93	31.98	635 I	593, 447, 285	FG	Kaempferol O-acetyl-O-p-coumaroyl-O-hexoside L [30–32]	+/+/+
94	32.86	693 I	651, 609, 463, 301	FG	Quercetin di-O-acetyl-O-p-coumaroyl-O-hexoside L [30–32]	+/+/+
95	34.26	737 I	695, 651, 609, 463, 301	FG	Quercetin O-acetyl-O-malonyl-O-p-coumaroyl-O-hexoside L [30–32]	+/+/+

a Groups of compounds: CO—coumarins; CR—carbohydrates; CY—anthocyanins; ET—ellagitannins; FG—flavonols and flavonol glycosides; GA—gallic acid derivatives; HC—hydroxycinnamates; OA—organic acids; PC—procyanidins; and TR—triterpenes. b Compound identification was based on comparison of retention time, UV and MS spectral data with reference standard (S), or interpretation of UV and MS spectral data and comparison with literature data (L). c Compounds were detected (+) or not (−) in unripe/intermediate ripe/fully ripe *F. viridis* fruits; if compound was previously reported in *F. viridis* fruits, the reference no. is mentioned.

2.1.1. Carbohydrates

Two types of carbohydrates were discovered in *F. viridis* fruits including hexosyl-hexose (*m/z* 341; **1**) and hexose (*m/z* 179; **2**). The HPLC-MS method used does not allow for identification of the nature of carbohydrates, so we used the HPLC-DAD procedure demonstrating the presence of three compounds identified as glucose, fructose, and saccharose (Figure S1), usual mono- and disaccharides of strawberry fruits [2].

2.1.2. Organic Acids

Citric (**3**), malic (**4**), tartaric (**5**), fumaric (**6**), ascorbic (**7**), and oxalic acids (**8**) were the organic acids found in *F. viridis* fruits. All mentioned compounds were shown previously in *F. ananassa* [33] and *F. vesca* [34].

2.1.3. Gallic Acid Derivatives

Gallic acid (**10**), 1-*O*-glucoside (**9**), and 1,2,3,4,6-penta-*O*-galloylglucose (**67**) were identified by comparison with reference standards. Gallic acid derivatives and gallotannins are not typical phenolics of *Fragaria* genus, but gallic acid is a metabolite found in *F. ananassa* [2] and compound **67** is detected in *F. ananassa* fruits [35] and *F. vesca* leaves [36].

2.1.4. Ellagic Acid Derivatives and Ellagitannins

Ellagic acid (**53**), four ellagic acid glycosides (**41**, **43**, **82**, and **86**), and eighteen ellagitannins (**11**, **14**, **16**, **18**, **30**, **33**–**35**, **40**, **42**, **44**, **46**, **47**, **51**, **52**, **54**, **62**, and **63**) were found in *F. viridis* fruits. The ellagic acid glycosides were ellagic acid *O*-pentoside (**41**), ellagic acid *O*-desoxyhexoside (**43**), ellagic acid *O*-methyl ester-*O*-desoxyhexoside (**82**), and ellagic acid di-*O*-methyl ester-*O*-desoxyhexoside (**86**) due to the presence of ions with m/z 301 typical for ellagic acid derivatives [18,23] and the size of loss particles with m/z 132 (*O*-pentose) or 146 (*O*-desoxyhexose) [16].

Known strawberry ellagitannins, lambertianin C (**47**), sanguiin H10 (**42**), sanguiin H6 (**52**; **46** as isomer), sanguiin H2 (**35**; **44** as isomer), and pedunculagin (**11**; **18** as isomer), were identified using reference standards [18]. The literature data gave additional identification of three *Fragaria* ellagitannin structures: strictinin (**14** and **16**), castalagin (**30** and **34**), and casuarictin (**33** and **40**) [18]. Agrimoniin (**62**) gave typical ions of deprotonated fragment [M-H]⁻ (m/z 1869) and double-charged particle [M-2H]²⁻ (m/z 934). The further MS/MS fragmentation of molecule **62** demonstrated the loss of fragments of hexahydroxydiphenoyl (HHDP; 302 Da), *bis*-HHDP-glucose (*bis*-HHDP-Glc; 784 Da), and galloyl-*bis*-HHDP-glucose (Gall-*bis*-HHDP-Glc; 934 Da), creating a cascade of ions with m/z 1567 [(M-H)-HHDP]⁻, 1265 [(M-H)-2×HHDP]⁻, 1085 [(M-H)-(*bis*-HHDP-Glc)]⁻, 935 [(M-H)-(Gall-*bis*-HHDP-Glc)]⁻, 633 [(M-H)-(Gall-*bis*-HHDP-Glc)-HHDP]⁻, and 481 [((*bis*-HHDP-Glc)-H)-HHDP]⁻ [23,29]. Agrimoniin was previously identified as the main ellagitannin of strawberry fruits from *F. vesca* and *F. ananassa* [24] and were found in *F. viridis* for the first time in this study. Compound **63** with a [M-2H]²⁻ ion with m/z 1018 gave the weak deprotonated ion [M-H]⁻ (m/z 2037); after decarboxylation (−44 Da) and loss of HHDP, gave the fragment with m/z 1691; and then degraded to fragments with m/z 1567 (loss of trihydroxy benzene) and 1265 (loss of HHDP). The alternative pathway of fragmentation of the particle with m/z 1691 led to the formation of de-HHDP-glucosylated ion with m/z 1209 and the fragments with m/z 935 [Gall-*bis*-HHDP-Glc–H]⁻, 783 [(*bis*-HHDP-Glc)-H]⁻, 633 [((Gall-*bis*-HHDP-Glc)-H)-HHDP]⁻, and 481 [((*bis*-HHDP-Glc)-H)-HHDP]⁻. The close mass spectrometric pattern gave the known strawberry ellagitannin fragariin A found in *F. ananassa* and has the structure of galloylated derivative of agrimoniin [29]. Two isomeric ellagitannins, **51** and **54**, were identified as biogenetic relatives to agrimoniin compounds, agrimonic acids A and B, respectively [28].

After all, only ellagic acid was mentioned previously as a component of *F. viridis* [14], indicating that this is the first report describing the profile of ellagic acid derivatives from *F. viridis* fruits. Traditionally used strawberries, such as *F. ananassa* and *F. vesca*, are a good source of ellagitannins and ellagic acid glycosides [2,18]. Lambertianin C, saguiins, and agrimoniin were also found in many varieties of cultivated strawberries, demonstrating their obligate position in the *Fragaria* metabolome [2,18,26,27].

2.1.5. Hydroxycinnamates and Coumarins

Four known hydroxycinnamates were identified by comparison with reference standards, including 4-*O*-caffeoylquinic acid (**13**), 5-*O*-caffeoylquinic acid (**15**), 3-*O*-caffeoylquinic acid (**17**), and *p*-coumaric acid 4-*O*-glucoside (**25**). Only 5-*O*-caffeoylquinic acid was previously found in *F. viridis* [15]. Component **24** produced a deprotonated ion with m/z 325 and dehexosylated fragment with m/z 163 characteristic for *p*-coumaric acid *O*-hexoside [22]. One coumarin umbelliferone (**12**) was also identified by comparison with a reference standard.

2.1.6. Catechins and Procyanidins

Catechin (**23**) and procyanidins B2 (**19**), B4 (**21**), and C2 (**31**) as well as an isomer to **31** catechin/epicatechin trimer **36** were detected in *F. viridis* fruits. Monomer **23** was already found in whole plant *F. viridis* [14].

2.1.7. Anthocyanins

Derivatives of cyanidin (**20**, **26**, **27**, **32**, and **38**) and pelargonidin (**22**, **28**, **29**, **37**, and **48**) were found in *F. viridis* fruits based on UV-Vis patterns (525–535 nm for cyanidins and 498–505 nm for pelargonidins) and mass spectral behaviour of aglycone fragments (m/z 285 for cyanidins and 269 for pelargonidins). Five phenolics were identified after comparing spectra with reference standards: cyanidin-3-*O*-sophoroside (**20**), cyanidin-3-*O*-rutinoside (**26**), cyanidin-3-*O*-glucoside (**27**), pelargonidin-3-*O*-rutinoside (**28**), and pelargonidin-3-*O*-glucoside (**29**). Anthocyanin *O*-glucosides **27** and **29** are the most frequent phenolic pigments of *Fragaria* fruits [2,14,26], and *O*-rutinoside **28** was found in *F. ananassa* [26]. Compound **22** gave an [M-2H]⁻ ion with m/z 593 and two dehexosylated fragments with m/z 431 [(M-2H)-hexose]⁻ and 269 [(M-2H)-2×hexose]⁻ and was determined as pelargonidin di-*O*-hexoside. The closest phenolic to **22** is pelargonidin-3-*O*-sophoroside detected in *F. ananassa* [27]. Two compounds, **32** and **37**, have additional maxima in UV spectra at approximately 312 nm characteristic to acylic anthocyanins with *p*-coumaroyl fragments [37], and they were preliminary determined as cyanidin *O*-*p*-coumaroyl-*O*-hexoside (**32**) and pelargonidin *O*-*p*-coumaroyl-*O*-hexoside (**37**). Two mono-acetylated *O*-hexosides, **38** and **48**, gave mass spectral ion fragments with m/z 42 and 162 and were identified as cyanidin *O*-acetyl-*O*-hexoside (**38**) and pelargonidin *O*-acetyl-*O*-hexoside (**48**). The known acylated anthocyanins of *Fragaria* species traditionally have moieties of acetic and malonic acids [2,26,27,34] so the *p*-coumaroyl esters of anthocyanins were found in *Fragaria* fruits for the first time.

2.1.8. Flavonols

Flavonols were defined by their specific UV spectral patterns with absorption at 256/268/360 nm for quercetin derivatives and 265/343 nm for kaempferol derivatives [17]. Thirty-four compounds were flavonols found in *F. viridis* fruits including two aglycones—quercetin (**74**) and kaempferol (**76**)—and 32 glycosides with non-acylated and acylated fragments linked with carbohydrate moieties.

Quercetin glycosides were the most diverse group of *F. viridis* phenolics with 19 members, some of which were identified using standard references. There are non-acylated compounds, such as quercetin-3-*O*-sophoroside (**39**), quercetin-3-*O*-rutinoside (**45**; rutin), quercetin-3-*O*-glucoside (**49**; isoquercitrin), quercetin-3-*O*-glucuronide (**50**; miquelianin), quercetin-3-*O*-xyloside (**55**; reynoutrin), and quercetin-3-*O*-arabinoside (**56**; avicularin) as well as acylated derivatives quercetin-3-*O*-(6''-*O*-*p*-coumaroyl)-glucoside (**60**; helichrysoside), quercetin-3-*O*-(6''-*O*-malonyl)-glucoside (**65**), quercetin-3-*O*-(2''-*O*-acetyl)-glucoside (**70**), quercetin-3-*O*-(6''-*O*-acetyl)-glucoside (**71**), and quercetin-3-*O*-(2'',6''-di-*O*-acetyl)-glucoside (**79**). Compounds **45**, **49**, and **74** were reported in *F. viridis* by Raudonis et al. [14] and in *F. ananassa* by many authors [26,27,35]. The remaining quercetin glycosides were acylated derivatives of quercetin *O*-hexoside giving the same MS/MS fragments with m/z 463 (quercetin *O*-hexoside) and 301 (aglycone). Compound **61** had [M-H]⁻ at m/z 609 and MS/MS fragmentation close to **60**, making it an isomer with the most likely structure of quercetin *O*-*p*-coumaroyl-*O*-hexoside. Glycoside **64** gave deprotonated ions with m/z 549 and is an isomer of quercetin 3-*O*-(6''-*O*-malonyl)-glucoside (**65**) or quercetin *O*-malonyl-*O*-hexoside.

A series of mixed *O*-acylated quercetin *O*-hexosides had higher retention times than quercetin. Their specific MS patterns showed the loss of fragments with m/z 42 (acetyl), 86 (malonyl), and/or 146 (*p*-coumaroyl). Five combinations of acylated quercetin *O*-hexosides were found, such as acetyl/malonyl (**80**), malonyl/*p*-coumaroyl (**84** and **85**), acetyl/*p*-coumaroyl (**88**), di-acetyl/*p*-coumaroyl

(**94**), and acetyl/malonyl/*p*-coumaroyl (**95**). To date, there are no known analogues of compounds **80**, **84**, **85**, **88**, **94**, and **95**, but most likely, structures are quercetin-3-*O*-glucosides with a substituted glucose moiety at positions 2″, 3″, 4″, and 6″.

Thirteen kaempferol glycosides were found in *F. viridis* fruits, and four were partially identified using a comparison of t_R, UV, and mass spectrometric data with reference standards. There were kaempferol-3-*O*-rutinoside (**57**; nicotiflorin), kaempferol-3-*O*-glucoside (**58**; astragalin), kaempferol-3-*O*-glucuronide (**59**), kaempferol-3-*O*-(6″-*O*-*p*-coumaroyl)-glucoside (**66**; tiliroside), and kaempferol-3-*O*-(6″-*O*-malonyl)-glucoside (**69**). No kaempferol glycosides were previously found in *F. viridis*, but other *Fragaria* species were reported to contain compounds **57**, **58**, **59**, and **66** (*F. ananassa*, *F. vesca*, and *F. chiloensis*) [2]. Non-mixed acylated kaempferol *O*-hexosides were defined as kaempferol *O*-malonyl-*O*-hexosides (**68**), kaempferol *O*-acetyl-*O*-hexosides (**72**,**73**), and kaempferol di-*O*-acetyl-*O*-hexoside (**87**). Among the possible known analogs of observed flavonols, kaempferol-3-*O*-(2″-*O*-malonyl)-glucoside (for **68**), kaempferol-3-*O*-(6″-*O*-acetyl)-glucoside (for **72**,**73**), and kaempferol-3-*O*-(3″,4″-di-*O*-acetyl)-glucoside (for **87**) should be mentioned [38]. Mixed acylated kaempferol *O*-hexosides were also found in *F. viridis* extract and identified using the same principle as quercetin *O*-hexosides; these compounds include kaempferol *O*-acetyl-*O*-malonyl-*O*-hexoside (**89**), kaempferol *O*-malonyl-*O*-*p*-coumaroyl-*O*-hexosides (**90** and **92**), and kaempferol *O*-acetyl-*O*-*p*-coumaroyl-*O*-hexoside (**93**). Contrary to mixed quercetin *O*-hexosides, there are some known variants of mixed kaempferol *O*-hexosides like kaempferol-*O*-3-(3″/4″-*O*-acetyl-6″-*O*-*p*-coumaroyl)-glucosides as an alternative for **93** [38].

2.1.9. Triterpenes

Six compounds were triterpenes, and two reference standard defined compounds were tormentic acid (**81**) and pomolic acid (**91**). Both compounds are the usual Rosaceous metabolites [39,40] but were not found in *Fragaria* fruits early studies. Glycosidic derivatives of **81** and **91** were described as two *O*-hexosides, **78** and **83**, and two di-*O*-hexosides, **75** and **77**, and are unusual components of strawberry fruits.

2.2. Quantitative Content and LS-MS Profile Variation of F. viridis Fruits during Ripening

We studied *F. viridis* fruits at three different stages of ripening, including unripe fruits, the stage of technological ripeness (intermediate stage), and the stage of full ripeness (Table 2). The total simple carbohydrate (mono- and disaccharides) content in *F. viridis* fruits varied from 41.14 mg/g in the unripe stage to 45.17 mg/g in ripe fruits. The main components were monosaccharides, glucose, and fructose, with a concentration of 41.10–45.16 mg/g responsible for the sweet taste of *F. viridis* fruits. Monosaccharides are the dominant sugars of *F. ananassa* [33,41,42] and *F. vesca* [43], but in some strawberry varieties, it happens that saccharose shows the highest content [34,44]. The sugar content of *F. ananassa* fruits demonstrated the same trend during ripening, with the lowest content in unripe fruits (3.61–4.45 mg/g) rising to the ripe stage with 4.82–8.20 mg/g [33], indicating the close character of carbohydrates changing in strawberries.

The highest total content of organic acids was found in ripe fruits of *F. viridis* (7.88 mg/g) and the lowest was found in the unripe stage (4.25 mg/g) including the greatest share of citric acid in all stages of ripening (2.83–5.63 mg/g). The remaining organic acids were minor components with concentration values 0.42–0.59 mg/g for malic acid, 0.37–0.42 mg/g for tartaric acid, 0.01–0.07 mg/g for fumaric acid, and trace–0.05 mg/g for oxalic acid. This results in an increase in the acidity of *F. viridis* fruits during ripening, which had a positive impact on strawberry taste. The domination of citric acid was demonstrated previously in many *F. ananassa* cultivars grown in Slovenia (4.4–10.5 mg/g) [42], Pakistan (12.0–14.3 mg/g) [33], and Turkey (5–10 mg/g) [45] as well as in *F. vesca* (5.6 mg/g) [34]. Moreover, the fruit development resulted in an increase in organic acids in strawberries [33], and malic, tartaric, fumaric, and oxalic acids were the minor acids in other *Fragaria* fruits [33,34,45].

Particularly noteworthy was the presence of a high level of ascorbic acid, up to 1.12 mg/g in ripe *F. viridis* fruits, that was significantly more than found in *F. vesca* (0.4 mg/g) and *F. ananassa* (0.25–0.9 mg/g) [33,45].

Galic acid derivatives showed trace (gallic acid, 1,2,3,4,6-penta-*O*-galloylglucose) or low-level content (1-*O*-galloyl glucose) without significant variation during ripening (0.04–0.05 mg/g). In contrast to the gallic acid derivatives, hydroxycinnamates were important compounds of *F. viridis* fruits with medium content although the amount decreased during ripening from 0.97 mg/g to 0.60 mg/g. The highest level was found for the *p*-coumaric acid 4-*O*-glucoside (0.29–0.35 mg/g), its isomer **24** (0.08–0.14 mg/g), and 5-*O*-caffeoylquinic acid (0.14–0.28 mg/g). The early study of 5-*O*-caffeoylquinic acid content variation in dry strawberries showed it ranging from 1.8 to 2.9 mg/g for *F. vesca*, from 1.2 to 1.7 mg/g for *F. viridis*, and from 0.7 to 1.8 mg/g for *F. moschata* [15]. The level of coumaroyl glycosides in Norway *F. ananassa* cultivars varied from 0.02 mg/g to 0.14 mg/g with maximal content in fully ripe fruits [25], which is different from our findings.

The most significant groups of phenolics with the highest content in all stages of maturity of *F. viridis* fruits were ellagitannins and ellagic acid derivatives. The general rule of ellagitannin variation in *F. viridis* fruits (with few exceptions) was decreasing content during ripening. This was particularly manifested in dominant compounds of agrimoniin (2.63→1.41 mg/g), lambertianin C (1.86→1.20 mg/g), fragariin A (0.93→0.63 mg/g), and sanguiin H6 (0.36→0.22 mg/g), where values were maximal in unripe fruits. The decrease of ellagitannin level in strawberry fruits during development was previously shown in some Norway cultivars of *F. ananassa*; the variation of agrimoniin content in Blink, Polka, and Senga cultivars was 0.72→0.57, 0.66→0.58, and 0.68→0.55 mg/g, respectively [25]. The most drastic fall in ellagitannin content, from 1.14 to 0.30 mg/g, was found in Italian cultivars of *F. ananassa* [18]. The most likely reason for the ellagitannin changes is due to increasing activity of specific enzymes, such as tannases, reaching the highest values in ripening fruits [46].

This is further illustrated by the slight rising content of ellagic acid, some ellagic acid *O*-glycosides, and low molecular weight ellagitannins (as pedunculagin, strictinin, castalagin, and casuarictin) that can be considered the breakdown products of ellagitannin molecules, but of course, this issue needs to be discussed additionally.

Catechins and procyanidins are compounds with medium levels in *F. viridis* fruits, for which the total concentration decreased from unripe to the ripe stage (0.29→0.09 mg/g). The content of major components showed the same behaviour, including catechin (0.11→0.05 mg/g), procyanidin B2 (0.09→0.02 mg/g), and procyanidin C2 (0.05→0.01 mg/g). Aaby et al. [25] reported similar data for 27 cultivars of *F. ananassa* for the content of catechin (0.02–0.08 mg/g), procyanidin dimers (0.05–0.16 mg/g), and trimers (0.05–0.19 mg/g).

Anthocyanins, which are important phenolics of strawberries, were at a low level in *F. viridis* characterized by slight red pigmentation of the outer layer of fruits and depigmented pulp. It is for this reason that the unripe and pre-ripe fruits had trace anthocyanin content. In the ripe stage, the domination of pelargonidin 3-*O*-glucoside (0.06 mg/g), cyanidin 3-*O*-glucoside (0.05 mg/g), and pelargonidin 3-*O*-rutinoside (0.03 mg/g) was observed. The remaining pigments were found in trace levels. Pelargonidin and cyanidin glycosides were also found as components of phenolic pigments of all studied strawberries including *F. ananassa* [47], *F. vesca*, and *F. moschata* [14]. It is to be expected that the ripening of strawberry fruits resulted in intense pigmentation caused by the accumulation of anthocyanins, as in the case of Norway cultivars from 0.2 mg/g in the pre-ripe stage to 0.8 mg/g in fully ripe fruits of *F. ananassa* [25].

Table 2. Content of compounds in unripe, intermediate ripe, and fully ripe fruits of *F. viridis*, mg/g of fresh fruit weight ± S.D.

Compound	Stage of Ripeness		
	Unripe	Intermediate	Ripe
Carbohydrates			
Hexose (glucose+fructose)	41.10 ± 0.82	43.26 ± 0.90	45.16 ± 0.92

Table 2. *Cont.*

Compound	Stage of Ripeness		
	Unripe	Intermediate	Ripe
Hexosyl-hexose (saccharose)	0.04 ± 0.00	0.06 ± 0.00	0.11 ± 0.00
Total carbohydrates	41.14	43.32	45.27
Organic acids			
Ascorbic acid	0.62 ± 0.02	0.86 ± 0.02	1.12 ± 0.02
Citric acid	2.83 ± 0.06	3.18 ± 0.07	5.63 ± 0.11
Malic acid	0.42 ± 0.01	0.45 ± 0.01	0.59 ± 0.02
Tartaric acid	0.37 ± 0.01	0.40 ± 0.01	0.42 ± 0.01
Fumaric acid	0.01 ± 0.00	0.03 ± 0.00	0.07 ± 0.00
Oxalic acid	traces	traces	0.05 ± 0.00
Total organic acids	4.25	4.92	7.88
Gallic acid derivatives			
Gallic acid	traces	0.01 ± 0.00	0.01 ± 0.00
1-*O*-Galloyl glucose	0.05 ± 0.00	0.03 ± 0.00	0.03 ± 0.00
1,2,3,4,6-Penta-*O*-galloylglucose	traces	traces	traces
Total gallic acid derivatives	0.05	0.04	0.04
Hydroxycinnamates and coumarins			
p-Coumaric acid 4-*O*-glucoside	0.35 ± 0.01	0.33 ± 0.01	0.29 ± 0.00
p-Coumaric acid *O*-hexoside **24**	0.14 ± 0.00	0.11 ± 0.00	0.08 ± 0.00
3-*O*-Caffeoylquinic acid	0.12 ± 0.00	0.08 ± 0.00	0.04 ± 0.00
4-*O*-Caffeoylquinic acid	0.08 ± 0.00	0.07 ± 0.00	0.05 ± 0.00
5-*O*-Caffeoylquinic acid	0.28 ± 0.00	0.21 ± 0.00	0.14 ± 0.00
Umbelliferone	traces	traces	traces
Total hydroxycinnamates and coumarins	0.97	0.80	0.60
Ellagic acid derivatives and ellagitannins			
Ellagic acid	0.10 ± 0.00	0.10 ± 0.00	0.12 ± 0.00
Ellagic acid *O*-pentoside **41**	0.05 ± 0.00	0.09 ± 0.00	0.11 ± 0.00
Ellagic acid *O*-desoxyhexoside **43**	0.01 ± 0.00	0.04 ± 0.00	0.07 ± 0.00
Ellagic acid *O*-methyl ester-*O*-desoxyhexoside **82**	0.14 ± 0.00	0.16 ± 0.00	0.24 ± 0.00
Ellagic acid di-*O*-methyl ester-*O*-desoxyhexoside **86**	0.10 ± 0.00	0.18 ± 0.00	0.30 ± 0.00
Pedunculagin	0.26 ± 0.00	0.30 ± 0.01	0.32 ± 0.01
Pedunculagin isomer **18**	0.05 ± 0.00	0.07 ± 0.00	0.11 ± 0.00
Strictinin isomer **14**	0.10 ± 0.00	0.10 ± 0.00	0.12 ± 0.00
Strictinin isomer **16**	0.11 ± 0.00	0.12 ± 0.00	0.18 ± 0.00
Castalagin isomer **30**	traces	0.02 ± 0.00	0.04 ± 0.00
Castalagin isomer **34**	traces	traces	0.01 ± 0.00
Casuarictin isomer **33**	traces	traces	0.02 ± 0.00
Casuarictin isomer **40**	0.06 ± 0.00	0.08 ± 0.00	0.14 ± 0.00
Sanguiin H2	traces	0.01 ± 0.00	0.05 ± 0.00
Sanguiin H2 isomer **44**	0.09 ± 0.00	0.05 ± 0.00	0.02 ± 0.00
Sanguiin H6	0.36 ± 0.01	0.25 ± 0.00	0.22 ± 0.00
Sanguiin H6 isomer **46**	0.45 ± 0.01	0.43 ± 0.01	0.40 ± 0.01
Sanguiin H10	0.21 ± 0.00	0.15 ± 0.00	0.08 ± 0.00
Lambertianin C	1.86 ± 0.04	1.42 ± 0.03	1.20 ± 0.02
Agrimonic acid A	0.02 ± 0.00	0.05 ± 0.00	0.08 ± 0.00
Agrimonic acid B	0.01 ± 0.00	0.03 ± 0.00	0.10 ± 0.00
Agrimoniin	2.63 ± 0.05	2.03 ± 0.04	1.41 ± 0.03
Fragariin A	0.93 ± 0.02	0.69 ± 0.02	0.63 ± 0.01
Total ellagic acid derivatives and ellagitannins	7.54	6.37	5.97
Catechins and procyanidins			
Catechin	0.11 ± 0.00	0.05 ± 0.00	0.05 ± 0.00
Procyanidin B2	0.09 ± 0.00	0.05 ± 0.00	0.02 ± 0.00
Procyanidin B4	0.02 ± 0.00	0.01 ± 0.00	traces
Procyanidin C2	0.05 ± 0.00	0.03 ± 0.00	0.01 ± 0.00
Procyanidin trimer **36**	0.02 ± 0.00	0.01 ± 0.00	0.01 ± 0.00
Total catechins and procyanidins	0.29	0.15	0.09
Anthocyanins			
Pelargonidin 3-*O*-glucoside	traces	0.02 ± 0.00	0.06 ± 0.00
Pelargonidin 3-*O*-rutinoside	n.d.	n.d.	0.03 ± 0.00
Pelargonidin di-*O*-hexoside **22**	n.d.	n.d.	traces

Table 2. *Cont.*

Compound	Stage of Ripeness		
	Unripe	Intermediate	Ripe
Pelargonidin *O*-acetyl-*O*-hexoside **48**	n.d.	n.d.	traces
Pelargonidin *O*-*p*-coumaroyl-*O*-hexoside **37**	n.d.	n.d.	traces
Cyanidin 3-*O*-glucoside	n.d.	0.01 ± 0.00	0.05 ± 0.00
Cyanidin 3-*O*-rutinoside	n.d.	n.d.	traces
Cyanidin 3-*O*-sophoroside	n.d.	n.d.	traces
Cyanidin *O*-acetyl-*O*-hexoside **38**	n.d.	n.d.	traces
Cyanidin *O*-*p*-coumaroyl-*O*-hexoside **32**	n.d.	n.d.	traces
Total anthocyanins	traces	0.03	0.14
Flavonols and flavonol glycosides			
Kaempferol	traces	traces	0.01 ± 0.00
Kaempferol 3-*O*-glucoside	traces	0.05 ± 0.00	0.09 ± 0.00
Kaempferol 3-*O*-glucuronide	traces	traces	0.08 ± 0.00
Kaempferol 3-*O*-rutinoside	0.28 ± 0.00	0.23 ± 0.00	0.11 ± 0.00
Kaempferol *O*-acetyl-*O*-hexoside **72**	traces	traces	traces
Kaempferol *O*-acetyl-*O*-hexoside **73**	traces	traces	traces
Kaempferol di-*O*-acetyl-*O*-hexoside **87**	traces	traces	traces
Kaempferol *O*-malonyl-*O*-hexoside **68**	0.01 ± 0.00	traces	traces
Kaempferol *O*-malonyl-*O*-hexoside **69**	0.02 ± 0.00	0.01 ± 0.00	traces
Kaempferol 3-*O*-(6″-*O*-*p*-coumaroyl)-glucoside	0.08 ± 0.00	0.04 ± 0.00	0.04 ± 0.00
Kaempferol *O*-acetyl-*O*-malonyl-*O*-hexoside **89**	0.02 ± 0.00	0.01 ± 0.00	0.01 ± 0.00
Kaempferol *O*-malonyl-*O*-*p*-coumaroyl-*O*-hexoside **90**	traces	traces	traces
Kaempferol *O*-malonyl-*O*-*p*-coumaroyl-*O*-hexoside **92**	traces	traces	traces
Kaempferol *O*-acetyl-*O*-*p*-coumaroyl-*O*-hexoside **93**	0.01 ± 0.00	0.01 ± 0.00	0.01 ± 0.00
Total kaempferol derivatives	0.42	0.35	0.35
Quercetin	traces	traces	0.02 ± 0.00
Quercetin 3-*O*-xyloside	traces	traces	0.03 ± 0.00
Quercetin 3-*O*-arabinoside	traces	traces	0.01 ± 0.00
Quercetin 3-*O*-glucoside	traces	0.04 ± 0.00	0.08 ± 0.00
Quercetin 3-*O*-glucuronide	traces	0.05 ± 0.00	0.11 ± 0.00
Quercetin 3-*O*-rutinoside	0.32 ± 0.00	0.28 ± 0.00	0.25 ± 0.00
Quercetin 3-*O*-sophoroside	0.11 ± 0.00	0.08 ± 0.00	0.03 ± 0.00
Quercetin 3-*O*-(2″-*O*-acetyl)-glucoside	0.06 ± 0.00	0.03 ± 0.00	0.01 ± 0.00
Quercetin 3-*O*-(6″-*O*-acetyl)-glucoside	0.03 ± 0.00	0.02 ± 0.00	0.02 ± 0.00
Quercetin 3-*O*-(2″,6″-di-*O*-acetyl)-glucoside	0.03 ± 0.00	0.01 ± 0.00	0.01 ± 0.00
Quercetin 3-*O*-(6″-*O*-malonyl)-glucoside	0.04 ± 0.00	0.04 ± 0.00	0.02 ± 0.00
Quercetin *O*-malonyl-*O*-hexoside **64**	0.01 ± 0.00	traces	traces
Quercetin 3-*O*-(6″-*O*-*p*-coumaroyl)-glucoside	0.11 ± 0.00	0.06 ± 0.00	0.05 ± 0.00
Quercetin *O*-*p*-coumaroyl-*O*-hexoside **61**	0.02 ± 0.00	0.02 ± 0.00	0.01 ± 0.00
Quercetin *O*-acetyl-*O*-malonyl-*O*-hexoside **80**	0.01 ± 0.00	0.01 ± 0.00	traces
Quercetin *O*-malonyl-*O*-*p*-coumaroyl-*O*-hexoside **84**	0.02 ± 0.00	0.01 ± 0.00	traces
Quercetin *O*-malonyl-*O*-*p*-coumaroyl-*O*-hexoside **85**	0.01 ± 0.00	0.01 ± 0.00	traces
Quercetin *O*-acetyl-*O*-*p*-coumaroyl-*O*-hexoside **88**	0.01 ± 0.00	traces	traces
Quercetin di-*O*-acetyl-*O*-*p*-coumaroyl-*O*-hexoside **94**	traces	traces	traces
Quercetin *O*-acetyl-*O*-malonyl-*O*-*p*-coumaroyl-*O*-hexoside **95**	0.04 ± 0.00	0.02 ± 0.00	0.01 ± 0.00
Total quercetin derivatives	0.82	0.68	0.66
Total flavonols and flavonol glycosides	1.24	1.03	1.01
Triterpenes			
Pomolic acid	traces	traces	0.01 ± 0.00
Pomolic acid *O*-hexoside **83**	traces	traces	traces
Pomolic acid di-*O*-hexoside **77**	traces	traces	traces
Tormentic acid	traces	traces	0.02 ± 0.00
Tormentic acid *O*-hexoside **78**	traces	traces	0.01 ± 0.00
Tormentic acid di-*O*-hexoside **75**	traces	traces	traces
Total triterpenes	traces	traces	0.04

The total concentration of flavonols in *F. viridis* demonstrated decreasing levels during fruit development from 1.24 mg/g in unripened fruits to 1.01 mg/g in ripened fruits. Quercetin derivatives (0.66–0.82 mg/g) prevailed over kaempferol derivatives (0.35–0.42 mg/g) in all stages of ripening; this was also found in *F. ananassa* (0.01–0.05 mg/g for quercetin derivatives vs. 0.01–0.02 mg/g for kaempferol derivatives) [9]. The main components of flavonol complex of *F. viridis* were quercetin 3-*O*-rutinoside (0.25–0.32 mg/g) and kaempferol 3-*O*-rutinoside (0.11–0.28 mg/g), followed by two acylated compounds: quercetin 3-*O*-(6″-*O*-*p*-coumaroyl)-glucoside (0.05–0.11 mg/g) and kaempferol 3-*O*-(6″-*O*-*p*-coumaroyl)-glucoside (0.04–0.08 mg/g). The gradual decline of flavonoid concentration was found for flavonol di-*O*-glycosides and acylated flavonol *O*-glycosides in contrast to aglycones and flavonol mono-*O*-glycosides accumulated in ripe fruits. Again, the variation of enzymatic activity of hydrolases may be relevant in the progress of *F. viridis* fruits ripening. This phenomenon has not been mentioned previously in any strawberries and needs additional experimental data to confirm this finding.

Triterpenes found in *F. viridis* fruits were trace compounds, but despite this, the quantifiable levels of tormentic acid, its *O*-hexoside, and pomolic acid were found in the stage of full ripening. The variation of triterpenoids in any *Fragaria* species was not discussed previously, but it is known that the accumulation of triterpenoids reaches the maximal level in the fully ripe stage of fruits; this was also declared for Chardonnay grape [48], olive fruits [49], and tomato [50].

2.3. Antioxidant Potential of F. viridis Fruits: Comparision with Other Strawberries

The activity of fruit total extracts of *F. viridis* in three stages of ripening was studied in four antioxidant assays including the scavenging capacity against 2,2-diphenyl-1-picrylhydrazyl radical (DPPH), and 2,2′-azino-bis(3-ethylbenzothiazoline-6-sulfonic acid) cation radical (ABTS), ferric reducing antioxidant power (FRAP), and oxygen radical absorbance capacity (ORAC) (Table 3). In comparison, the activity of two extracts from commercially available ripe fruits of *F. vesca* (wild strawberry, *Regina* cultivar) and *F. ananassa* (garden strawberry, *Senga Sengana* cultivar) was also studied. Both species are much more common strawberries, and their antioxidant potential has been analysed many times [2].

Table 3. Antioxidant activity of *Fragaria* extracts in four assays, μM trolox-eq./g of dry weight ± S.D.

Assay [a]	F. viridis			F. vesca (Ripe)	F. ananassa (Ripe)
	Unripe	Intermediate	Ripe		
DPPH	29.2 ± 0.6 [d,e]	28.4 ± 0.5 [c]	27.5 ± 0.5 [c,d]	15.2 ± 0.3 [b]	9.3 ± 0.2 [a]
ABTS	35.1 ± 0.8 [h,i]	35.3 ± 0.8 [h]	36.2 ± 0.9 [i]	19.7 ± 0.4 [f,g]	14.7 ± 0.3 [f]
FRAP	42.6 ± 1.0 [l]	45.4 ± 1.0 [l,m]	47.1 ± 1.0 [m]	27.1 ± 0.5 [k]	21.1 ± 0.4 [j]
ORAC	33.6 ± 0.8 [p,q]	32.8 ± 0.7 [o,p]	33.0 ± 0.8 [p]	25.1 ± 0.5 [n,o]	18.9 ± 0.4 [n]

[a] DPPH—scavenging capacity against 2,2-diphenyl-1-picrylhydrazyl radical; ABTS—scavenging capacity against 2,2′-azino-bis(3-ethylbenzothiazoline-6-sulfonic acid) cation radical; FRAP—ferric reducing antioxidant power; and ORAC—oxygen radical absorbance capacity. Averages ± standard deviation (S.D.) were obtained from five different experiments. Values with different letters (a–q) indicate statistically significant differences among groups at $p < 0.05$ by one-way ANOVA.

The extracts of *F. viridis* fruits in all stages of ripening were effective radical scavengers against both radicals DPPH and ABTS. Variations of the antioxidant potential values were 27.53–29.18 μM trolox-eq./g in the DPPH assay and 35.07–36.22 μM trolox-eq./g in the ABTS assay, while the more active scavenger in the DPPH assay was the extract of unripe fruits and the ABTS assay gave the extract of ripe fruits as more active. The extracts of *F. vesca* and *F. ananassa* were less effective in DPPH/ABTS scavenging assays with values of trolox-equivalent content 15.21/19.73 and 9.33/14.67 μM/g, respectively. An early research of *F. ananassa* extracts in the DPPH assay showed a wide range of fluctuation of antiradical activity from 9.75–12.83 μM BHT-eq./g for Brazil cultivars [4] to 3.00–13.15 μM trolox-eq./g for Polish cultivars [10]. Sikmilar characteristics were found for ABTS assay data varying from

1.50–2.27 μM trolox-eq./g for Japan varieties [51] to 7.06–29.73 μM trolox-eq./g for Polish cultivars [10]. Raudonis et al. [14] analysed the activity of *F. vesca* and *F. moschata* extracts using HPLC-assisted ABTS assay, which gave the values of protection 25.11 and 8.24 μM trolox-eq./g, respectively.

The FRAP assay is one of the most popular assays to estimate antioxidant activity for analysis of edible fruits, and strawberries are not an exception. The level of ferric reducing antioxidant power of *F. viridis* extracts was high and increased during fruit ripening from 42.63 μM trolox-eq./g in the unripe stage to 47.11 μM trolox-eq./g in ripe fruit extract. The parameters of *F. vesca* (27.14 μM trolox-eq./g) and *F. ananassa* (21.06 μM trolox-eq./g) extracts were lower but close to known data (24.84 μM trolox-eq./g for *F. vesca* [14]). The level of antioxidant activity in the ORAC assay for *F. viridis* fruit extracts was similar to ABTS data and slightly decreased in ripening progress from 33.62 μM trolox-eq./g (unripe fruits) to 32.98 μM trolox-eq./g (ripe fruits). The ORAC data of *F. vesca* extract 25.05 μM trolox-eq./g was higher than for *F. ananassa* extract (18.87 μM trolox-eq./g) but at a level lower than *F. viridis*. The known information about ORAC potential of strawberries demonstrated high effectiveness of anthocyanins fraction of *F. ananassa* (2.7–24.46 mM trolox-eq./g) [52], opposite the activity of the total fruit extract (8.90–16.63 μM trolox-eq./g) [53].

Applying the DPPH-radical scavenging-assisted HPLC-PDA-ESI-tQ-MS assay, we identified the compounds responsible for the antioxidant defence of *F. viridis* extracts. For that to happen, an aliquot of the total extract was separated with chromatography and portions of the eluates were collected. A part of the eluates was used for the DPPH decolouration assay, and the remainder were used for HPLC-PDA-ESI-tQ-MS assay for the qualitative confirmation of compounds (Figure S2). The results showed that the majority of compounds found in *F. viridis* were involved in the process of radical scavenging (most likely because of their phenolic nature), but 12 sites of elution gave more pronounced decolouration of the DPPH solution. There were ascorbic acid, ellagic acid, five ellagitannins (pedunculagin, sanguiin H6, lambertianin C, agrimoniin, and fragariin A), two anthocyanins (pelargonidin 3-*O*-glucoside, and cyanidin 3-*O*-glucoside), and three flavonols (quercetin 3-*O*-glucoside, quercetin 3-*O*-glucuronide, and quercetin 3-*O*-rutinoside). Three compounds, ascorbic acid, lambertianin C, and agrimoniin, were the most active due to their high content so they were the principal antioxidants of *F. viridis* fruits.

In brief, the information obtained in four in vitro assays demonstrates the high effectiveness of *F. vesca* fruit extracts as antioxidant agents, exceeding the activity of two well-known strawberries: *F. vesca* and *F. ananassa*. In light of the obtained results about the activity of *F. vesca* fruits, checking its usefulness in antioxidant protection of the human organisms was considered. To this end, this was done by pilot experiment by analysing total antioxidant capacity (TAC) of blood serum of healthy male volunteers after a 1-week intake of *F. viridis* fresh ripe fruits at doses of 100, 250, and 400 g/day. The level of TAC before *F. vesca* fruit intake was 510–516 μM trolox-eq./L. The week-long consumption of *F. viridis* fresh fruits gave a statistically significant increase of serum TAC level in all dose groups up to 524, 544, and 557 μM trolox-eq./L, respectively, for groups with 100, 250, and 400 g/day consumption (Figure 3).

By comparison, the results of *F. vesca* and *F. ananassa* fruit groups (both 250 g/day) were also positive—the consumption of both kinds of strawberries resulted in increases in serum TAC levels, but to a lesser degree (535 μM trolox-eq./L for *F. vesca*, 525 μM trolox-eq./L for *F. ananassa*).

This illustrates the good antioxidant potential of *F. viridis* fruits in any dose applied. To date, it is known that the consumption of *F. ananassa* resulted in increases in serum TAC by 7–25% [54]. The possible reasons for that phenomenon may be an increase in human serum of strawberry-related metabolites such as pelargonidin-glucuronide, urolithin A-glucuronide [55] and *p*-hydroxybenzoic acid [56] possessing high antioxidant potential and also the rising of serum antioxidants (glutathione) and serum level of antioxidant enzyme activity (catalase, glutathione peroxidase, and glutathione reductase) [57]. The metabolite profile of *F. viridis* is qualitatively and quantitatively close to *F. ananassa*; therefore, it is logical to assume that the increase of serum TAC after *F. viridis* consumption is caused by enhancement of the serum level of antioxidant metabolites of phenolic nature, serum antioxidants, and antioxidant enzymes.

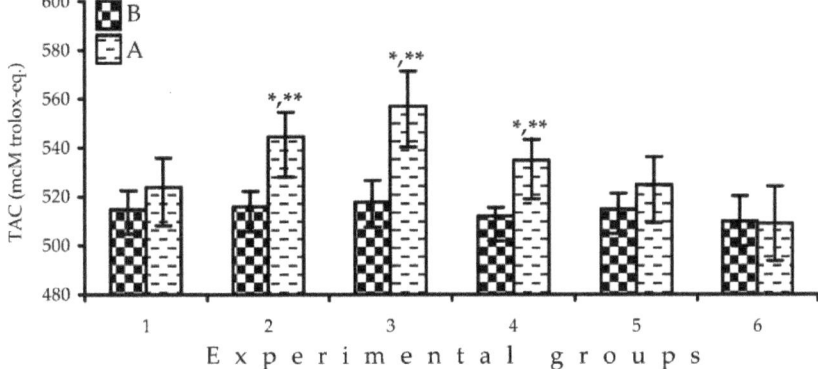

Figure 3. Changes in serum total antioxidant capacity (TAC) before (B) and after (A) 1-week intake of *Fragaria* fresh ripe fruits (group 1—*F. viridis*, 100 g/day, $n = 5$; group 2—*F. viridis*, 250 g/day, $n = 5$; group 3—*F. viridis*, 400 g/day, $n = 5$; group 4—*F. vesca*, 250 g/day, $n = 4$; and group 5—*F. ananassa*, 250 g/day, $n = 6$) and 10 g/day fructose (group 6, control group; $n = 3$). * $p < 0.05$ vs. control group after intake; ** $p < 0.05$ vs. same group before intake.

2.4. Storage Stability of Antioxidants and Antioxidant Potential of F. viridis Ripe Fruits

Twenty compounds with the most pronounced antioxidant effects were quantified in *F. viridis* fruits in two series of storage experiments (Table 4). Primarily, we studied the change in concentration of ripe fruits stored at two temperatures, 4 °C (cool temperature) and 20 °C (room temperature), to define the stability of antioxidants in fresh fruits for a short period.

Results from HPLC data show that the storage of ripe *F. viridis* fruits at 4 °C caused a decrease of ascorbic acid content by 55.2% (1.14→0.51 mg/g), anthocyanin content by 28.6–60.0% (0.07→0.05 mg/g for pelargonidin 3-*O*-glucoside and 0.05→0.02 mg/g for cyanidin-3-*O*-glucoside), ellagitannin polymers content by 20.4–26.2% (1.26→0.93 mg/g for lambertianin C, 1.47→1.17 mg/g for agrimoniin, and 0.65→0.51 mg/g for fragariin A), and quercetin 3-*O*-rutinoside content by 16.7% (0.24→0.20 mg/g). There has also been an increase in the concentration of ellagic acid by 90% (0.10→0.19 mg/g), ellagitannin monomers and dimers by 17.5–25.0% (0.33→0.40 mg/g for pedunculagin and 0.20→0.25 mg/g for sanguiin H6), and flavonol monoglucosides by 10.0–13.3% (0.10→0.11 mg/g for quercetin 3-*O*-glucoside and 0.15→0.17 mg/g for quercetin 3-*O*-glucuronide). As a result of chemical changes, the reduction of bioactivity of fruits was also observed, and the loss of total antioxidant potential was 20.6% (4.12→3.27 μmol trolox-eq./g).

The seven-day storage of ripe *F. viridis* fruits at 4 °C and three-day storage at 20 °C were the maximal periods of storage without external damage (browning, rotting, untypical smell, and taste) [58].

The storage of fresh *F. viridis* fruits at room temperature (20 °C) resulted in more drastic changes within a shorter period. The level of ascorbic acid declined from 1.14 mg/g to 0.36 mg/g (68.4%) for three days; additionally, anthocyanins became a trace compound. The strong reduction of content was detected for the polymeric ellagitannins, lambertianin C (42.6%), agrimoniin (36.7%), and fragariin A (66.2%) in opposition to ellagic acid, pedunculagin, and sanguiin H6, which increased at 150.0, 48.5, and 50.0%, respectively. The flavonoid biocide quercetin 3-*O*-rutinoside showed a statistically significant decrease of content from 0.24 mg/g to 0.18 mg/g (25%) coupled with a rising level of quercetin 3-*O*-glucoside and quercetin 3-*O*-glucuronide.

Table 4. Content of selected antioxidants in ripe fruits of *F. viridis* (mg/g of fresh fruit weight ± S.D.) and its total antioxidant potential (coulometric titration assay; μmol trolox-eq./g of fresh fruit weight ± S.D.) after storage at 4 °C (1 week) and 20 °C (3 days).

Compound	T, °C	Day of Storage							
		0	1	2	3	4	5	6	7
Ascorbic acid	4	1.14 ± 0.02	1.02 ± 0.02	0.95 ± 0.02	0.89 ± 0.02	0.86 ± 0.02	0.73 ± 0.02	0.55 ± 0.02	0.51 ± 0.02
	20		0.85 ± 0.02	0.54 ± 0.01	0.36 ± 0.01	n.a.	n.a.	n.a.	n.a.
Ellagic acid	4	0.10 ± 0.00	0.10 ± 0.00	0.10 ± 0.00	0.12 ± 0.00	0.14 ± 0.00	0.15 ± 0.00	0.17 ± 0.00	0.19 ± 0.00
	20		0.10 ± 0.00	0.12 ± 0.00	0.25 ± 0.00	n.a.	n.a.	n.a.	n.a.
Pedunculagin	4	0.33 ± 0.01	0.34 ± 0.01	0.34 ± 0.01	0.35 ± 0.01	0.35 ± 0.01	0.38 ± 0.01	0.38 ± 0.01	0.40 ± 0.01
	20		0.35 ± 0.01	0.38 ± 0.01	0.49 ± 0.01	n.a.	n.a.	n.a.	n.a.
Sanguiin H6	4	0.20 ± 0.00	0.20 ± 0.00	0.20 ± 0.00	0.21 ± 0.00	0.22 ± 0.00	0.24 ± 0.00	0.25 ± 0.00	0.25 ± 0.00
	20		0.20 ± 0.00	0.21 ± 0.00	0.30 ± 0.00	n.a.	n.a.	n.a.	n.a.
Lambertianin C	4	1.26 ± 0.02	1.24 ± 0.02	1.20 ± 0.02	1.15 ± 0.02	1.11 ± 0.02	0.99 ± 0.02	0.97 ± 0.02	0.93 ± 0.02
	20		1.04 ± 0.02	0.90 ± 0.02	0.72 ± 0.02	n.a.	n.a.	n.a.	n.a.
Agrimoniin	4	1.47 ± 0.03	1.45 ± 0.03	1.40 ± 0.03	1.37 ± 0.03	1.35 ± 0.03	1.25 ± 0.02	1.22 ± 0.02	1.17 ± 0.02
	20		1.33 ± 0.03	1.08 ± 0.02	0.93 ± 0.02	n.a.	n.a.	n.a.	n.a.
Fragariin A	4	0.65 ± 0.02	0.65 ± 0.02	0.62 ± 0.02	0.60 ± 0.02	0.59 ± 0.01	0.55 ± 0.01	0.53 ± 0.02	0.51 ± 0.01
	20		0.42 ± 0.01	0.34 ± 0.01	0.22 ± 0.00	n.a.	n.a.	n.a.	n.a.
Pelargonidin 3-*O*-glucoside	4	0.07 ± 0.00	0.07 ± 0.00	0.07 ± 0.00	0.07 ± 0.00	0.06 ± 0.00	0.06 ± 0.00	0.05 ± 0.00	0.05 ± 0.00
	20		0.04 ± 0.00	0.02 ± 0.00	traces	n.a.	n.a.	n.a.	n.a.
Cyanidin 3-*O*-glucoside	4	0.05 ± 0.00	0.05 ± 0.00	0.05 ± 0.00	0.04 ± 0.00	0.04 ± 0.00	0.02 ± 0.00	0.02 ± 0.00	0.02 ± 0.00
	20		0.02 ± 0.00	traces	traces	n.a.	n.a.	n.a.	n.a.
Quercetin 3-*O*-glucoside	4	0.10 ± 0.00	0.10 ± 0.00	0.10 ± 0.00	0.10 ± 0.00	0.10 ± 0.00	0.10 ± 0.00	0.11 ± 0.00	0.11 ± 0.00
	20		0.10 ± 0.00	0.11 ± 0.00	0.12 ± 0.00	n.a.	n.a.	n.a.	n.a.
Quercetin 3-*O*-glucuronide	4	0.15 ± 0.00	0.15 ± 0.00	0.15 ± 0.00	0.16 ± 0.00	0.17 ± 0.00	0.17 ± 0.00	0.17 ± 0.00	0.17 ± 0.00
	20		0.15 ± 0.00	0.15 ± 0.00	0.17 ± 0.00	n.a.	n.a.	n.a.	n.a.
Quercetin 3-*O*-rutinoside	4	0.24 ± 0.00	0.24 ± 0.00	0.24 ± 0.00	0.24 ± 0.00	0.24 ± 0.00	0.22 ± 0.00	0.21 ± 0.00	0.20 ± 0.00
	20		0.24 ± 0.00	0.20 ± 0.00	0.18 ± 0.00	n.a.	n.a.	n.a.	n.a.
Total antioxidant potential	4	4.12 ± 0.09	4.10 ± 0.08	4.07 ± 0.08	4.02 ± 0.08	3.97 ± 0.08	3.86 ± 0.08	3.59 ± 0.07	3.27 ± 0.07
	20		2.88 ± 0.05	1.72 ± 0.04	0.52 ± 0.02	n.a.	n.a.	n.a.	n.a.

n.a.—not analyzed.

The parameter of total antioxidant potential decreased from 4.12 to 0.52 μmol trolox-eq./g or 87.4% less antioxidant potential. Postharvest storage of ripe fruits is inextricably linked to senescence causing changes in biochemical profiles, biomolecules and polymers degradation, cell dysfunction and disintegration, and the leaking of enzymes [58]. Not long after, the fruits begin rotting, which reduces its alimentary value. In our study, the ripe *F. viridis* fruits after storage showed negative changes in content of ascorbic acid and anthocyanins, which are environmentally unstable plant compounds diminished in light and high humidity [59,60], just like polymeric ellagitannins and rutin typically degrading after contact with oxygen and esterase-like enzymes [61,62]. The preservative value of cool temperature (4 °C) was higher than room temperature (20 °C), saving antioxidants and the antioxidant potential of fruits longer. The decrease in phenolic compounds and ascorbic acid content in strawberries was shown in the number of papers. Anthocyanin content decreased in *F. ananassa* fruits during refrigerated storage at 4 °C in cultivars Camarosa (385→46 mg/kg) [63,64] and Elsanta (40→20 mg/g) [65]. The ascorbic acid level was also unstable at 0–20 °C with a loss of about 40% (cultivars Dover, Campineiro, and Mazi) [3] or more (cultivar Camarosa) [63]. The content of ellagic acid and flavonol monoglucosides in cool storage (5 °C) of *F. ananassa* fruits tends to rise as in the Selva cultivar from 19.9 to 26.8 μg/g for ellagic acid, from 40.1 to 44.1 μg/g for quercetin derivatives, and from 13.7 to 15.8 μg/g for kaempferol derivatives [66]. Our findings revealed that various strawberries (*F. viridis* and *F. ananassa*) have the same response during storage at cool and room temperature conditions.

3. Materials and Methods

3.1. Plant Materials and Chemicals

Samples of *Fragaria viridis* fruits were collected in Sakha (Yakutia) Republic (Aldanskii ulus, 58°37′27.1″ N, 125°17′17.5″ E, 15–25 July 2019) in three ripening stages (unripe—green fruits, intermediate ripe—half red fruits, and fully ripe—red fruits). The species was authenticated by N.I. Kashchenko (IGEB SB RAS, Ulan-Ude, Russia). The fruits were conditioned in plastic boxes and transported to the laboratory at 4 °C within 2–3 h. The ripe fruits of *F. vesca* (*Regina* cultivar) and *F. ananassa* (*Senga Sengana* cultivar) were purchased via a local market. The reference compounds were purchased from BioCrick (Chengdu, PRC), BOC Sciences (Shirley, NY, USA), Carbosynth Ltd. (Compton, UK), ChemFaces (Wuhan, PRC), Extrasynthese (Lyon, France), Funakoshi Co. Ltd. (Tokyo, Japan), Sigma-Aldrich (St. Louis, MO, USA), Toronto Research Chemicals (North York, ON, Canada), and TransMIT GmbH (Gießen, Germany) (Table S1). Ellagitannins sanguiins H2, H6, and H10; agrimonic acids A and B; and agrimoniin were isolated previously in our laboratory from Rosaceous species (purity 90–95%) [28,67,68], and flavonols quercetin 3-*O*-(2″-*O*-acetyl)-glucoside, quercetin 3-*O*-(2″-*O*-acetyl)-glucoside, and quercetin 3-*O*-(2″,6″-di-*O*-acetyl)-glucoside were isolated from *Calendula officinalis* [32]. Selected chemicals were from Sigma-Aldrich—acetonitrile for HPLC (Cat. No 34851, ≥99.9%), 2,2′-azino-bis(3-ethylbenzothiazoline-6-sulfonic acid) diammonium salt (Cat. No A1888, ≥98%), 2,2′azobis(2-methylpropionamidine) dihydrochloride (Cat. No 440914, ≥97%), 2,2-diphenyl-1-picrylhydrazyl radical (Cat. No 281689, ≥97%), formic acid (Cat. No 33015, ≥98%), fructose (Cat. No 47739, ≥99%), hydrogen peroxide (Cat. No H1009, ≥30%), methanol (Cat. No 322415, ≥99.8%), myoglobin (Cat. No M0630, ≥95%), potassium bromide (Cat. No 243418, ≥99%), sulphuric acid (Cat. No 339741, ≥99%), 2,4,6-tri(2-pyridyl)-1,3,5-triazine (Cat. No 93285, ≥99%), and trolox (Cat. No 238813, ≥97%).

3.2. Total Extract Preparation from Fragaria Fruits

For preparation of the total extract of *Fragaria* fruits, the fresh material was homogenized in a Grindomix GM 200 grinder (Retsch GmbH, Haan, Germany) and 100 g was extracted twice with stirring in a glass flask (0.5 L) with methanol (100 mL) using an ultrasonic bath Sapphire 2.8 (Sapphire Ltd., Moscow, Russia) for 30 min and at 50 °C (ultrasound power 100 W and frequency 35 kHz).

The extracts were filtered through cellulose, concentrated in vacuo until dryness, and stored at 4 °C before use for chemical analysis and biological activity study. The yields of total extracts of *Fragaria* fruits were 10.63 g (*F. viridis* unripe fruits), 11.02 g (*F. viridis* intermediate ripe fruits), 12.43 g (*F. viridis* fully ripe fruits), 15.63 g (*F. vesca* fully ripe fruits), and 17.33 g (*F. ananassa* fully ripe fruits).

3.3. High-Performance Liquid Chromatography with Photodiode Array Detection and Electrospray Ionization Triple Quadrupole Mass Spectrometric Detection (HPLC-PDA-ESI-tQ-MS): Metabolite Profiling

Metabolite profiling of *F. viridis* extracts was realized using high-performance liquid chromatography with photodiode array detection and electrospray ionization triple quadrupole mass spectrometric detection (HPLC-PDA-ESI-tQ-MS) performed on a liquid chromatograph LC-20 Prominence coupled photodiode array detector SPD-M30A (wavelength range 200–600 nm), triple-quadrupole mass spectrometer LCMS 8050 (all Shimadzu, Columbia, MD, USA) and C18 column (GLC Mastro; 150 × 2.1 mm, Ø 3 µm; Shimadzu, Kyoto, Japan) at the column temperature 30 °C. Gradient elution was implemented with two eluents A (0.5% HCOOH in water) and B (0.5% HCOOH in MeCN) and the following gradient program: 0–5 min 5–7% B, 5–7 min 7–8% B, 7–10 min 8–19% B, 10–14 min 19–29% B, 14–20 min 29–52% B, 20–25 min 52–73% B, 25–35 min 73–90% B, and 35–45 min 90–5% B. The values of injection volume and elution flow were 1 µL and 100 µL/min, respectively. The UV-Vis spectra were obtained in the spectral range of 200–600 nm. MS detection was performed in negative ESI mode using the parameters as follows: temperature levels of ESI interface, desolvation line, and heat block were 300 °C, 250 °C, and 400 °C, respectively. The flow levels of nebulizing gas (N_2), heating gas (air), and collision-induced dissociation gas (Ar) were 3 L/min, 10 L/min, and 0.3 mL/min, respectively. The MS spectra were recorded in the negative mode (−3––5 kV source voltage) by scanning in the range of *m/z* 50–2000 at the collision energy of 5–40 eV. The system was managed under LabSolution's workstation software with the inner LC-MS library. The identification of compounds was done by the analysis of their retention time, ultraviolet, and mass-spectrometric data, comparing the same parameters with the reference samples and/or literature data. Before analysis, the sample of *F. viridis* fruits dry extract (10 mg) was dissolved in 50% MeCN (25 mL), filtered (0.22-µm PTFE syringe filter), and injected (1 µL) into the HPLC-DAD-ESI-tQ-MS system for analysis.

3.4. High-Performance Liquid Chromatography with Diode Array Detection (HPLC-DAD): Carbohydrate Analysis

The composition of free carbohydrates was analyzed by high-performance liquid chromatography with diode array detection (HPLC-DAD) using the procedure described previously [69]. To prepare the sample, dry extracts of *F. viridis* fruits (5 mg) were dissolved in 20 mL of deionized water and passed sequentially through a series of two cartridges Dowex® 50WX8 (H+-form; 10 mL) and Dowex® 1 × 8 (Cl−-form; 10 mL) eluted with water (20 mL). The final eluates were reduced in vacuo (20 mL) and filtered using 0.22-µm PTFE syringe filter before injection into the HPLC-DAD system for analysis.

3.5. HPLC-ESI-tQ-MS: Metabolite Quantification

To quantify compounds **1–95** in *F. viridis* fruits, we used HPLC-MS data (MS peak area) obtained in early conditions (Section 3.3). The reference standards (48 compounds; Table S2) were accurately weighed (10 mg) and individually dissolved in DMSO-50% methanol mixture (1:10) in a volumetric flask (10 mL). The stock solutions were used to build external standard calibration curves generated using six data points, 100, 50, 25, 10, 5, and 1 µg/mL followed by plotting the MS peak area vs. the concentration levels. The validation criteria (correlation coefficients, r^2; standard deviation, S_{YX}; limits of detection, LOD; limits of quantification, LOQ; and linear ranges) were calculated using the previous recommendations [70] (Table S2). All analyses were carried out in triplicate, and the data were expressed as mean value ± standard deviation (S.D.). The sample solution was prepared from homogenized *F. viridis* fruits (50 mg) and 5 mL of methanol in an Eppendorf tube. The mixture was sonicated for 30 min at 50 °C (ultrasound power 100 W, frequency 35 kHz), centrifuged (6000× *g*), filtered (using 0.22-μm PTFE syringe filter), and transferred to the volumetric flask (10 mL), and the final volume was reduced to 10 mL by 50% MeOH before HPLC-ESI-tQ-MS analysis. Genkwanin was used as the internal standard (final concentration 25 μg/mL in acetonitrile).

3.6. Antioxidant Activity: In Vitro Assays

Radical scavenging activity of *Fragaria* extracts against the 2,2-diphenyl-1-picrylhydrazyl radical (DPPH) and the 2,2′-azino-bis(3-ethylbenzothiazoline-6-sulfonic acid) cation radical (ABTS) was studied using microplate spectrophotometric decoloration assays as described previously [71,72]. The value of the ferric reducing antioxidant power (FRAP) was measured by spectrophotometric assay based on the reduction of the Fe^{3+}-2,4,6-tri(2-pyridyl)-1,3,5-triazine complex to the ferrous form at low pH [73]. To determine the level of oxygen radical absorbance capacity (ORAC), we used an assay based on peroxyl radical generation by thermal decomposition of 2,2′-azobis(2-amidino-propane) dihydrochloride followed by fluorimetric detection [74]. All assays used trolox as a reference standard (methanolic solution 0.5–100 μg/mL), and the calibration curve was created by plotting the trolox concentration (μg/mL) vs. the absorbance (or fluorescence). The values of antioxidant parameters were expressed as μmol trolox-equivalents/g of dry weight. All the analyses were carried out five times and the data were expressed as mean value ± standard deviation (SD).

3.7. DPPH Radical Scavenging Assisted HPLC-PDA-ESI-tQ-MS Assay

High-performance liquid chromatography with photodiode array detection and electrospray ionization triple quadrupole mass spectrometric detection (HPLC-PDA-ESI-tQ-MS) assisted with spectrophotometric DPPH radical scavenging assay was realized in the chromatographic conditions described in Section 3.3 with enlarged injection volume at 30 μL. The eluates (50 μL) were collected every 30 s using an automated fraction collector (Econova, Novosibirsk, Russia) in 96-well microplates, then dried under a N_2-stream, and redissolved in 50 μL of 50% methanol. An aliquot (25 μL) of the methanolic solution was mixed with DPPH solution (50 μg/mL in methanol) and absorbance was measured at 520 nm fifteen minutes later by a Bio-Rad microplate reader Model 3550 UV (Bio-Rad Labs, Richmond, CA, USA). The most active antioxidants gave strong decoloration of the DPPH solution, and corresponding eluates were separated in known HPLC-PDA-ESI-tQ-MS conditions again in order to confirm the presence of separate compounds.

3.8. Serum Total Antioxidant Capacity

Twenty-eight men, aged 20–25 years, were recruited. All were free from hypertension, cardiovascular disorders, and alcohol abuse; none smoked or took any other drug and oral medication. We had the guarantee that all subjects had a similar diet and lifestyle because they were recruited from the same community with a refectory service. All subjects gave their informed consent for inclusion before they participated in the study. The study was conducted in accordance with the Declaration of Helsinki, and the protocol was approved by the Ethics Committee of Institute of General and Experimental Biology (protocol No. LM-0324, 27 January 2012). The volunteers were divided on six experimental groups: group 1—*F. viridis* fruits, 100 g/day (*n* = 5); group 2—*F. viridis* fruits, 250 g/day (*n* = 5); group 3—*F. viridis* fruits, 400 g/day (n = 5); group 4—*F. vesca* fruits, 250 g/day (*n* = 4); group 5—*F. ananassa* fruits, 250 g/day (*n* = 6); and group 6—fructose, 10 g/day (*n* = 3). Then, they took *Fragaria* fruits or fructose for 1 week (3 times a day in equal portions). Before and after the test, blood was drawn from the antecubital vein into a heparinized syringe, and immediately after blood drawing, serum was prepared by centrifugation (6000× *g*) and the serum total antioxidant capacity was estimated. Phosphate buffer (10 mM, pH 7.2; 100 μL), myoglobin solution (5 μM; 50 μL), ABTS solution (3 mM; 20 μL), and serum sample (20 μL) were mixed in 96-well microplate and incubated 3 min at 25 °C. Then H_2O_2 solution (250 μM; 20 μL) was added and immediately measured at 600 nm for 5 min at 25 °C. A lag time (in sec) was estimated as the suppression period of ABTS oxidation (or absorbance increasing). The reference compound (trolox; 1, 2.5, 5, and 10 μM) was analyzed using the same protocol, and the calibration curve was created by plotting the lag time (in s) vs. the absorbance at 600 nm. The value of the serum total antioxidant capacity was expressed as μmol trolox-equivalents/L. All the analyses were carried out in triplicate, and the data were expressed as mean value ± standard deviation (SD).

3.9. F. viridis Fruit Storage Experiment

Seven and three portions of the fresh *F. viridis* fruits (200 g) were placed into individual polystyrene bags (300 mL) and incubated at 4 °C (7 days) or 20 °C (3 days), respectively, in a ventilated MK 53 thermostat (BINDER GmbH, Tuttlingen, Germany). Five portions (20 g each) of fresh *F. viridis* fruits were taken out of storage for analysis every 24 h, extracted as described previously (Section 3.5), and analyzed using HPLC-ESI-tQ-MS quantitative procedure (Section 3.5) or used without pre-extraction for the total antioxidant potential determination by coulometric assay (Section 3.10).

3.10. Total Antioxidant Potential of Fresh F. viridis Fruits: Coulometric Assay

The total antioxidant potential of fresh *F. viridis* fruits was found using a sightly modified bromine radical scavenging assay based on the coulometric titration method with electrogenerated bromine radicals [17,75]. Potentiostat Expert-006 (Econics Expert Ltd., Moscow, Russia) with a four-electrode two-compartment electrochemical cell was used for measurements. The working electrode was a bare platinum foil (surface area 1 cm^2), and the auxiliary electrode was a platinum wire isolated from the anodic cell with a semipermeable diaphragm. To detect the titration end-point ($\Delta E = 200$ mV), a pair of polarized platinum electrodes was used and the electrochemical generation was carried out from the supporting electrolyte (0.25 M KBr in 0.1 M H_2SO_4) at a current density 5 mA·cm^{-2}, providing 100% current yield. To start the measurement, the portion fruit of *F. viridis* (50 g) with various storage periods was homogenized and 10 mg of homogenate was inserted into the coulometric cell (50 mL) containing 20.0 mL of supporting electrolyte. The time of titration was used for the total antioxidant potential calculation expressed in units of the quantity of electricity (Coulombs (C)) spent for titration of the full probe of homogenized fruits. The trolox solutions were used as a reference compound (500, 250, 100, 50, and 10 μg/mL in methanol) titrated coulometrically, and a calibration curve was plotted in coordinates "concentration (μg/mL)—the quantity of electricity (C)". Finally, the value of the total antioxidant potential was calculated as mg trolox-equivalents per g of fresh fruits. Values are expressed as mean obtained from ten independent experiments.

3.11. Statistical Analysis

Statistical analyses were performed using a one-way analysis of variance (ANOVA), and the significance of the mean difference was determined by Duncan's multiple range test. Differences at $p < 0.05$ were considered statistically significant. The results are presented as mean values ± S.D. (standard deviations) of some (3–10) replicates.

4. Conclusions

The current study reported the metabolic profile of fruits of *Fragaria viridis* in various stages of ripening using the HPLC-DAD-ESI-tQ-MS technique not applied previously to this strawberry species. About a hundred compounds were characterized, and this is many more than the previously reported amount of *F. viridis* metabolites [14,15]. The largest number of components were phenolics, particularly ellagitannins and flavonol glycosides, forming the basis of *F. viridis* metabolome in all stages of ripening. In addition, derivatives of gallic acid, ellagic acid, hydroxycinnamates, coumarins, procyanidins, catechins, and anthocyanins were also found. Non-phenolic compounds, such as carbohydrates and organic acids, were quantitatively predominant, opposite triterpenes, with trace levels found. The concentrations of all compounds were affected by the ripening process with increased (anthocyanins and non-phenolics) or decreased (the majority of phenolic compounds) values to a fully ripe stage. This indicates that the ripening of *F. viridis* fruits is a complex process impacting the quantitative profile of metabolites. The high content of ascorbic acid and selected phenolics in *F. viridis* fruits were the source of strong antioxidant properties of fruit extracts, in particular free radical scavenging capacity, ferric reducing antioxidant power, and oxygen radical absorbance capacity studied in in vitro models. The same is true for human experiments, which demonstrated that the serum total antioxidant capacity increased significantly after a week's consumption of *F. viridis* fruits. Changes in antioxidant content and total antioxidant potential of fresh *F. viridis* fruits was found during storage at 4 °C and 20 °C, with the safest condition at 4 °C storage used within a week. The information received in our study highlighted the potential of *F. viridis* fruits as a source of antioxidant metabolites that need more scientific attention and wider implementation in the human diet.

Supplementary Materials: The following are available online at http://www.mdpi.com/1424-8247/13/9/262/s1, Figure S1: High-performance liquid chromatography with diode array detection chromatogram of free sugars in F. viridis ripe fruits, Figure S2: High-performance liquid chromatography with electrospray ionization triple quadrupole mass spectrometric detection chromatogram of F. viridis ripe fruits extract coupled with spectrophotometric DPPH radical scavenging assay, Table S1: Reference standards used for the qualitative and quantitative analysis by HPLC-DAD-ESI-tQ-MS assays, Table S2: Regression equations, correlation coefficients, standard deviation, limits of detection, limits of quantification, and linear ranges for 48 reference standards.

Author Contributions: Conceptualization, D.N.O.; methodology, D.N.O. and N.K.C.; software, D.N.O.; validation, D.N.O. and N.K.C.; formal analysis, A.G.V.; investigation, D.N.O. and N.K.C.; resources, N.K.C., and A.G.V.; data curation, N.K.C. and A.G.V.; writing—original draft preparation, D.N.O.; writing—review and editing, N.K.C.; visualization, D.N.O.; supervision, D.N.O.; project administration, N.K.C.; funding acquisition, D.N.O. and N.K.C. All authors have read and agreed to the published version of the manuscript.

Funding: This research was funded by Ministry of Education and Science of the Russian Federation, grant numbers AAAA-A17-117011810037-0 and FSRG-2020-0019, and by the Russian Foundation for Basic Research, grant number 19-09-00361.

Acknowledgments: The authors acknowledge the Buryat Research Resource Center for the technical support in chromatographic and mass-spectrometric research.

Conflicts of Interest: The funders had no role in the design of the study; in the collection, analyses, or interpretation of data; in the writing of the manuscript; or in the decision to publish the results.

References

1. Liston, A.; Cronn, R.; Ashman, T.L. *Fragaria*: A genus with deep historical roots and ripe for evolutionary and ecological insights. *Am. J. Bot.* **2014**, *101*, 1686–1699. [CrossRef] [PubMed]
2. Fierascu, R.C.; Temocico, G.; Fierascu, I.; Ortan, A.; Babeanu, N.E. *Fragaria* genus: Chemical composition and biological activities. *Molecules* **2020**, *25*, 498. [CrossRef] [PubMed]
3. Cordenunsi, B.R.; Nascimento, J.R.O.; Lajolo, F.M. Physico-chemical changes related to quality of five strawberry fruit cultivars during cool-storage. *Food Chem.* **2003**, *83*, 167–173. [CrossRef]
4. Pineli, L.L.O.; Moretti, C.L.; dos Santos, M.S.; Campos, A.B.; Brasileiro, A.V.; Cordova, A.C.; Chiarello, M.D. Antioxidants and other chemical and physical characteristics of two strawberry cultivars at different ripeness stages. *J. Food Compos. Anal.* **2011**, *24*, 11–16. [CrossRef]
5. Gasparrini, M.; Giampieri, F.; Forbes-Hernandez, T.Y.; Afrin, S.; Cianciosi, D.; Reboredo-Rodriguez, P.; Varela-Lopez, A.; Zhang, J.; Quiles, J.L.; Mezzetti, B.; et al. Strawberry extracts effiently counteract inflammatory stress induced by the endotoxin lipopolysaccharide in human dermal fibroblast. *Food Chem. Toxicol.* **2018**, *114*, 128–140. [CrossRef]
6. Cardoso, O.; Donato, M.M.; Luxo, C.; Almeida, N.; Liberal, J.; Figueirinha, A.; Batista, M.T. Anti-*Helicobacter pylori* potential of *Agrimonia eupatoria* L. and *Fragaria vesca*. *J. Funct. Food.* **2018**, *44*, 299–303. [CrossRef]
7. Ninomiya, M.; Itoh, T.; Ishikawa, S.; Saiki, M.; Narumiya, K.; Yasuda, M.; Koshikawa, K.; Nozawa, Y.; Koketsu, M. Phenolic constituents isolated from *Fragaria ananassa* Duch. inhibit antigen-stimulated degranulation through direct inhibition of spleen tyrosine kinase activation. *Bioorg. Med. Chem.* **2010**, *18*, 5932–5937. [CrossRef]
8. Abdulazeez, S.S. Effects of freeze-dried *Fragaria × ananassa* powder on alloxan-induced diabetic complications in Wistar rats. *J. Taibah Univ. Med. Sci.* **2014**, *9*, 268–273. [CrossRef]

9. Somasagara, R.R.; Hegde, M.; Chiruvella, K.K.; Musini, A.; Choudhary, B.; Raghavan, S.C. Extracts of strawberry fruits induce intrinsic pathway of apoptosis in breast cancer cells and inhibits tumor progression in mice. *PLoS ONE* **2012**, *7*, e47021. [CrossRef]

10. Nowicka, A.; Kucharska, A.Z.; Sokół-Łętowska, A.; Fecka, I. Comparison of polyphenol content and antioxidant capacity of strawberry fruit from 90 cultivars of *Fragaria × ananassa* Duch. *Food Chem.* **2019**, *270*, 32–46. [CrossRef]

11. Komarov, V.L. *Flora of USSR*; AN SSSR: Moscow, Russia, 1941; Volume X, pp. 58–67.

12. Gruner, P.; Ulrich, D.; Neinhuis, C.; Olbricht, K. *Fragaria viridis* Weston: Diversity and breeding potential of an underutilised strawberry species. *Acta Horticult.* **2017**, *1156*, 203–208. [CrossRef]

13. Kirillov, V.; Stikhareva, T.; Atazhanova, G.; Makubayeva, A.; Serafimovich, M.; Kabanova, S.; Rakhimzhanov, A.; Adekenov, S. Composition of essential oil of leaves and fruits of green strawberry (*Fragaria viridis* Weston) growing wild in Northern Kazakhstan. *J. Appl. Bot. Food Qual.* **2019**, *92*, 39–48. [CrossRef]

14. Raudonis, R.; Raudone, L.; Jakstas, V.; Janulis, V. Comparative evaluation of post-column free radical scavenging and ferric reducing antioxidant power assays for screening of antioxidants in strawberries. *J. Chromatogr. A* **2012**, *1233*, 8–15. [CrossRef] [PubMed]

15. Bagdonaite, E.; Jakstas, V.; Raudonis, R.; Janulis, V. Chlorogenic acid, rutin and hyperoside content in *Fragaria vesca*, *F. viridis* and *F. moschata* in Lithuania. *Nat. Prod. Res.* **2013**, *27*, 181–184. [CrossRef] [PubMed]

16. Olennikov, D.N.; Gadimli, A.I.; Isaev, J.I.; Kashchenko, N.I.; Prokopyev, A.S.; Katayeva, T.N.; Chirikova, N.K.; Vennos, C. Caucasian *Gentiana* species: Untargeted LC-MS metabolic profiling, antioxidant and digestive enzyme inhibiting activity of six plants. *Metabolites* **2019**, *9*, 271. [CrossRef] [PubMed]

17. Olennikov, D.N.; Chirikova, N.K.; Vasilieva, A.G.; Fedorov, I.A. LC-MS profile, gastrointestinal and gut microbiota stability and antioxidant activity of *Rhodiola rosea* herb metabolites: A comparative study with subterranean organs. *Antioxidants* **2020**, *9*, 526. [CrossRef]

18. Gasperotti, M.; Masuero, D.; Guella, G.; Palmieri, L.; Martinatti, P.; Pojer, E.; Mattivi, F.; Vrhovsek, U. Evolution of ellagitannin content and profile during fruit ripening in *Fragaria* spp. *J. Agric. Food Chem.* **2013**, *61*, 8597–8607. [CrossRef]

19. Olennikov, D.N.; Chirikova, N.K.; Kashchenko, N.I.; Nikolaev, V.M.; Kim, S.-W.; Vennos, C. Bioactive phenolics of the genus *Artemisia* (Asteraceae): HPLC-DAD-ESI-TQ-MS/MS profile of the Siberian species and their inhibitory potential against α-amylase and α-glucosidase. *Front. Pharmacol.* **2018**, *9*, 756. [CrossRef]

20. Clifford, M.N.; Wu, W.; Kuhnert, N. The chlorogenic acids of *Hemerocallis*. *Food Chem.* **2006**, *95*, 574–578. [CrossRef]

21. Sun, J.; Lin, L.; Chen, P. Study of the mass spectrometric behaviors of anthocyanins in negative ionization mode and its applications for characterization of anthocyanins and non-anthocyanin polyphenols. *Rapid Commun. Mass Spectrom.* **2012**, *26*, 1123–1133. [CrossRef]

22. Schuster, B.; Winter, M.; Herrmann, K. 4-O-β-D-Glucosides of hydroxybenzoic and hydroxycinnamic acids—Their synthesis and determination in berry fruit and vegetable. *Z. Naturforsch. C.* **1986**, *41*, 511–520. [CrossRef]

23. Moilanen, J.; Sinkkonen, J.; Salminen, J.-P. Characterization of bioactive plant ellagitannins by chromatographic, spectroscopic and mass spectrometric methods. *Chemoecology* **2013**, *23*, 165–179. [CrossRef]

24. Vrhovsek, U.; Guella, G.; Gasperotti, M.; Pojer, E.; Zancato, M.; Mattivi, F. Clarifying the identity of the main ellagitannin in the fruit of the strawberry, *Fragaria vesca* and *Fragaria ananassa* Duch. *J. Agric. Food Chem.* **2012**, *60*, 2507–2516. [CrossRef]

25. Aaby, K.; Mazur, S.; Nes, A.; Skrede, G. Phenolic compounds in strawberry (*Fragaria × ananassa* Duch.) fruits: Composition in 27 cultivars and changes during ripening. *Food Chem.* **2012**, *132*, 86–97. [CrossRef]

26. Aaby, K.; Ekeberg, D.; Skrede, G. Characterization of phenolic compounds in strawberry (*Fragaria x ananassa*) fruits by different HPLC detectors and contribution of individual compounds to total antioxidant capacity. *J. Agric. Food Chem.* **2007**, *55*, 4395–4406. [CrossRef] [PubMed]

27. Kajdžanoska, M.; Gjamovski, V.; Stefova, M. HPLC-DAD-ESI-MSn identification of phenolic compounds in cultivated strawberries from Macedonia. *Macedon. J. Chem. Chem. Eng.* **2010**, *29*, 181–194. [CrossRef]

28. Olennikov, D.N.; Kashchenko, N.I.; Chirikova, N.K. Phenolic profile of *Potentilla anserina* L. (Rosaceae) herb of Siberian origin and development of a rapid method for simultaneous determination of major phenolics in *P. anserina* pharmaceutical products by microcolumn RP-HPLC-UV. *Molecules* **2015**, *20*, 224–248. [CrossRef]

29. Karlińska, E.; Pecio, Ł.; Macierzyński, J.; Stochmal, A.; Kosmala, M. Structural elucidation of the ellagitannin with a molecular weight of 2038 isolated from strawberry fruit (*Fragaria ananassa* Duch.) and named fragariin A. *Food Chem.* **2019**, *296*, 109–115. [CrossRef]

30. Olennikov, D.N.; Kashchenko, N.I. New acylated apigenin glycosides from edge flowers of *Matricaria chamomilla*. *Chem. Nat. Comp.* **2016**, *52*, 996–999. [CrossRef]

31. Olennikov, D.N.; Chirikova, N.K.; Kim, E.; Kim, S.W.; Zul'fugarov, I.S. New glycosides of eriodictyol from *Dracocephalum palmatum*. *Chem. Nat. Comp.* **2018**, *54*, 860–863. [CrossRef]

32. Olennikov, D.N.; Kashchenko, N.I. New isorhamnetin glycosides and other phenolic compounds from *Calendula officinalis*. *Chem. Nat. Comp.* **2013**, *49*, 833–840. [CrossRef]

33. Mahmood, T.; Anwar, F.; Abbas, M.; Boyce, M.C.; Saari, N.S. Compositional variation in sugars and organic acids at different maturity stages in selected small fruits from Pakistan. *Int. J. Mol. Sci.* **2012**, *13*, 1380–1392. [CrossRef] [PubMed]

34. Dias, M.I.; Barros, L.; Morales, P.; Cámara, M.; Alves, M.J.; Oliveira, M.B.P.P.; Santos-Buelga, C.; Ferreira, I.C.F.R. Wild *Fragaria vesca* L. fruits: A rich source of bioactive phytochemicals. *Food Funct.* **2016**, *7*, 4523–4532. [CrossRef] [PubMed]

35. Kosińska, A.; Diering, S.; Prim, D.; Héritier, J.; Andlauer, W. Phenolic compounds profile of strawberry fruits of Charlotte cultivar. *J. Berry Res.* **2013**, *3*, 15–23. [CrossRef]

36. Liberal, J.; Costa, G.; Carmo, A.; Vitorino, R.; Marques, C.; Domingues, M.R.; Domingues, P.; Gonçalves, A.C.; Alves, R.; Sarmento-Ribeiro, A.B.; et al. Chemical characterization and cytotoxic potential of an ellagitannin-enriched fraction from *Fragaria vesca* leaves. *Arab. J. Chem.* **2019**, *12*, 3652–3666. [CrossRef]

37. Jordheim, M.; Måge, F.; Andersen, Ø.M. Anthocyanins in berries of *Ribes* including Gooseberry cultivars with high content of acylated pigments. *J. Agricult. Food Chem.* **2007**, *55*, 5529–5535. [CrossRef]

38. Williams, C.A. Flavone and flavonol *O*-glycosides. In *Flavonoids: Chemistry, Biochemistry, and Applications*; Andersen, Ø.M., Markham, K.R., Eds.; CRC Press: Boca Raton, FL, USA, 2006; pp. 749–856.

39. Zuo, G.-Y.; Liu, S.-L.; Xu, G.-L.; Wang, G.-C.; Zhang, Y.-L.; Zheng, D. Triterpenoids from the Roots of *Rubus obcordatus* (Rosaceae). *Plant Divers.* **2008**, *30*, 381–382.

40. Yean, M.-H.; Kim, J.-S.; Hyun, Y.-J.; Hyun, J.-W.; Bae, K.-H.; Kang, S.-S. Terpenoids and phenolics from *Geum japonicum*. *Korean J. Pharmacogn.* **2012**, *43*, 107–121.

41. Basson, C.E.; Groenewald, J.H.; Kossmann, J.; Cronje, C.; Bauer, R. Sugar and acid-related quality attributes and enzyme activities in strawberry fruits: Invertase is the main sucrose hydrolysing enzyme. *Food Chem.* **2010**, *121*, 1156–1162. [CrossRef]

42. Sturm, K.; Koron, D.; Stampar, F. The composition of fruit of different strawberries varieties depending on maturity stage. *Food Chem.* **2003**, *83*, 417–422. [CrossRef]

43. Blanch, M.; Sanchez-Ballesta, M.T.; Escribano, M.I.; Merodio, C. The relationship between bound water and carbohydrate reserves in association with cellular integrity in *Fragaria vesca* stored under different conditions. *Food Bioprocess. Technol.* **2015**, *8*, 875–884. [CrossRef]

44. Castro, I.; Goncalves, O.; Teixeira, J.A.; Vicente, A.A. Comparative study of *selva* and *camarosa* strawberries for the commercial market. *J. Food Sci.* **2002**, *67*, 2132–2137. [CrossRef]

45. Kouyncu, M.A.; Dilmacunal, T. Determination of vitamin C and organic acid changes in strawberry by HPLC during cold storage. *Not. Bot. Hort. Agrobot. Cluj* **2010**, *38*, 95–98. [CrossRef]

46. Palma, J.M.; Corpas, F.J.; Freschi, L.; Valpuesta, V. Fruit ripening: From present knowledge to future development. *Front. Plant Sci.* **2019**, *10*, 545. [CrossRef]

47. Mazur, S.P.; Nes, A.; Wold, A.-B.; Remberg, S.F.; Martinsen, B.K.; Aaby, K. Effects of ripeness and cultivar on chemical composition of strawberry (*Fragaria × ananassa* Duch.) fruits and their suitability for jam production as a stable product at different storage temperatures. *Food Chem.* **2014**, *146*, 412–422. [CrossRef]

48. Le Fur, Y.; Hory, C.; Bard, M.H.; Olsson, A. Evolution of phytosterols in Chardonnay grape berry skins during last stages of ripening. *Vitis* **1994**, *33*, 127–131.

49. Stiti, N.; Triki, S.; Hartmann, M.A. Formation of triterpenoids throughout *Olea europaea* fruit ontogeny. *Lipids* **2007**, *42*, 55–67. [CrossRef]

50. Kosma, D.K.; Parsons, E.P.; Isaacson, T.; Lü, S.; Rose, J.K.C.; Jenks, M.A. Fruit cuticle lipid composition during development in tomato ripening mutants. *Physiol. Plant.* **2010**, *139*, 107–117. [CrossRef]

51. Zhu, Q.; Nakagawa, T.; Kishikawa, A.; Ohnuki, K.; Shimizu, K. In vitro bioactivities and phytochemical profile of various parts of the strawberry (*Fragaria × ananassa* var. Amaou). *J. Funct. Food* **2015**, *13*, 38–49. [CrossRef]
52. Cerezo, A.B.; Cuevas, E.; Winterhalter, P.; Garcia-Parrilla, M.C.; Troncoso, A.M. Isolation, identification, and antioxidant activity of anthocyanin compounds in Camarosa strawberry. *Food Chem.* **2010**, *123*, 574–582. [CrossRef]
53. Álvarez-Fernández, M.A.; Hornedo-Ortega, R.; Cerezo, A.B.; Troncoso, A.M.; García-Parrilla, M.C. Effects of the strawberry (*Fragaria ananassa*) purée elaboration process on non-anthocyanin phenolic composition and antioxidant activity. *Food Chem.* **2014**, *164*, 104–112. [CrossRef] [PubMed]
54. Cao, G.; Russell, R.M.; Lischner, N.; Prior, R.L. Serum antioxidant capacity is increased by consumption of strawberries, spinach, red wine or vitamin C in elderly women. *J. Nutr.* **1998**, *128*, 2383–2390. [CrossRef] [PubMed]
55. Henning, S.M.; Seeram, N.P.; Zhang, Y.; Li, L.; Gao, K.; Lee, R.-P.; Wang, D.C.; Zerlin, A.; Karp, H.; Thames, G.; et al. Strawberry consumption is associated with increased antioxidant capacity in serum. *J. Med. Food* **2010**, *13*, 116–122. [CrossRef] [PubMed]
56. Azzini, E.; Vitaglione, P.; Intorre, F.; Napolitano, A.; Durazzo, A.; Foddai, M.S.; Fumagalli, A.; Catasta, G.; Rossi, L.; Venneria, E.; et al. Bioavailability of strawberry antioxidants in human subject. *Brit. J. Nutr.* **2010**, *104*, 1165–1173. [CrossRef]
57. Basu, A.; Morris, S.; Nguyen, A.; Betts, N.M.; Fu, D.; Lyons, T.J. Effects of dietary strawberry supplementation on antioxidant biomarkers in obese adults with above optimal serum lipids. *J. Nutr. Metabol.* **2016**, *2016*, 3910630. [CrossRef]
58. Pott, D.M.; Vallarino, J.G.; Osorio, S. Metabolite changes during postharvest storage: Effects on fruit quality traits. *Metabolites* **2020**, *10*, 187. [CrossRef]
59. Gazdik, Z.; Zitka, O.; Petrlova, J.; Adam, V.; Zehnalek, J.; Horna, A.; Reznicek, V.; Beklova, M.; Kizek, R. Determination of vitamin C (ascorbic acid) using high performance liquid chromatography coupled with electrochemical detection. *Sensors* **2008**, *8*, 7097–7112. [CrossRef]
60. Rubinskiene, M.; Jasutiene, I.; Venskutonis, P.R.; Viskelis, P. HPLC determination of the composition and stability of blackcurrant anthocyanins. *J. Chromatogr. Sci.* **2005**, *43*, 478–482. [CrossRef]
61. Sójka, M.; Janowski, M.; Grzelak-Błaszczyk, K. Stability and transformations of raspberry (*Rubus idaeus* L.) ellagitannins in aqueous solutions. *Eur. Food Res. Technol.* **2019**, *245*, 1113–1122. [CrossRef]
62. Szőke, É.; Petroianu, G.; Tekes, K.; Benkő, B.; Szegi, P.; Laufer, R.; Veress, G. HPLC monitoring of the microsomal stability of rutin and quercetin. *Acta Chromatogr.* **2009**, *21*, 399–410. [CrossRef]
63. Octavia, L.; Choo, W.S. Folate, ascorbic acid, anthocyanin and colour changes in strawberry (*Fragaria × annanasa*) during refrigerated storage. *LWT* **2017**, *86*, 652–659. [CrossRef]
64. Hernández-Herrero, J.A.; Frutos, M.J. Colour and antioxidant capacity stability in grape, strawberry and plum peel model juices at different pHs and temperatures. *Food Chem.* **2014**, *154*, 199–204. [CrossRef] [PubMed]
65. Gössinger, M.; Moritz, S.; Hermes, M.; Wendelin, S.; Scherbichler, H.; Halbwirth, H.; Stich, K.; Berghofer, E. Effects of processing parameters on colour stability of strawberry nectar from puree. *J. Food Eng.* **2009**, *90*, 171–178. [CrossRef]
66. Gil, M.I.; Holcroft, D.M.; Kader, A.A. Changes in strawberry anthocyanins and other polyphenols in response to carbon dioxide treatments. *J. Agric. Food Chem.* **1997**, *45*, 1662–1667. [CrossRef]
67. Kashchenko, N.I.; Olennikov, D.N.; Chirikova, N.K. Ellagitannins in Rosaceous plants from the flora of Sakha (Yakutia) Republic. *Butl. Commun.* **2014**, *39*, 127–138.
68. Olennikov, D.N.; Kruglova, M.Y. New quercetin glucoside and other phenolic compounds from *Filipendula* genus. *Chem. Nat. Comp.* **2013**, *49*, 524–529. [CrossRef]
69. Olennikov, D.N. Free carbohydrates, glucofructans, and other polysaccharides from *Rhaponticum uniflorum*. *Chem. Nat. Comp.* **2018**, *54*, 751–754. [CrossRef]
70. Olennikov, D.N.; Zilfikarov, I.N.; Penzina, T.A. Use of microcolumn HPLC for analysis of aloenin in *Aloe arborescens* raw material and related drugs. *Pharm. Chem. J.* **2013**, *47*, 494–497. [CrossRef]
71. Olennikov, D.N.; Kashchenko, N.I.; Chirikova, N.K.; Gornostai, T.G.; Selyutina, I.Y.; Zilfikarov, I.N. Effect of low temperature cultivation on the phytochemical profile and bioactivity of Arctic plants: A case of *Dracocephalum palmatum*. *Int. J. Mol. Sci.* **2017**, *18*, 2579. [CrossRef]

72. Olennikov, D.N.; Chirikova, N.K.; Okhlopkova, Z.M.; Zulfugarov, I.S. Chemical composition and antioxidant activity of *Tánara Ótó* (*Dracocephalum palmatum* Stephan), a medicinal plant used by the North-Yakutian nomads. *Molecules* **2013**, *18*, 14105–14121. [CrossRef]

73. Pellegrini, N.; Serafini, M.; Colombi, B.; Del Rio, D.; Salvatore, S.; Bianchi, M.; Brighenti, F. Total antioxidant capacity of plant foods, beverages and oils consumed in Italy assessed by three different in vitro assays. *J. Nutr.* **2003**, *133*, 2812–2819. [CrossRef] [PubMed]

74. Thaipong, K.; Boonprakob, U.; Crosby, K.; Cisneros-Zevallos, L.; Byrne, D.H. Comparison of ABTS, DPPH, FRAP, and ORAC assays for estimating antioxidant activity from guava fruit extracts. *J. Food Comp. Anal.* **2006**, *19*, 669–675. [CrossRef]

75. Olennikov, D.N.; Kashchenko, N.I.; Chirikova, N.K. Meadowsweet teas as new functional beverages: Comparative analysis of nutrients, phytochemicals and biological effects of four *Filipendula* species. *Molecules* **2017**, *22*, 16. [CrossRef] [PubMed]

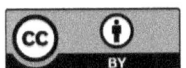

MDPI

St. Alban-Anlage 66

4052 Basel

Switzerland

Tel. +41 61 683 77 34

Fax +41 61 302 89 18

www.mdpi.com

Pharmaceuticals Editorial Office

E-mail: pharmaceuticals@mdpi.com

www.mdpi.com/journal/pharmaceuticals

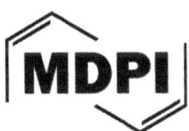

www.ingramcontent.com/pod-product-compliance
Lightning Source LLC
Chambersburg PA
CBHW060622070526

44654CB00012B/217